CANCER METASTASIS AND THE LYMPHOVASCULAR SYSTEM: BASIS FOR RATIONAL THERAPY

Cancer Treatment and Research

Steven T. Rosen, M.D., *Series Editor*

CANCER METASTASIS AND THE LYMPHOVASCULAR SYSTEM: BASIS FOR RATIONAL THERAPY

edited by

STANLEY P. L. LEONG, MD, FACS
Professor and Director of Sentinel Lymph Node Program
University of California San Francisco
and UCSF Comprehensive Cancer Center at Mount Zion
San Francisco, CA, USA

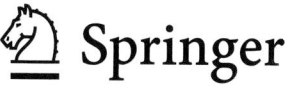

Stanley P. L. Leong
Department of Surgery
University of California San Francisco
and UCSF Comprehensive Cancer Center at Mount Zion
1600 Divisadero Street
San Francisco, CA 94143
leongs@surgery.ucsf.edu

Series Editor:
Steven T. Rosen
Robert H. Lurie Comprehensive Cancer Center
Northwestern University
Chicago, IL
USA

Cancer Metastasis and the Lymphovascular System: Basis for rational therapy

Library of Congress Control Number: 2006939419

ISBN-13: 978-0-387-69218-0   e-ISBN-13: 978-0-387-69219-7

Printed on acid-free paper.

9 8 7 6 5 4 3 2 1

springer.com

CONTENTS

CONTRIBUTORS

J. L. Albérini, MD, Centre Rene Huguenin, 92210 Saint-Cloud, France

Mauro Andrade, MD, PhD, Department of Surgery, University of Sao, Paulo Sao Paulo, Brazil

Athanassios Argiris, MD, Division of Hematology-Oncology, University of Pittsburgh School of Medicine, Head and Neck Cancer Program, University of Pittsburgh Cancer Institute, Pittsburgh, Pennsylvania, USA

Jürgen Becker, MD, Children's Hospital, Pediatrics I, University of Goettingen, Robert-Koch-Strasse 40, 37075 Goettingen, Germany

D. Bellet, MD, PhD, Centre Rene Huguenin, 92210 Saint-Cloud, France

Michael Bernas, MS, Department of Surgery, University of Arizona, Tucson, Arizona, USA

David Berz, MD, PhD, Fellow, Hematology and Oncology, Brown University, Providence, Rhode Island, USA

Kerstin Buttler, DB, Children's Hospital, Pediatrics I, University of Goettingen, Robert-Koch-Strasse 40, 37075 Goettingen, Germany

Blake Cady, MD, Department of Surgery, Brown Medical School, Rhode Island Hospital, Providence, Rhode Island, USA

Ann F. Chambers, PhD, London Regional Cancer Program, 790 Commissioners Road East, London, Ontario, Canada N6A 4L6

R. V. Cluzan, MD, Centre Rene Huguenin, 92210 Saint-Cloud, France

Peter A. Cohen, MD, Center for Surgery Research, Cleveland Clinic, Cleveland, Ohio, USA

Michael Dictor, MD, PhD, Department of PathologyLund University Hospital, Sölvegatan 25, SE 22185, Lund, Sweden

Katharina E. Effenberger, PhD, Institute of Tumor Biology, University Medical Center, Hamburg-Eppendorf, 20246 Hamburg, Germany

Claus Garbe, MD, Division of Dermatooncology, Department of Dermatology, University Medical Center, Tuebingen, Germany

Julio Garcia-Aguilar, MD, Department of Surgery, University of California, San Francisco, San Francisco, California, USA

Edwin Glass, MD, VA Greater Los Angeles Healthcare System, John Wayne Cancer Institute, Santa Monica, California, USA

Axel Hauschild, MD, Department of Dermatology, University of Kiel, D-24105 Kiel, Germany

Peter Hirnle, MD, PhD, Department of Radiation Oncology, Central Academic Hospital, Bielefeld, Germany

David S. B. Hoon, PhD, Department of Molecular Oncology, John Wayne Cancer Institute, Saint Johns Health Center, Santa Monica, California, USA

David M. Jablons, MD, Department of Surgery, University of California, San Francisco, San Francisco, California, USA

David G. Jackson B.A. (Mod.), PhD, MRC Human Immunology Unit, University of Oxford, Headington, Oxford OX3 9DS, UK

Alfredo Jacomo, PhD, Department of Surgery, University of Sao Paulo, Sao Paulo, Brazil

Kimberly Jones, MD, Department of Medicine (Oncology), University of Utah, Salt Lake City, Utah, USA

Katharina C. Kähler, MD, Department of Dermatology, University of Kiel, Kiel, Germany

Michalis V. Karamouzis, MD, PhD, Division of Hematology-Oncology, Department of Medicine, University of Pittsburgh School of Medicine, Head and Neck Cancer Program, University of Pittsburgh Cancer Institute, Pittsburgh, Pennsylvania, USA

Yuko Kitagawa, MD, PhD, Department of Surgery, Keio University School of Medicine, Tokyo, Japan

Minoru Kitago, MD, Department of Molecular Oncology, John Wayne Cancer Institute, Saint Johns Health Center, Santa Monica, California, USA

Jorgen Kjaergaard, PhD, New England Inflammation and Tissue Protection Institute, Northeastern University, Boston, Massachusetts, USA

Walter T. Lee, MD, Center for Surgery Research, Cleveland Clinic, Cleveland, Ohio, USA

Stanley P. L. Leong, MD, Department of Surgery, University of Californi, San Francisco, UCSF Comprehensive Cancer Center, San Francisco, California, USA

Michael M. Lizardo, MSc, Department of Medical Biophysics, University of Western Ontario, Medical Sciences Building, London, Ontario, Canada N6A 5C1

Zerina Lokmic, PhD, Department of Experimental Pathology, Lund University Hospital, Sölvegatan 25, SE 22185, Lund, Sweden

Ian C. MacDonald, PhD, Department of Medical Biophysics, University of Western Ontario, Medical Sciences Building, London, Ontario, Canada N6A 5C1

Sofia Mebrahtu, BSc, Department of Pathology, Lund University Hospital, Sölvegatan 25, SE 22185, Lund, Sweden

Anthony Mega, MD, Medical Oncology, Brown University, Providence, Rhode Island, USA

Martin C. Mihm, Jr., MD, Departments of Pathology and Dermatology, Massachusetts General Hospital, Harvard Medical School, Boston, Massachusetts, USA

S. David Nathanson, MD, Henry Ford Health System, Detroit, Michigan, USA

Klaus Pantel, MD, PhD, Institute of Tumor Biology, University Medical Center Hamburg-Eppendorf, 20246 Hamburg, Germany

Maria Papoutsi, PhD, Children's Hospital, Pediatrics I, University of Goettingen, Robert-Koch-Strasse 40, 37075 Goettingen, Germany

Alain P. Pecking, MD, Centre Rene Huguenin, 92210 Saint-Cloud, France

Adriano Piris, MD, Department of Dermatopathology, Massachusetts General Hospital, Harvard Medical School, Boston, Massachusetts, USA

Douglas Reintgen, MD, Lakeland Regional Cancer Center, Lakeland, Florida, USA

Dirk Schadendorf, PhD, Skin Cancer Unit, German Cancer Research Centre Heidelberg, Department of Dermatology, University Hospital of Mannheim, D-68167 Mannheim, Germany

Manuel Selg, PhD, Department of Experimental Pathology, Lund University Hospital, Sölvegatan 25, SE 22185, Lund, Sweden

Suyu Shu, PhD, Center for Surgery Research, Cleveland Clinic, Cleveland, Ohio, USA

Wulf Sienel, MD, Department of Thoracic Surgery, Albert-Ludwigs-University Freiburg, 79106 Freiburg, Germany

Lydia Sorokin, PhD, Department of Experimental Pathology, Lund University Hospital, Sölvegatan 25, SE 22185, Lund, Sweden

Hiroya Takeuchi, MD, Department of Surgery, Keio University School of Medicine, Tokyo, Japan

Alan B. Tuck, MD, PhD, Department of Pathology, London Health Sciences Center, London, Ontario, Canada N6A 5A5

Selma Ugurel, MD, Skin Cancer Unit, German Cancer Research Centre & University Hospital Mannheim, University of Heidelberg, Mannheim, Germany

Harold J. Wanebo, MD, Boston University, Boston, Massachusetts, USA and, Roger Williams Hospital, Providence, Rhode Island, USA

M. Wartski, MD, Centre Rene Huguenin, 92210 Saint-Cloud, France

Jochen A. Werner, MD, PhD, Department of Otolaryngology, Head and Neck Surgery, Philipps-University Marburg, Marbug, Germany

Jörg Wilting, PhD, Children's Hospital, Pediatrics I, University of Goettingen, Robert-Koch-Strasse 40, 37075 Goettingen, Germany

Charles L. Witte, MD, Department of Surgery, University of Arizona College of Medicine, Tucson, Arizona, USA

Marlys H. Witte, MD, Department of Surgery, University of Arizona College of Medicine, Tucson, Arizona, USA

Rongxiu Zheng, MD, Center for Surgery Research, Cleveland Clinic, Cleveland, Ohio, USA

FOREWORD

The major cause of death from cancer is metastases that are resistant to conventional therapy. Advances in the study of the biology of cancer metastasis have reached two general conclusions. First, primary neoplasms are heterogeneous for a large number of properties, including invasion, metastasis, and ability to proliferate in distant organs. Second, the process of metastasis is sequential and selective, with every step of the process containing stochastic elements. The growth of metastases represents the end-point of many lethal events that only few tumor cells can survive. In fact, the successful metastatic cell, that some years ago I named the "decathlon champion", is a cell able to exploit homeostatic factors in its new environment.

Early clinical observations led to the impression that carcinomas spread mainly by the lymphatic route, whereas tumors of mesenchymal origin spread mainly by the bloodstream. The reality, however, invalidates this belief. The lymphatic and vascular systems have numerous connections, and disseminating tumor cells may pass from one circulatory system to the other. For these reasons, the division of metastatic routes into lymphatic spread and hematogenous spread is arbitrary. During invasion, tumor cells can easily penetrate small lymphatic vessels and can be passively transported in the lymph. Tumor emboli may be trapped in the first lymph node encountered on their route, or they may bypass regional draining lymph nodes to form distant nodal metastases ("skip metastasis"). Although this phenomenon was recognized by Stephen Paget in 1889, its implications for treatment were frequently ignored in the development of surgical approaches to treating cancers.

Regional lymph nodes (RLN) in the area of a primary neoplasm may become enlarged as a result of reactive hyperplasia or growth of tumor cells. Lymphocyte-depleted lymph nodes indicate a less favorable prognosis than those demonstrating reactive inflammatory characteristics. Whether the RLN can retain tumor cells and serve as a temporary barrier for cell dissemination has been controversial. In many experimental animal systems used to investigate this question, normal lymph nodes were subjected to a single challenge with a large number of tumor cells, a situation that is not analogous to the early stages of cancer spread in cancer patients, when small numbers of cancer cells continuously enter the lymphatics. This issue is important because of practical considerations for surgical management of specific types of cancer. For example, some evidence exists that patients with melanomas of intermediate thickness (1-4 mm) have an improved survival rate subsequent to elective lymph node dissection. In colorectal cancers, more radical operations that include removal of RLN have been associated with improved survival rates. In contrast, in breast cancer, removal of the axillary lymph nodes in a randomized prospective study was not associated with improved survival rates.

Advances in mapping of the lymphatics draining cutaneous melanoma (by the use of dyes or radioactive tracers) have allowed surgeons to identify the lymph node draining the tumor site (i.e., the sentinel lymph node). The presence of melanoma micrometastases in sentinel lymph nodes is correlated with poor prognosis and hence indicates wide-field dissection.

The recent discovery of several lymphatic markers has facilitated a more extensive study of lymphangiogenesis and lymphatic metastasis. For example, it is now known that activation of VEGFR-3 by VEGF-C and VEGF-D signals for survival and cell division in lymphatic endothelial cells growing in cell culture. VEGF-C and -D have also been shown to induce lymphangiogenesis *in vivo* and to enhance lymphatic metastasis in some tumor models. Other growth factors, including VEGF-A, bFGF, PDGF-BB, HGF, IGF-1, IGF-2, and EGF, have also been shown to promote lymphangiogenesis, indicating the complexity of lymphatic endothelial cell biology.

Biology is the foundation for therapy. The need to improve our understanding of the pathogenesis of cancer metastasis and the lymphovascular system stimulated Dr. Stanley P.L. Leong to organize the first international symposium on this topic. Participants in this successful meeting have contributed a series of excellent chapters addressing a variety of topics dealing with basic translational and clinical issues of lymphatic metastasis. The chapters contain a succinct review of the literature and exciting new data that the reader will find important.

For many years, all of our efforts to treat cancer have concentrated on the inhibition or destruction of tumor cells. Strategies to modulate the host microenvironment could provide an additional approach for eradicating a cancer. The recent advancements in our understanding of the role of the lymphovascular system in cancer metastasis present unprecedented possibilities for translating basic research to the clinical reality of cancer treatment.

Isaiah J. Fidler, D.V.M., Ph.D.
Houston, TX
USA

PREFACE

Sentinel lymph node procedures have opened a window of opportunity for the study of tumor metastasis. In about 80% of metastasis, there is an orderly pattern of progression through the lymphatic system network, whereas 20% of the time, systemic metastasis occurs directly presumably bypassing the lymphatic system. During the past several decades, substantial progress has been achieved in understanding the anatomical, functional, cellular, and molecular aspects of the integrated lymphovascular system and relationships to the process of metastasis.

Advanced multimodal molecular imaging now localizes early cancers more precisely. Immune responses against cancer in the draining lymph nodes are under scrutiny. New paradigms of early cancer growth, proliferation, and overcoming apoptosis are being exploited in the development of anticancer treatment. And the array of ligand–receptor interactions between vascular endothelium and tumors is being uncovered along with the underlying molecular pathways.

The basic mechanisms of cancer metastasis through the lymphovascular system should form the basis for rational therapy against cancer, but we are not yet there. To address this crucial gap between theory and practice, upon which our patients' lives and well-being depend, the first international symposium on Cancer Metastasis and the Lymphovascular System: Basis for Rational Therapy was held in San Francisco from April 28 to 30, 2005. Basic scientists and clinicians gathered from around the world to exchange ideas across disciplines and specialties so that laboratory findings can be translated into explanations of clinical dilemmas, and pressing clinical problems can be targeted for research in the laboratory.

Stanley P. L. Leong, M.D.
San Francisco, CA
USA

ACKNOWLEDGMENTS

We appreciate the effort of Regina Hopkins of the UCSF Department of Surgery in the preparation of the manuscripts. We also would like to thank the staff at Springer, Laura Walsh and Maureen Tobin, for their advice and expertise in making this book possible.

1. LANDMARKS AND ADVANCES IN TRANSLATIONAL LYMPHOLOGY

MARLYS H. WITTE, KIMBERLY. JONES*, MICHAEL BERNAS, AND CHARLES L. WITTE

Department of Surgery, University of Arizona, Tucson, AZ, USA
*Department of Medicine (Oncology), University of Utah, Salt Lake City, UT, USA

INTRODUCTION

The lymph vascular system parallels the blood vasculature and as one of its key functions, returns liquid and solute to the bloodstream, including macromolecules that have escaped from blood capillaries and entered the interstitium. In conjunction with interspersed lymph nodes and lymphoid organs, the lymphatic vasculature also acts as a conduit for trafficking immune cell populations. Lymphatics are involved in diverse developmental, growth, repair, and pathologic processes similar to but distinct from those affecting the blood vasculature. Interference with the blood–lymph circulatory loop produces edema, scarring, nutritional, and immunodysregulatory disorders as well as disturbances in lymph(hem)angiogenesis (lymphedema–angiodysplasia syndromes). The lymphatic system – encompassing lymphatics, lymph, lymph nodes, and lymphocytes – is also the stage on which key events in tumor biology and cancer progression are played out, and historically, also has formed the basis for evaluation, prognostication, and both operative and nonoperative treatment of most cancers. Interpreted in the light of landmark discoveries about the structure and function of the lymphatic system during the last century, recent advances in molecular lymphology combined with fresh insights and refined tools in clinical lymphology, including noninvasive lymphatic imaging, are fueling translation to the clinical arena, i.e., translational lymphology.

HISTORIC LANDMARKS (TABLE 1)

By odd coincidence, Gaspar Aselli of Padua in 1627 described the milky "chyliferous vessels" of the intestinal lymph circulation (3) at almost precisely the same moment that William Harvey, King Charles I of England's physician, demonstrated the circulation of blood (21). In contrast to the immediate interest and rapid advances that followed the latter discovery, the inaccessible barely visible lymphatic system, except for postmortem anatomic dissections, entered centuries of neglect. Even Harvey in his later years declined to work on the "other" circulation. It was not until the 1890s that British physiologist Ernest Starling, imbued with French experimentalist Claude Bernard's milieu interieur (the "lymph suffusing the tissue spaces"), set out to investigate the forces governing transcapillary movement of fluid from blood into tissues by monitoring changes in lymph flow from cannulated central and regional lymphatic vessels. His observations on the effect of altering hydrostatic and colloid osmotic pressure gradients established the physiologic principles controlling transcapillary fluid flux and lymph formation (52) (Fig. 1; (56)), demonstrated the dynamic flow responses of the lymph circulation to perturbations in the blood vasculature and tissues, and further led him to conclude that all edemas in the final analysis represent an imbalance between lymph formation and lymph absorption (51). Decades later, once again largely through central and regional lymphatic cannulation and lymph sampling studies in experimental animals, the transcapillary movement, molecular sieving, and recirculation of plasma proteins and macromolecules (10, 36) were

Table 1. Landmarks in lymphology

1. Discovery of "chyliferous vessels" – Aselli, 1627
2. Lymph as the milieu interieur – Bernard, 1878
3. Transcapillary exchange of liquid, lymph formation, and edema – Starling, 1896
4. Embryology and phylogeny of lymphatic system – Sabin and Kampmeier, 1902
5. Transcapillary protein movement and lymph absorption – Krogh, Drinker, Mayerson, Courtice, 1925
6. Lymphangiogenesis in vivo – Clark and Florey, 1932; and in vitro – Witte, Johnston, Gnepp, Leak, 1984
7. Lymphocyte migrant streams – Yoffey, Morris, Gowans, 1939
8. Oil contrast lymphography/lymphatic disease classification – Kinmonth, Servelle, Kaindl, 1950
9. Intrinsic lymphatic contractility – Hall and Roddie; and distinctive lymphatic ultrastructure – Casley-Smith and Leak, 1962
10. Lymphostatic disorders – Rusznyák, Szabo, M/E Földi, Olszewski, Dumont, Witte, 1960
11. Lymphoscintigraphy – Sage, 1960
12. Founding of International Society of Lymphology – 1965
13. Sentinel lymph node intraoperative mapping and biopsy – Morton, 1992
14. Specific lymphatic immunohistochemical markers (Lyve-1, Prox-1, 5′ nucleotidase, VEGFR-3, Podoplanin) – Jackson, Oliver, Kato, Alitalo, Breiteneder-Geleff, 1990s
15. Vascular/lymphatic growth factors: VEGF-A – Ferrara and Dvorak, 1989/VEGF-C – Alitalo, 1996; angiopoietins – Gale and Yancopoulos, 2002
16. Human lymphvascular genomics (VEGFR3, FOXC2, SOX18 mutations) – teams U Pittsburgh/U Helsinki; U Arizona/U Michigan; U Connecticut/St George's Medical School; U Leuven, 1998

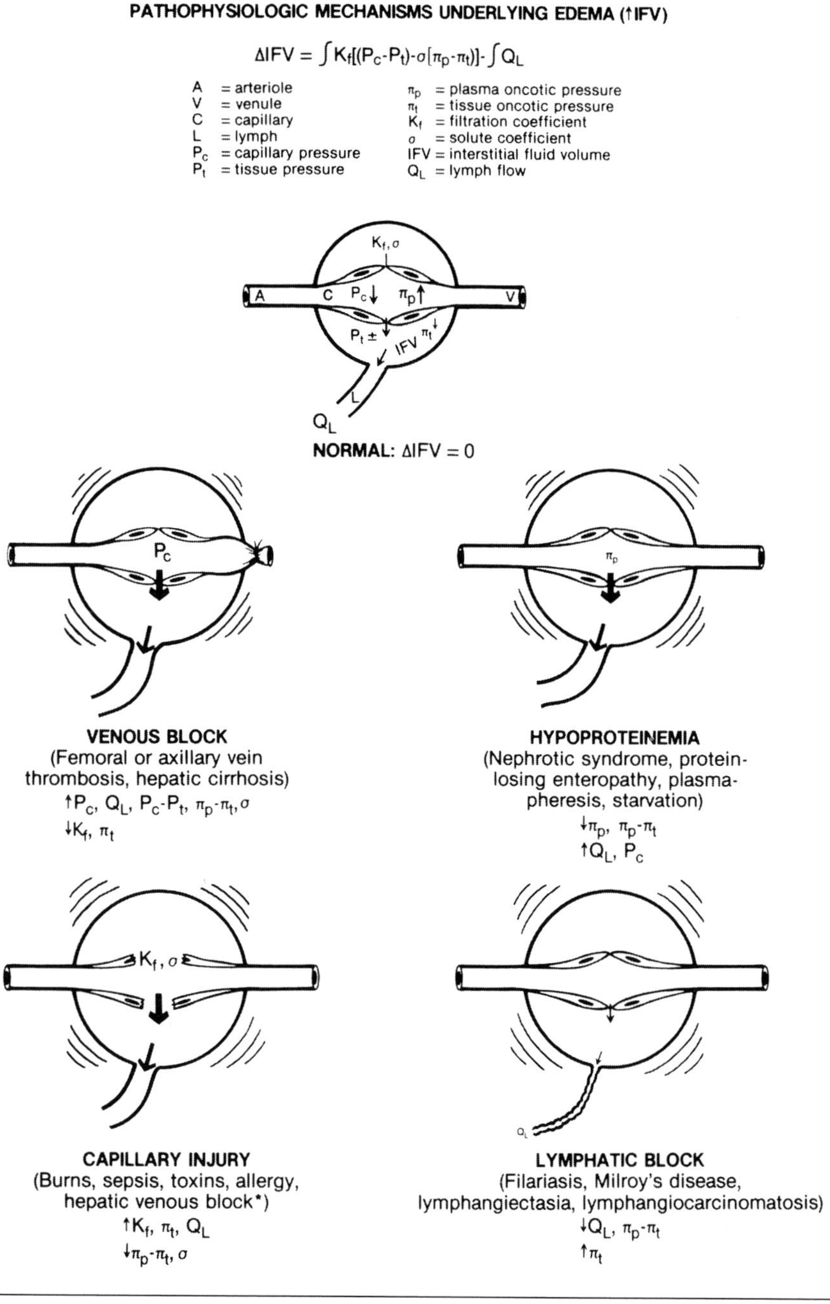

PATHOPHYSIOLOGIC MECHANISMS UNDERLYING EDEMA (↑IFV)

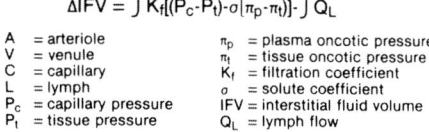

$$\Delta IFV = \int K_f[(P_c - P_t) - \sigma(\pi_p - \pi_t)] - \int Q_L$$

A	= arteriole	π_p	= plasma oncotic pressure
V	= venule	π_t	= tissue oncotic pressure
C	= capillary	K_f	= filtration coefficient
L	= lymph	σ	= solute coefficient
P_c	= capillary pressure	IFV	= interstitial fluid volume
P_t	= tissue pressure	Q_L	= lymph flow

NORMAL: ΔIFV = 0

VENOUS BLOCK
(Femoral or axillary vein
thrombosis, hepatic cirrhosis)
↑P_c, Q_L, P_c-P_t, π_p-π_t, σ
↓K_f, π_t

HYPOPROTEINEMIA
(Nephrotic syndrome, protein-
losing enteropathy, plasma-
pheresis, starvation)
↓π_p, π_p-π_t
↑Q_L, P_c

CAPILLARY INJURY
(Burns, sepsis, toxins, allergy,
hepatic venous block*)
↑K_f, π_t, Q_L
↓π_p-π_t, σ

LYMPHATIC BLOCK
(Filariasis, Milroy's disease,
lymphangiectasia, lymphangiocarcinomatosis)
↓Q_L, π_p-π_t
↑π_t

Figure 1. Schematic diagram of the major processes initiating increased water flux into the interstitium. Because physiologic disturbances are often complex, the primary abnormality is highlighted and directional changes in each factor in the Starling equilibrium are also indicated where known. Each of these mechanisms alone or in combination may be involved in edema and effusion during the course of cancer and its treatment. Edema represents an imbalance between lymph formation and lymph absorption, either in a high–lymph output (Q_L) or a low–output state (classical lymphedema). Treatment works by restoring the balance by either reducing lymph formation or enhancing lymph absorption. Reproduced with permission from Witte and Witte (56)

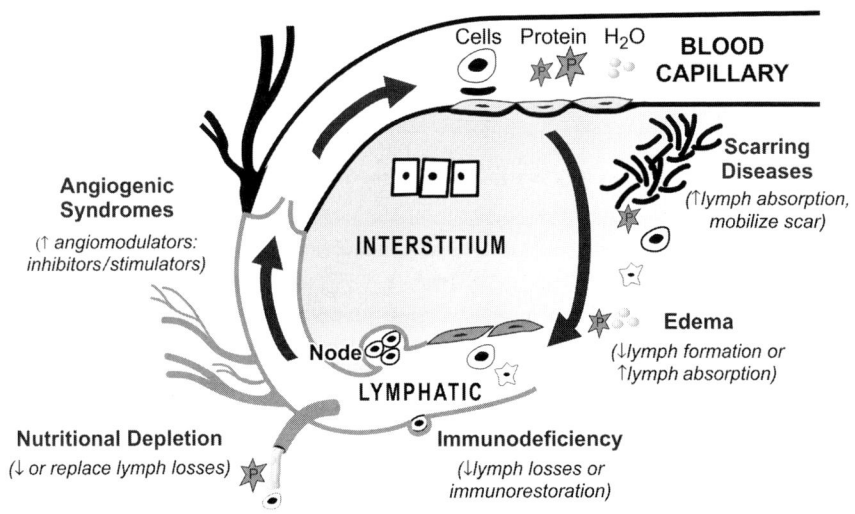

Figure 2. Blood–lymph circulatory loop. Within the bloodstream, liquid flows rapidly as a plasma suspension of erythrocytes; outside the bloodstream, it flows slowly as a tissue fluid–lymph suspension of immunocytes through lymphatics and lymph nodes. Small and large molecules including plasma protein, trafficking cells, particulates, and respiratory gases cross the blood capillary endothelial barrier, percolate through the tissues, enter the lymph stream, and return to the central venous system to complete the loop. Clinical disorders of the blood–lymph circulatory loop manifest as swelling, scarring, immunodeficiency, nutritional depletion, and uncontrolled lymphangiogenesis (along with hemangiogenesis) and angiotumorigenesis. The phrases in parentheses designate current and potential future therapeutic approaches. Reprinted with permission from Witte et al. (71)

elucidated in a variety of organ systems (e.g., liver, intestine, kidney, lung, limbs, and heart), and in addition, trafficking lymphocytes were traced in their travels through the lymphatic network of vessels and lymph nodes (Fig. 2). These observations and principles were later confirmed and extended by monitoring central thoracic duct and regional lymph flow and composition in man under both normal (43) and pathologic conditions including hepatic cirrhosis (58, 59, 66), congestive heart failure (67), and organ transplantation (11, 53).

Almost contemporaneously with Starling's landmark observations on the physiology of lymph formation, Florence Sabin's meticulous anatomical studies (49) of human and pig embryos and evolving primordial lymph sacs opened a window on the origin and development of the lymphatic system. These findings stirred a vigorous still unresolved controversy over whether the lymphatic system arises centrifugally by budding from central veins or de novo in the periphery from primitive mesenchymal precursors spreading centripetally (27). Subsequent investigators compared morphologic differences and similarities between blood and lymphatic vessels in various organ systems, the boundaries between the two, and the pathologic processes in which they were involved. Electron microscopic studies (8, 31) uncovered distinctive ultrastructural features of lymphatics including discontinuous basement membrane, open interendothelial junctions, anchoring filaments, and valves, and the lymphangion's intrinsic contractility became the basis for the "lymphatic pump" (15, 20, 35, 37). In 1984, following up earlier observations on the regeneration of lymphatic vessels after surgical disruption (9) and proliferation during inflammation (47) ("lymphangiogenesis in vivo"), in vitro culture of cells from lymphatic vessels was reported by several groups. Normal, dysplastic, and neoplastic lymphatic endothelial cells from various animal species and man (6, 19, 25) were isolated, propagated, and phenotypically characterized with subsequent documentation of spontaneous and induced "lymphangiogenesis in vitro" (32, 63).

The era of lymphatic imaging (Fig. 3) suitable for living human subjects began with McMaster's vital dye injections in the skin of edematous limbs (38) demonstrating selective uptake of protein-bound colored dyes exclusively into the highly permeable lymphatic capillaries. Guided by these blue "streamers," Kinmonth (29) and others subsequently introduced direct oil contrast lymphography via cannulated lymphatic collectors in the distal limbs. The resulting vivid images provided the first navigable map of the peripheral and central lymphatic system in a wide variety of clinical disorders afflicting lymphatic vessels and lymph nodes either primarily (e.g., congenital lymphedema and lymphoma) or secondarily (e.g., lymphatic obstruction from filariasis or from cancer and its treatment) and also visualized a route for

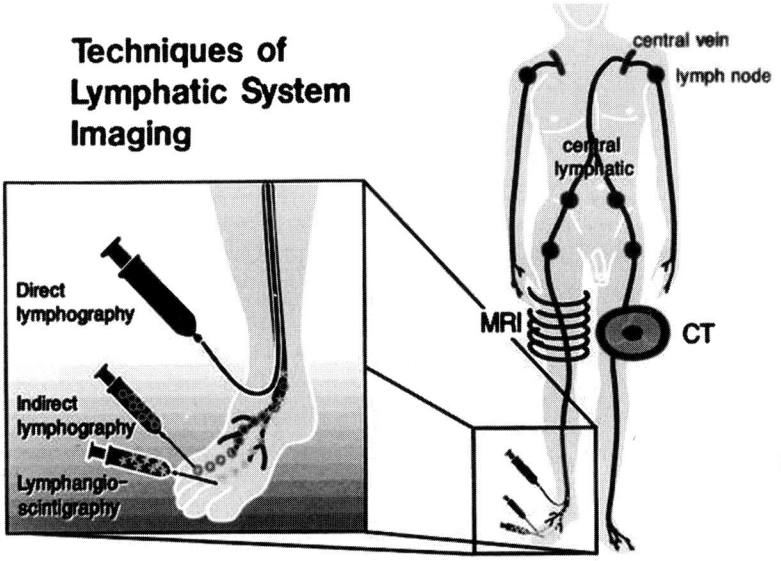

Figure 3. Lymphatic vessels and lymph nodes have been imaged experimentally and clinically by both direct (intralymphatic infusion) and a variety of indirect (interstitial injection) methods alone or in combination with other imaging modalities (multimodal, fusion imaging). See text for further details

administering endolymphatic therapy. Subsequently, noninvasive imaging of lymph nodes by computed tomography and magnetic resonance imaging and of lymphatic vessels and nodal pathways by radioisotopic lymphangio/adenoscintigraphy (LAS) was introduced into the evaluation of patients. Initially, interstitially deposited Au198 was used for lymphscintigraphy (50), and in combination with colored tracers (vital blue dyes), became the foundation for sentinel lymph node intraoperative mapping and biopsy (34, 39). Subsequent refinements of LAS with improved short-lived radiotracers, highly sophisticated gamma camera detection systems, and standardized protocols have made this noninvasive technique the current gold standard for lymphatic system imaging of both peripheral and central lymphatic vessels and nodal drainage pathways (Fig. 4). Noninvasive techniques currently in use or under development to dynamically image the peripheral and central lymphatic system (60) include magnetic resonance contrast imaging (lymphangiomagnetograms), indirect lymphography, laser-Doppler ultrasound, computed tomography, fluorescent microlymphangiography, and positron emission tomography. Simultaneous multimodal combinations of these different imaging modalities are being refined for more precise spatial and temporal resolution. LAS alone or in combination with these other noninvasive imaging methods has replaced the cumbersome and invasive conventional lymphography and provided dynamic details of lymphatic system structure, lymph reflux, and soft tissue changes in lymphedema, angiodysplastic syndromes, lymphoma, and lymphogenous cancer spread.

Between 1960 and 1970, two comprehensive seminal texts on the lymphatic system were published: Rusznyák, Földi, and Szabo's *Lymphatics and Lymph Circulation* (Rusznyák et al. (48) and subsequent updates of *Földi's Textbook of Lymphology*) detailing the normal function and pathophysiologic sequelae of lymph stasis in various organ systems and treatment approaches, and Yoffey and Courtice's encyclopedic *Lymphatics, Lymph, and the Lymphomyeloid Complex* (72) that continued the tradition of Cecil Drinker's pioneering work. In 1965, the International Society of Lymphology (ISL) was founded exclusively devoted to the study of the integrated system of lymph, lymphatics, lymph nodes, and lymphocytes in health and disease. The ISL's quarterly journal *Lymphology* (33) and its biennial international scientific congresses (46) defined the new discipline, involved lymphologists from around the word, and chronicled the progress and transformation of basic and clinical lymphology since that time. During the past decade, the era of "molecular lymphology" has been ushered in with the discovery of lymphatic-specific growth factor ligands and receptor systems along with a constellation of genes implicated in the development and growth of the lymphatic system, some mutated in human lymphedema syndromes (Table 3) (65).

LYMPHATIC SYSTEM BIOLOGY AND PATHOBIOLOGY

The foregoing landmarks and the past century of lymphology have led to the concept of the "blood–lymph loop" (Fig. 2) (71) – a continuous, dynamic, exchanging circulation of extracellular fluid (plasma, interstitial fluid, and lymph) passing back

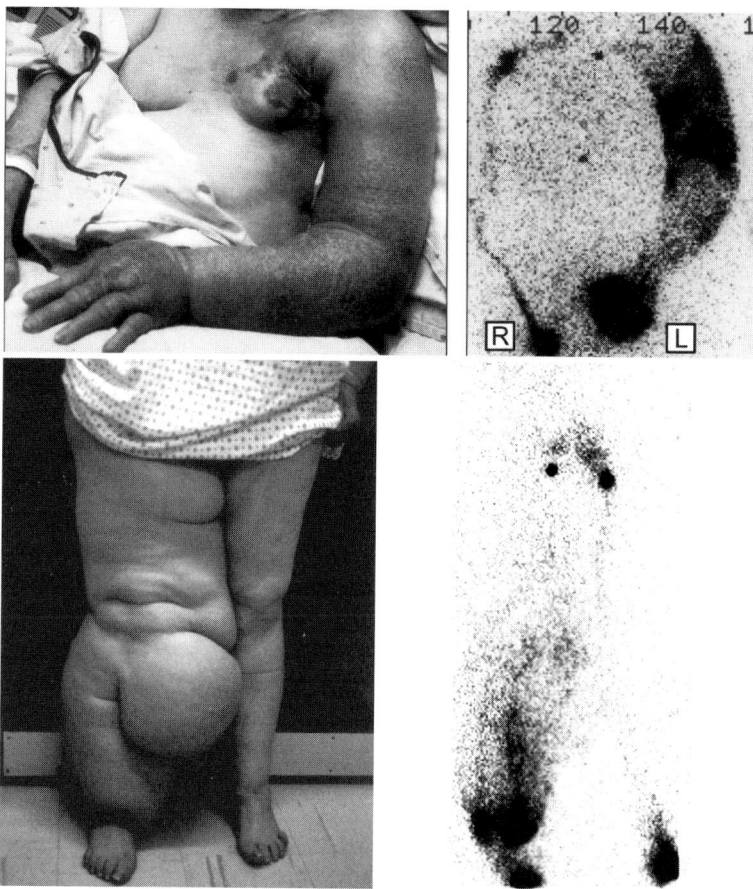

Figure 4. Whole body lymphangioscintigraphy in patients with lymphedema from untreated and treated cancer. Seventy-three-year-old woman (*upper left*) with advanced intractable lymphedema of the arm and shoulder from "untreated" locally aggressive breast carcinoma over a 4-year period extending into the axilla and invading the adjacent left chest and lung. Radionuclide lymphangioscintigram (*upper right*) depicts high-grade lymphatic obstruction in the left arm (*L*) with extensive dermal backflow (radiotracer dispersion) as compared with the normal right arm (*R*), which displays patent lymphatic trunks and several paraclavicular lymph nodes ("hot spots"). Fifty-eight-year-old woman (*lower left*) with advanced elephantiasis of the right leg 25 years after radical groin lymphadenectomy for malignant melanoma of the right calf (excised lymph nodes were all negative and there was no recurrence of melanoma). Lymphangioscintigram (*lower right*) shows severe lymphatic obstruction with extensive dermal tracer reflux/diffusion in the right leg without visualization of right groin nodes. *Left leg* shows normal lymphatic trunk clearing tracer, no dermal reflux diffusion, and well-visualized left groin nodes

and forth from the bloodstream to the tissues and lymphatic system, traversing lymph nodes and returning to the bloodstream the fluid, proteins, macromolecules, and migrant cells that have leaked from blood microvessels into the interstitium. Among the ingredients added along the way are products of tissue metabolism, "absorbents" such as chylomicra from the gut, and immune cells arising and

Table 2. Circulatory dynamics of vascular conduits

	Lymphatic	Vein	Artery
First propulsive unit	Lymphangion	Heart	Heart
Second propulsive force	Haphazard[a]	Skeletal muscle	Vasomotion
Distal (upright) pressure (mmHg)	2–3	90–100	20
Central pressure (mmHg)	6–10	0–2	100
Flow rate	Very low	High	High
Vascular resistance	Relatively high	Very low	High
Intraluminal valves	Innumerable	Several	None
Impediment to flow	Lymph nodes	None	None
Conduit fluid column	Incomplete	Complete	Complete
Conduit failure	Edema protein high (>1.5 g dl^{-1})	Edema protein low (<1.0 g dl^{-1})	Claudication
	Brawny induration	Skin pigmentation	Rest pain
	Acanthosis	"Stasis" ulceration	Tissue necrosis

[a]Breathing, sighing, yawning, peristalsis, transmitted arterial pulsation; skeletal muscle contraction also increases the amplitude and frequency of lymphatic contractions and squeezes interstitial fluid into initial lymphatics (i.e., lymph capillaries). Reproduced with permission from Witte and Witte (57).

trafficking in lymphoid tissues (72). Flow-pressure dynamics within this larger circulation is distinct and compartmentalized (Table 2) (45, 57).

Furthermore, the lymph circulation is a mirror of tissue events, a route of entry/dissemination of microorganisms and tumor cells, and, when damaged or diseased, the source of common chronic, vexing disorders, and less common life-threatening ones characterized by edema, fibrosis, immunodysregulation, nutritional depletion, and/or disturbed lymphangiogenesis and hemangiogenesis (64, 70, 71) (Fig. 2). As Starling surmised, edema and its sequelae in different organs ultimately represent a failure of the lymph circulation to maintain the balance between lymph formation and lymph absorption (Fig. 1). This failure may occur in either a high-lymph output (e.g., ascites from hepatic cirrhosis and portal hypertension) (59), low output (classical lymphedema), or mixed state (e.g., congestive heart failure (67) where venous hypertension both provokes increased lymph formation but also constitutes an impediment to its return to the central veins) of "dynamic" or mechanical failure of the lymph circulation, where lymph formation exceeds lymph absorption. Accordingly, treatment of edema works when it restores lymph balance through reducing lymph formation and/or enhancing lymph absorption. Therapeutic options for patients with lymphedema have expanded to include a variety of nonoperative (largely physical rather than pharmacologic) and operative methods, including bypass microsurgery on the delicate lymphatic vessels. New molecular and cellular therapeutic approaches are on the horizon to restore or modulate lymphatic system structure, function, and growth. And noninvasive lymphatic imaging technology provides a safe, reproducible dynamic means for defining, localizing, and monitoring the course of lymphatic disease and its treatment, and also a route of selective lymphatic administration of therapeutic agents.

MOLECULAR LYMPHOLOGY AND LYMPHVASCULAR GENOMICS (TABLE 3)

Culminating in the past decade, revolutionary advances in molecular biology have impacted lymphology by identifying some of the key molecules underlying lymphatic vascular growth and development and reigniting the century long Sabin–Kampmeier controversy over the centrifugal vs. centripetal embryonic development of the lymphatic system. These molecules (Table 3) include among others (1) VEGF-C and -D, new members of the vascular endothelial growth factor (VEGF) family which are predominantly lymphatic endothelial-specific growth factors (26) and earlier, what would be their corresponding receptor VEGFR-3 (*flt4*) (18) located on the surface of lymphatic endothelial cells (and also some hematopoietic precursor cells); (2) Prox-1 transcription factor crucial to the development of the embryonic lymph sacs (55); (3) angiopoietin 1 and 2 of the angiopoietin family of vascular growth-remodeling factors (17); and (4) podoplanin (7), a transmembrane sialomucoprotein highly expressed on lymphatic vessel endothelia with uncertain function perhaps relating to maintaining permeability of lymphatics as well as glomerular capillaries, pulmonary epithelium, and the choroid plexus. Of particular interest as a lymphatic-specific marker is the LYVE-1 hyaluronan receptor (5), the primary lymphatic endothelial receptor for hyaluronan, a mucopolysaccharide abundant in lymph. This receptor is structurally similar to CD44, the leukocyte inflammatory homing receptor, suggesting a possible role in lymphatic trafficking.

Accordingly, a host of new lymphatic-specific markers have thereby become available for investigation and application. The neglected phenomenon of lymphatic growth and regeneration, newly termed "lymphangiogenesis" in contradistinction to hemangiogenesis (64, 70), has been brought to the fore for reexamination in molecular terms in embryogenesis, tissue repair, and neoplasia (1, 2, 22, 42). Indeed, lymphangiogenesis has become a "hot topic" with important clinical implications (e.g., prenatal diagnosis, angiomodulator drugs, and gene therapy). Tissue engineering to regenerate lymphatic vessels as scaffolds is also in the developmental stage.

Using forward (candidate gene) genetic approaches, various transgenic mouse models have been engineered to delineate the genetic control of specific steps in lymphatic growth and development (65). Beginning in 1998 (12, 14, 68), reverse (family pedigree/linkage) genetic approaches using genome-wide searches

Table 3. Growth factor ligands, endothelial receptors, and transcription factors implicated in lymphatic vascular growth and development

Growth factors (GFs)	Endothelial receptors	Transcription factors
VEGF-A, -C, -D	VEGFR-2, -3	PROX-1
Angiopoeitin 1, 2	Tie2	FOXC2
Ephrin-B2	EphB4	SOX18
IGF-1, -2	Neuropilin2	Net
FGF-1, -2		
PDGF-BB		

reported linkage of familial autosomal dominant congenital Milroy lymphedema to the distal arm of chromosome 5 (q35.3) in some but not all families. The identification of VEGFR3 and the subsequent finding of specific mutations (28) in this coding region previewed the probability of a constellation of "lymphangiogenesis genes." In 2000, autosomal dominant lymphedema–distichiasis (LD) syndrome (pubertal onset lymphedema, lymphatic and lymph node hyperplasia, lymph reflux, and a double row of eyelashes) was linked to a mutation in FOXC2 (13), a forkhead transcription factor located on chromosome 16 that is important in embryogenesis as early as somite formation and specifically involved in tissues derived from mesenchyme. With striking similarity, the FOXC2 haploinsufficient (+/−) transgenic mouse (30, 40) typically exhibits not only a double row of eyelashes, but also a similar hyperplastic refluxing lymphatic system phenotype, and the embryonic lethal FOXC2 knockout (FOXC2$^{-/-}$) mouse displays aortic arch and ventricular septal defects and cleft palate (23) like some LD patients and also defective lymphatic valve formation (44). Lymphedema–hypotrichosis–telangiectasia syndrome has been linked to mutations in the transcription factor SOX18 on chromosome 20 (24). These collective findings underscore the phenotypic and genotypic heterogeneity among the nearly 40 Mendelian inherited lymphedema–angiodysplasia syndromes where specific mutated genes have not been identified (41) as well as in the more common chromosomal aneuploidies, such as trisomy 21 (Down), Turner XO, and Klinefelter XXY syndromes, which may present with lethal prenatal lymphatic malformations and hydrops. Taken together, these forward and reverse lymphvascular genomic studies point to a genome-wide distribution of growth factors, endothelial receptors, and transcription factors (Table 3), as well as other lymphatic-associated proteins concerned with lymphatic growth, development, structure, and function.

CANCER AND THE LYMPHATIC SYSTEM (FIG. 5)

For the past several centuries, it has been recognized that the lymphatic system is the stage on which cancer development and progression are played out, and historically up to the present time, lymphatic system involvement has also formed the basis for evaluation, prognostication, and operative and nonoperative treatment of most cancers. Indeed, in the one notable exception to the centuries-long neglect of the lymphatic system following Aselli's report of the chyliferous vessels in 1627, cancer theorists of his day seized upon the newly discovered lymphatic system to promulgate the "lymph theory" of cancer's origin from a tissue gel of lymph (54). The "lymph theory" replaced the discredited "black bile" theory of Galen, which had held sway for thousands of years, and remained popular until it, too, was displaced this time by Virchow's cell theory of cancer. In addition, even in the 1700s, surgeons, observing gross lymph node involvement in common cancers such as those arising in the breast, warned that once the cancer bulk reached regional lymph glands, the prognosis was poor. Later, within the context of Virchow's cell theory, it was thought that removal of all areas of tumor involvement had the

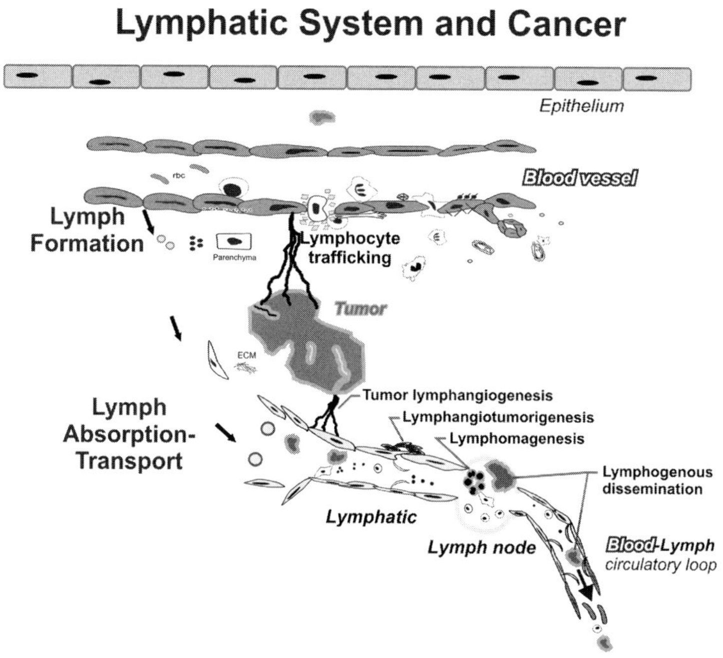

Lymphatic System and Cancer

Figure 5. Points of interplay between a developing tumor and ongoing processes within the interstitium and lymphatic system: lymph formation, lymphangiogenesis, lymph absorption–transport, lymphogenous tumor spread, tumor-generated immune response. These structural–functional interactions play a crucial role in the pathogenesis, clinical manifestations, evaluation, and prognosis as well as the treatment of cancer. Questions abound and need exploration. Reproduced with permission from Witte et al. (69)

highest chance for cure, and, accordingly, in the late 1800s, this view culminated in extensive Halstedian operations with radical lymphadenectomy. With the development of vital blue dye lymphatic imaging in 1937, lymphography by cannulation in the 1950s, and expanding application of lymphoscintigraphy to sentinel lymph node intraoperative mapping and biopsy (39), progressively less radical procedures could be planned to assess spread to lymph nodes and, when appropriate, to debulk adjacent tumor spread. As the significance of lymph nodes and lymphocytes in immune defense and surveillance became apparent in the latter half of the twentieth century, questions have lingered about the balance of beneficial and harmful influences of the lymphatic system in cancer (72) and how and when tumor cells gain entry (4) and spread through the lymphatic system.

Recent insights in molecular lymphology reveal that the growth factors, receptors, and transcription factors involved in development and function of the lymphatic system overlap and interdigitate with those involved in cancer development and spread. Members of the VEGF family are overexpressed in several tumors with some studies showing a positive correlation with lymphatic spread and tumor vasculogenesis. Angiopoietins 1 and 2 play a context dependent agonist and antagonist role in vascular remodeling probably through the recruitment and sustenance of perioendothelial cells and thus may modulate tumor cell invasion. Receptors for lymphatic growth factors are in the tyrosine kinase family, of which several others have been implicated in cancer growth and appear to have overlapping downstream signaling pathways. Other receptors and growth factors with lymphatic specificity are already in use as lymphatic markers within and around tumors. For example, LYVE1 also is expressed in a large variety of tumors. The D6 proinflammatory beta chemokine receptor has been identified in some malignant vascular tumors that show phenotype overlapping with lymphatic endothelial cells. Although there is limited understanding of these markers, their functional properties may or may not play a role in cancer metastasis.

Thus, the perturbations in lymphatic system processes in cancer (Fig. 5) (69) have remained largely inaccessible and unexplored. Some elements of long abandoned theories and unexplained clinical observations surrounding the lymphatic system persist until the present day and comprise key unanswered questions about cancer development, lymphogenous spread, and clinical course (62, 69).

TRANSLATIONAL LYMPHOLOGY

Whereas "translational medicine," i.e., basic scientists and clinicians coming together to expedite the close linking and application of advances in the laboratory from the "bench to the trench," i.e., from the laboratory to the bedside/clinic and community, may be a new movement for some medical specialties, it is nothing new for lymphology and lymphologists (61) (Table 1). As reviewed in this chapter, since before the official founding of the 44-member nation ISL, clinical lymphology has transcended the barriers of medical specialization, language, and geography. There is hardly a lymphologist, exemplified by pioneers such as Ernest Starling exploring the physiologic principles governing lymph formation and edema or Florence Sabin meticulously dissecting the lymphatic sacs of the human embryo, who was not looking, either as a basic scientist for the clinical implications of their findings, or, on the other hand, astute clinicians, like British surgeon John Kinmonth seeking out geneticists and imaging scientists for better explanations of the inheritance patterns and dysfunctional lymphographic images he was seeing for the first time in patients with lymphedema–angiodysplasia syndromes and better ways to visualize the barely visible lymphatic system and its hidden processes, or the Földis, framing the boundaries of lymphology with their ideas, experiments, teachings, and clinical practice (Table 1) (16). And collaborations in the field have contributed to better understanding and control of lymphatic filariasis, which afflicts hundreds of millions worldwide.

Recent advances in molecular lymphology and lymphangiogenesis research, particularly lymphvascular structural and functional genomics, proteomics, and lymphatic system biology, combined with fresh insights in clinical lymphology, especially those provided by noninvasive lymphatic system imaging including sentinel node mapping, should continue to shed light and lead to new management approaches for congenital and acquired lymphedema–angiodysplasia syndromes, tumors primarily and secondarily involving the lymphatic system as well as a variety of perplexing multisystem disorders.

EPILOGUE

In the words of "evo–devo" (evolution/development) expert of his day, Kampmeier, summing up his life immersed in "lympha" (the divine clear fluid captured by nymphs to fill the vessels of the gods but never mortals), "The lymph vessels, so unimpressive when they were first pointed out to me in 1909 under the microscope – but, I was soon to discover, so elusive or baffling to everyone who had studied them – have lost none of their tantalizing nature in all these years" (27).

ACKNOWLEDGMENTS

Supported by grants NIH RO1HL48493 (subcontract), R13HL64615, R21AT00405, Arizona Disease Control Research Commission Contracts 8277-000000-1-1-AT-6625, ZB-7492, I-103, and American Cancer Society RSGTL-05-090-01-CCE.

REFERENCES

1. Achen MG, McColl BK, Stacker SA (2005) Focus on lymphangiogenesis in tumor metastasis. Cancer Cell 7: 121-127
2. Alitalo K, Tammela T, Petrova T (2005) Lymphangiogenesis in development and human disease. Nature 438: 946-953
3. Aselli G (1627) De Lactibus sive Lacteis Venis, Quarto Vasorum Mesarai corum Genere novo invento. J.B. Biddellium, Mediolani, Milano
4. Azzali G (2003) Transendothelial transport and migration in vessels of the apparatus lymphaticus peripherics absorbens (ALPA). Int Rev of Cytology 230: 41-87
5. Banerji S, Ni J, Wang S-X, Clasper S, Su J, Tammi R, Jones M, Jackson DG (1999) LYVE-1, a new homologue of the CD44 glycoprotein, is a lymph-specific receptor for hyaluronan. J Cell Biology 144: 789-801
6. Bowman C, Witte MH, Witte CL, Way D, Nagle R, Copeland J, Daschbach C (1984) Cystic hygroma reconsidered: hamartoma or neoplasm? Primary culture of an endothelial cell line from a massive cervicomediastinal cystic hygroma with bony lymphangiomatosis. Lymphology 17: 15-22
7. Breiteneder-Geleff, S, Soleiman A, Kowalski H, Horvat R, Amann G, Kreihuber E, Diem K, Weninger W, Tschachler E, Alitalo K, Kerjaschki D (1999) Angiosarcomas express mixed endothelial phenotypes of blood and lymphatic capillaries: podoplanin as a specific marker for lymphatic endothelium. Am J Path 154: 385-394
8. Casley-Smith JR, Florey HL (1961) The structure of normal small lymphatics. Quart J Exp Physiol 46: 101-106
9. Clark ER, Clark EL (1932) Observations on the new growth of lymphatic vessels as seen in transparent chambers introduced into the rabbit's ear. Am J Anat 51: 49-87
10. Drinker CK, Yoffey JM (1941) Lymph flow and lymph pressure. In: Lymphatics, lymph and lymphoid Tissue. Harvard University Press, Cambridge, pp. 112-145
11. Dumont AE, Witte MH (1969) Clinical usefulness of thoracic duct cannulation. In: Stollerman GH (ed), Advances in internal medicine, vol. XV, Year Book Medical Publ., Inc., pp. 51-72
12. Evans AL, Brice G, Sotirova V, Mortimer P, Beninson J, Burnand K, Rosbotham J, Child A, Sarfarazi M (1999) Mapping of primary congenital lymphedema to the 5q35.3 region. Am J Hum Genet 64: 547-555
13. Fang JM, Dagenais SL, Erickson RP, Arlt MF, Glynn MW, Gorski JL, Seaver LH, Glover TW (2000) Mutations in FOXC2 (MFH-1), a forkhead family transcription factor, are responsible for the hereditary lymphedema-distichiasis syndrome. Am J Hum Genet 67: 1382-1388
14. Ferrell RE, Levinson KL, Esman JH, Kimak MA, Lawrence EC, Barmada MM, Finegold DN (1998) Hereditary lymphedema: evidence for linkage and genetic heterogeneity. Hum Mol Genet 7: 2073-2078
15. Florey H (1927) Observations on the contractility of lacteals. Part II. J Physiol 63: 1-18

16. Földi M, Földi E, (eds) (2006) Földi's textbook of lymphology. Urban & Fischer Verlag, München, Germany, 2nd ed, pp. 735
17. Gale NW, Thurston G, Hackett SF, Renard R, Wang Q, McClain J, Martin C, Witte C, Witte MH, Suri C, Campochiaro PA, Wiegand SJ, Yancopoulos GD (2002) Angiopoietin-2 is required for postnatal angiogenesis and lymphatic patterning, and only the latter role is rescued by angiopoietin-1. Developmental Cell 3: 411-423
18. Galland F, Karamysheva A, Mattei MG, Rosnet O, Marchetto S, Birnbaum D (1992) Chromosomal localization of FLT4, a novel receptor-type tyrosine kinase gene. Genomics 13: 475-478
19. Gnepp DR, Chandler W (1985) Tissue culture of human and canine thoracic duct endothelium. In Vitro 21: 200-206
20. Hall JG, Morris B, Woolley G (1965) Intrinsic rhythmic propulsion of lymph in the unanaesthetised sheep. J Physiol (Lond) 180: 336-349
21. Harvey W (1628) Exertatio anatomico de motu cordis et sanguinis in animalibus. Frankfurt, Guilielmi Fitzeri
22. Hong YK, Shin JW, Detmar M (2004) Development of the lymphatic vascular system: a mystery unravels. Dev Dyn 231: 462-473
23. Iida K, Koseki H, Kakinuma H, Kato N, Mizutani-Koseki Y, Ohuchi H, Yoshioka H, Noji S, Kawamura K, Kataoka Y, Ueno F, Taniguchi M, Yoshida N, Sugiyama T, Miura N (1997) Essential roles of the winged helix transcription factor MFH-1 in aortic arch patterning and skeletogenesis. Development 124: 4627-4638
24. Irrthum A, Devriend K, Chitayat D, Matthijs G, Glade C, Steijlen PM, Fryns J-P, Van Steensel AM, Vikkula M (2003) Mutations in the transcription factor gene SOX18 underlie recessive and dominant forms of hypotrichosis-lymphedema-telangiectasis. Am J Hum Genet 72: 1470-1478
25. Johnston MG, Walker MA (1984) Lymphatic endothelial and smooth-muscle cells in tissue culture. In Vitro 20: 566-572
26. Joukov V, Pajusola K, Kaipainen A, Chilov D, Lahtinen I, Kukk E, Saksela O, Kalkkinen N, Alitalo K (1996) A novel vascular endothelial growth factor, VEGF-C, is a ligand for the Flt-4 (VEGFR-3) and KDR (VEGFR-2) receptor tyrosine kinases. EMBO 15: 290-298
27. Kampmeier OF (ed) (1969) Evolution and comparative morphology of the lymphatic system. Charles C. Thomas, Springfield, Illinois, 620 p
28. Karkkainen MJ, Ferrell RE, Lawrence EC, Kimak MA, Levinson KL, McTigue MA, Alitalo K, Finegold DN (2000) Missense mutations interfere with vascular endothelial growth factor receptor-3 signaling in primary lymphedema. Nature Genet 25: 153-159
29. Kinmonth JB (ed) (1972) The lymphatics: diseases, lymphography and surgery. Edward Arnold, London, 420 p
30. Krieaderman BM, Myloyde TL, Witte MH, Dagenais SL, Witte CL, Rennels M, Bernas MJ, Lynch MT, Erickson RP, Caulder MS, Miura N, Jackson D, Brooks BP, Glover TW (2003) Foxc2 haploinsufficient mice are a model for human autosomal dominant lymphedema-distichiasis syndrome. Hum Molec Genet 12: 1179-1185
31. Leak LV, Burke JF (1966) Fine structure of the lymphatic capillary and the adjoining connective tissue area. Am J Anat 118: 785-809
32. Leak LV, Jones M (1994) Lymphangiogenesis in vitro: formation of lymphatic capillary-like channels from confluent monolayers of lymphatic endothelial cells. In Vitro Cell Dev Biol 30A: 512-518
33. Lymphology 1-40, 1967-2007
34. Mansel RE, Khonji NI, Clarke D (2000) History, present status and future of sentinel node biopsy in breast cancer. Acta Oncologica 39: 265-268
35. Mawhinney HJ, Roddie IC (1973) Spontaneous activity in isolated bovine mesenteric lymphatics. J Physiol 229: 339-348
36. Mayerson HS, Wolfram CG, Shirley HH, Wasserman K (1960) Regional differences in capillary permeability. Am J Physiol 198: 155-160
37. McHale NG, Thornbury KD (1986) A method for studying lymphatic pumping activity in conscious and anaesthetised sheep. J Physiol 378: 109-118
38. McMaster PD (1937) The lymphatics and lymph flow in the edematous skin of human beings with cardiac and renal disease. J Exp Med 65: 373-397
39. Morton DL, Wien DR, Wong JH, Economou JS, Cagle LA, Storm FK, Foshag LJ, Cochran AJ (1992) Technical details of intraoperative lymphatic mapping for early stage melanoma. Arch Surgery 127: 392-399
40. Noon A, Hunter RJ, Witte MH, Krieaderman B, Bernas M, Rennels M, Percy D, Enerback S, Erickson RP (2006) Comparative lymphatic ocular and metabolic phenotypes of Foxc2 haploinsufficient and aP2-FOXC2 transgenic mice. Lymphology 39: 84-94

41. Northup KA, Witte MH, Witte CL (2003) Syndromic classification of hereditary lymphedema. Lymphology 36: 162-189
42. Oliver G (2004) Lymphatic vascular development. Nat Rev Immunol 4: 35-45
43. Olszewski WL (1991) Lymph pressure and flow in limbs. In: Lymph stasis: pathophysiology, diagnosis and treatment. Boca Raton, FL, CRC Press, pp. 109-156
44. Petrova TV, Karpanen T, Norrmén C, Mellor R, Tamakoshi T, Finegold D, Ferrell R, Kerjaschki D, Mortimer P, Ylä-Herttuala S, Miura N, Alitalo K (2004) Defective valves and abnormal mural cell recruitment underlie lymphatic vascular failure in lymphedema distichiasis. Nature Med 10: 974-981
45. Pippard C, Roddie IC (1987) Comparison of fluid transport systems in lymphatics and veins. Lymphology 20: 224-229
46. Progress in Lymphology I-XX (1967-2007) Proceedings of the International Congresses of Lymphology
47. Pullinger DB, Florey HW (1937) Proliferation of lymphatics in inflammation. J Path Bacter 45: 157-170
48. Rusznyák I, Földi M, Szabo G (1960) Lymphatics and lymph circulation. Pergamon Press, New York:Oxford, 853 p
49. Sabin FR (1902) On the origin and development of the lymphatic system from the veins and the development of the lymph hearts and the thoracic duct in the pig. Am J Anat 1: 367-389
50. Sage HH, Kizilay D, Miyazaki M, Shapiro G, Sinha B (1960) Lymph node scintigrams. Am J Roentgenol Radium Ther Nucl Med: 84: 606-672
51. Starling EH (1896) Physiologic factors involved in the causation of dropsy. Lancet 1: 1267-1270
52. Starling EH (1909) The fluids of the body. The Herter Lectures. Chicago, WT Keener, p 81
53. Tilney ML, Murray JE (1968): Chronic thoracic duct fistula: operative technic and physiologic effects in man. Ann Surg 167:1-8
54. Triola VA (1965) Nineteenth century foundations of cancer research. Advances in tumor pathology, nomenclature, and theories of oncogenesis. Cancer Res 25: 75-106
55. Wigle JT, Oliver G (1999) Prox1 function is required for the development of the murine lymphatic system. Cell 98: 769-778
56. Witte CL, Witte MH (1985) Lymphatics in pathophysiology of edema. In: Johnston MG (ed) Experimental biology of the lymph circulation. New York, pp. 165-188
57. Witte CL, Witte MH (2005) Lymph circulatory dynamics, lymphangiogenesis, and pathophysiology of the lymphvascular system. In: Rutherford RB (ed) Vascular surgery. 6th ed, W.B. Saunders Company, Philadelphia, Pennsylvania, Chapter 166, pp. 2379-2396
58. Witte CL, Myers J, Witte MH, Katz M (1983) Transcapillary water and protein flux in the canine intestine with chronic extrahepatic portal hypertension. Circulation Res 53: 622-629
59. Witte CL, Witte MH, Dumont AE (1980) Lymph imbalance in the genesis and perpetuation of the ascites syndrome in hepatic cirrhosis. Gastroenterology 78: 1059-1068
60. Witte CL, Witte MH, Unger EC, Williams WH, Bernas MJ, McNeill GC, Stazzone A (2000) Advances in imaging of lymph flow disorders. RadioGraphics 20:1697-1719
61. Witte MH (2007) Translational lymphology and the Földiklinik. Eur J Lymphology (in press)
62. Witte MH, Witte CL (1999) What we don't know about cancer. Epilogue. In: Otter W, Root-Bernstein R, Koten J-W (eds) What is cancer? Theories on carcinogenesis. Anticancer Research 19: 4919-4934
63. Witte MH, Witte CL (1986) Lymphangiogenesis and lymphologic syndromes. Lymphology 19:21-28
64. Witte MH, Bernas M, Martin C, Witte CL (2001) Lymphangiogenesis and lymphangiodysplasias: from molecular to clinical lymphology. In: Wilting J (guest ed) The biology of lymphangiogenesis. Microscopy Research and Techniques 55: 122-145
65. Witte MH, Dellinger M, Northup K, Bernas M, Witte CL (2006a) Molecular lymphology and genetics of lymphedema-angiodysplasia syndromes. In: Földi M, Földi E (eds) Földi's textbook of lymphology, 2th ed, Chapter 16. Urban & Fischer Verlag, München, Germany, pp. 498-523
66. Witte MH, Dumont AE, Clauss RH, Rader B, Levine N, Breed ES (1969a) Lymph circulation in congestive heart failure: effect of external thoracic duct drainage. Circulation 39: 723-733
67. Witte MH, Dumont AE, Cole WR, Witte CL, Kintner K (1969b) Lymph circulation in hepatic cirrhosis: effect of portacaval shunt. Ann Intern Med 70: 303-310
68. Witte MH, Erickson R, Bernas M, Andrade M, Reiser F, Conlon W, Hoyme HE, Witte CL (1998) Phenotypic and genotypic heterogeneity in familial Milroy lymphedema. Lymphology 31: 145-155
69. Witte MH, Jones K, Wilting J, Dictor M, Selg M, McHale N, Gershenwald JE, Jackson DG (2006b) Structure function relationships in the lymphatic system and implications for cancer biology. Cancer Metastasis Rev 25: 159-184

70. Witte MH, Way DL, Witte CL, Bernas M (1997) Lymphangiogenesis: mechanisms, significance and clinical implications. In: Goldberg ID, Rosen EM (eds) Regulation of angiogenesis, Birkhäuser Verlag Basel/Switzerland, pp. 65–112
71. Witte MH, Witte CL, Way DL (1990) Medical ignorance, AIDS-Kaposi sarcoma complex, and the lymphatic system. Western J Med 153: 17–23
72. Yoffey JM, Courtice, FC (eds) (1970) Lymphatics, lymph and the lymphomyeloid complex. Academic Press, London, 942 p

2. EMBRYONIC DEVELOPMENT OF THE LYMPHOVASCULAR SYSTEM AND TUMOR LYMPHANGIOGENESIS

JÖRG WILTING, MARIA PAPOUTSI, KERSTIN BUTTLER, AND JÜRGEN BECKER

Children's Hospital, Pediatrics I, University of Goettingen, Robert-Koch-Strasse, Goettingen, Germany

INTRODUCTION

The embryonic development of the lymphatic vascular system starts considerably later than the blood vascular system. In chick embryos, the first blood vessels can be seen after 1 day of incubation, whereas morphological evidence for lymphatic endothelial cells (LECs) is present around day 5. However, with specific marker molecules, such as the transcription factor Prox1, LEC precursors can be identified in day-3.5 embryos. In the mouse, blood vessel development starts at embryonic day (ED) 7.5, whereas the anlagen of lymph vessels can be seen in the jugular region at ED 10. In human embryos there is a period of 3–4 weeks between the appearance of the first blood vascular endothelial cells (BECs) and LECs. There is good evidence that LECs develop from specialized parts of the venous system; however, there is growing evidence that scattered mesenchymal cells integrate into the growing fetal lymphatics. Similarly, lymphatics induced by tumors are derived mainly from local vessels, but, to some extent, pathologic lymphatics seem to develop by integration of circulating cells with lymphendothelial characteristics. In embryos, like in tumors, the most potent inducers of lymphangiogenesis are vascular endothelial growth factor (VEGF)-C and -D, which act mainly via VEGF receptor-3 (flt-4) on LECs. We have shown that blocking of this interaction prevents lymphangiogenesis in experimental A375 melanomas, while blocking of VEGF-A greatly inhibits blood vessel development (hemangiogenesis) in such tumors. However, local invasive growth of A375 melanoma cells is not significantly inhibited, showing that this tumor cell line induces hemangiogenesis, lymphangiogenesis, and invasiveness by distinct mechanisms.

EMBRYONIC LYMPHANGIOGENESIS

Development of Embryonic Lymph Sacs

The first obvious morphological criteria of the developing lymphatics are the lymph sacs, which are located in close vicinity to deep embryonic veins. Studies on mammalian embryos have shown that there are eight lymph sacs: three paired and two unpaired (30). The first lymph sacs develop in the jugular region, which is the area where the cranial and caudal jugular veins fuse into the common cardinal vein. The LECs of the jugular lymph sacs develop considerably later than the first BECs. In the chick, the first blood vessels can be seen after 1 day of incubation (26), whereas jugular lymph sacs are present around day 5 (5). However, with specific markers, such as the transcription factor Prox1, their precursors can be identified in day-3.5 embryos (40). In the mouse, blood vessel development starts at ED 7.5 (2). The anlagen of the lymph vessels can be seen in the jugular region at ED 10 (34). The consecutive development of BECs and LECs has led to the hypothesis that LECs are derived from BECs, specifically from neighboring veins (29). Recently, Oliver and Harvey (22) have supported this hypothesis on the basis of the expression pattern of the homeobox transcription factor Prox1. Prox1–deficient mice die at ED 14.5. They possess a normal blood vascular system, but the development of the lymphatics is arrested at ED 10.5 (34). The first Prox1-positive endothelial cells (ECs) are located in the jugular segment of the cardinal veins, and it has been postulated that these venous ECs are the precursors for LECs in the embryo (22). In avian embryos, the expression pattern of Prox1 is identical with that of mice. The jugular segment of the cardinal veins is Prox1-positive, and labeling of the early (day 4) blood vessels results in a signal in day 6.5 jugular lymph sacs (40), suggesting a blood vascular origin of lymph sacs. The lymphangiogenic protein vascular endothelial growth factor-C (VEGF-C) is essential for the development of lymph sacs. Mice deficient for VEGF-C, which is the ligand of VEGF receptor-3 (VEGFR-3), do not form lymph sacs. This deficiency can be rescued by the application of VEGF-C (14). The studies are in line with the traditional view of the development of LECs from specific parts of the venous system, also called "centrifugal theory." The main representative of this theory was Sabin (29, 30), who had performed India ink injections into the JLS of pig embryos. At about the same time, an opposing theory, the "centripetal theory," had been set up by Huntington and McClure (10) and Kampmeier (13), who had studied cat and pig embryos. According to them, the lymphatics develop by confluence of mesenchymal cells, and only the lymph sacs might be of venous origin (13). By means of grafting experiments we have recently shown that LECs of quail embryos are able to integrate into the lymph sacs of chick embryos (38), suggesting an additional, mesenchymal source for lymph sac ECs.

Transdifferentiation of Venous into Lymphatic Endothelial Cells

The lymph vessels of the body wall in the head, neck, and thoracic region are derived from the jugular segment of the cardinal veins. ECs in the cardinal veins obviously have the potency to give rise to two subtypes of ECs: venous and lymphatic. There are two likely mechanisms behind this phenomenon. Either bipotential ECs develop into the two lineages after asymmetric cell division, or venous ECs transdifferentiate into lymphatic ECs. Both mechanisms could be regulated by the transcription factor Prox1, which was originally cloned in mice due to its homology to the *Drosophila* homeobox protein *prospero* (23). Asymmetric distribution of *prospero* in the cytoplasm of ganglion mother cells of *Drosophila* regulates asymmetric division into *prospero*-negative neuroblasts and *prospero*-positive neurons or glia cells (11). Alternatively, Prox1 may induce transdifferentiation of venous ECs into lymphatic ECs. Transcriptional profiling of BECs that were transfected with *Prox1* cDNA has provided evidence for a shift toward a lymphatic phenotype (9, 28). In the jugular region, a subpopulation of ECs in the cardinal veins start to express Prox1 in ED 10 mouse and ED 4 chick embryos (34, 40). VEGFR-3 expression becomes restricted to the Prox1-positive LECs. Before, VEGFR-3 is expressed in all blood vessels of the embryo and VEGFR-3 knockout (ko) mice die of cardiovascular failure before lymph vessels develop (6). The ECs of the lymph sacs downregulate BEC markers such as type IV collagen and laminin, and upregulate LEC markers such as secondary lymphoid chemokine (SLC/CCL21) and LYVE-1, a sialoglycoprotein receptor for hyaluronan (1, 35).

Mesenchymal Lymphangioblasts

In the early days of lymphangiogenesis research employing serial sectioning of embryos, it was suggested that lymph vessels develop from "mesenchymal clefts" (10). Using modern terminology, this means the authors assumed that lymph vessels develop from scattered lymphangioblasts in the embryonic mesenchyme. These cells aggregate into tubes and form a communicating vascular system. It is well established that the blood vascular system of higher vertebrates develops in such a way. The precursor cells of BECs are called *angioblasts* and *hemangioblasts*, according to their potential to form endothelial cells or both endothelial and blood cells (36). Experimental studies on chick and quail embryos have provided evidence that the paraxial and splanchnic mesoderm contain cells with lymphangiogenic potential. Cells derived from these compartments are capable of integrating into embryonic lymphatics, and lymphangiogenic potential of mesodermal cells is present even before Prox1 is expressed in any of these cells (25, 31, 40). During subsequent development, coexpression of Prox1 and the endothelial marker QH1 in scattered mesodermal cells of quail embryos seems to be a marker of lymphangioblasts (40). Like in avian embryos, expression of LEC markers can also be observed in scattered mesodermal cells of murine embryos (Fig. 1). These cells are located in various mesodermal compartments of the embryo, e.g., in the dermatomes along the body axis (3). Scattered cells in this region are positive for Prox1 and LYVE-1 (Fig. 1a,b). We assume that these cells integrate into the lymph vessels in the dermis of the back.

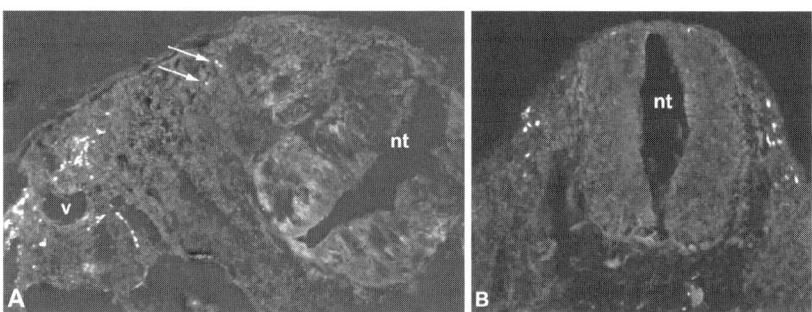

Figure 1. Staining of ED 11 mouse embryos with antibodies against markers of lymphendothelial cells. (a) Prox1 demarcates scattered cells (*arrows*) in the dermatomes and lymphatics close to the jugular vein (*v*). (b) LYVE-1 demarcates scattered cells in the dermatomes close to the neural tube (*nt*)

Evidence for the existence of embryonic lymphangioblasts in other vertebrate species has been provided recently. In *Xenopus* tadpoles, lymph vessels are obviously derived from both the venous system and from scattered mesenchymal cells (20). Like in other species, Prox1 and VEGF-C are essential for the development of lymph vessels in tadpoles. However, in the zebrafish, the primary source for lymph vessels seems to be the venous system (41).

TUMOR LYMPHANGIOGENESIS

Growth of tumors is largely dependent on active interactions of tumor cells with the blood vessels of the neighboring healthy tissue (7), and a high density of tumor microvessels is a high risk for hematogenic metastasis (33). However, in human solid cancer, the lymph node status is the most important prognostic indicator for the clinical outcome of patients (15, 16, 18, 19), but it has long been denied that tumors induce lymphangiogenesis (8, 32, 42), and it is still under debate if there is significant lymphangiogenesis in human tumors. An elaborated system of lymphatics has been observed in close proximity to invasive areas in breast cancer (4, 16), and *lymphangiosis carcinomatosa*, the destruction of the lymphatic endothelial lining by tumor cells, is an unfavorable prognostic finding (12). Although increased proliferation of LECs in the vicinity of human tumors can hardly be detected, numerous studies have reported on a positive correlation between expression of lymphangiogenic factors (VEGF-C and -D) and lymphatic vessel density or lymph node metastases (review: (27)). In small laboratory animals, tumors grow much faster and lymphangiogenesis can be measured. We have developed a model of tumor-induced lymphangiogenesis employing the chorioallantoic membrane (CAM) of avian embryos (24).

Tumor-Induced Lymphangiogenesis in the Avian Chorioallantoic Membrane

The CAM of reptiles and birds is an extraembryonic organ with respiratory functions. Furthermore, it serves as embryonic urinary bladder and mobilizes calcium from the eggshell. In chick embryos, the CAM develops on day 4, matures on day 12, and involutes on day 18–19. Hatching of chicks takes places around day 20–21. The CAM contains an almost two-dimensional blood vascular system of interdigitating arteries and veins connected to an intraepithelial capillary plexus. Additionally, there is a network of lymphatic capillaries, mostly along the arteries, but also surrounding larger veins. We have shown that VEGF-A applied on the CAM induces hemangiogenesis but not lymphangiogenesis, whereas VEGF-C induces lymphangiogenesis with a mild hemangiogenic side effect in higher doses (21, 37). VEGF-C-expressing human A375 melanoma cells induce development of lymphatics both at the tumor margins and within the tumor, with a BrdU labeling index of LECs of 11.6% (24). Huge dilated lymphatics can be seen at the tumor margins. These lymphatic capillaries are characterized by their extremely thin lining, which clearly distinguishes them from the blood capillaries. Within the tumors morphological criteria cannot be used to differentiate blood from lymphatic capillaries; however, with specific markers such as Prox1, LECs can be identified. Within the experimental melanomas, while the density of tumor cells increases, the lumina of the lymphatic vessels are lost. This is due to compression or destruction of the vessels. Also, preexisting lymphatic vessels become compressed or obstructed by the growing tumor mass, as shown by fluorescence microlymphangiography in the mouse (17). Proliferation of LECs is markedly reduced to 3.9% BrdU labeling, when A375 melanoma cells are stably transfected with cDNA for the soluble form of VEGFR-3 (sFlt4). Soluble VEGFR-3 markedly inhibits lymphangiogenesis in experimental A375 melanomas, but it does not inhibit hemangiogenesis, and the cells form huge vascularized tumors on the surface of the CAM (24, 39). This behavior completely changes after transfection of A375 melanoma cells with cDNA for the soluble form of VEGFR-1 (sFlt1), which binds VEGF-A with high affinity. The cells do not form vascularized solid tumors on the surface of the CAM. They remain avascular and become necrotic (Fig. 2a,b). However, the cells retain their high invasive potential. They invade the tumor stroma, interact with local vessels, and form tumor nodules (Fig. 2a,c–e). The nodules become surrounded by dilatated lymph capillaries, and finally the melanoma cells penetrate the lymphatics (Fig. 2e).

The data strongly suggest that:

1. VEGF-C is a lymphangiogenic factor that can be secreted by tumor cells. Inhibition of VEGFR-3 signaling strongly reduces tumor lymphangiogenesis, but not hemangiogenesis and tumor growth, and the high invasive potential of A375 melanoma cells also remains unaffected.
2. VEGF-A is a hemangiogenic factor secreted by A375 melanoma cells. Its inhibition greatly reduces formation of solid, vascularized tumors, but does not prevent interaction of the cells with the vascularized stroma of the host and formation of metastases.

In sum, tumor-hemangiogenesis, -lymphangiogenesis, and -invasiveness are distinct, although partially overlapping, mechanisms.

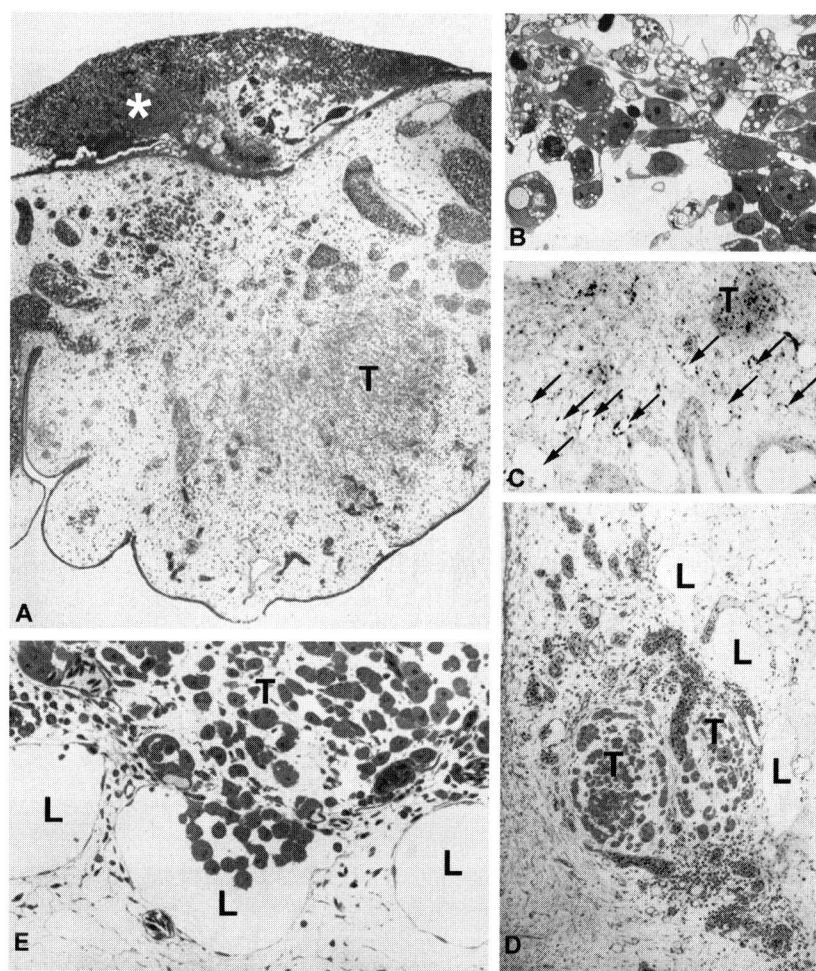

Figure 2. Human A375 melanoma cells were transfected with cDNA encoding soluble VEGFR-1 (sFlt1) and grown on the CAM of chick embryos. (**a**) Overview showing tumor cells (*asterisk*) on top of the CAM. Some tumor cells have invaded the stroma of the CAM and formed tumor nodules (*T*). (**b**) Melanoma cells on top of the CAM do not form solid tumors, remain avascular and become necrotic. (**c**) Tumor nodules (*T*) in the CAM stroma induce numerous VEGFR-3-positive lymphatics (*arrows*). (**d**) Semithin section showing tumor nodules (*T*) and adjacent, dilatated lymphatics (*L*). (**e**) Note invasion of melanoma cells into lymphatic vessels (*L*)

REFERENCES

1. Banerji S, Ni J, Wang SX, Clasper S, Su J, Tammi R, Jones M, Jackson DG (1999) LYVE-1, a new homologue of the CD44 glycoprotein, is a lymph-specific receptor for hyaluronan. J Cell Biol 144: 789-801
2. Breier G, Breviario F, Caveda L, Berthier R, Schnurch H, Gotsch U, Vestweber D, Risau W, Dejana E (1996) Molecular cloning and expression of murine vascular endothelial-cadherin in early stage development of cardiovascular system. Blood 87: 630-641

3. Buttler K, Kreysing A, von Kaisenberg CS, Schweigerer L, Gale N, Papoutsi M, Wilting J (2006) Mesenchymal cells with leukocyte and lymphendothelial characteristics in murine embryos. Dev Dyn 235: 1554-1562

4. Cann SA, van Netten JP, Ashby TL, Ashwood-Smith MJ, van der Westhuizen NG (1995) Role of lymphangiogenesis in neovascularization. Lancet 346: 903

5. Clark ER, Clark EL (1920) On the origin and early development of the lymphatic system of the chick. Contr Embryol 9: 447-482

6. Dumont DJ, Fong G, Puri PC, Gradwohl G, Alitalo K, Breitman ML (1995) Vascularisation of the mouse embryo: A study of flk-1, tek, tie and vascular endothelial growth factor expression during development. Dev Dyn 203: 80-92

7. Folkman J (1974) Tumor angiogenesis factors. Cancer Res 34: 2109-2113

8. Folkman J (1996) Angiogenesis and tumor growth. New England J Med 334: 921

9. Hong YK, Harvey N, Noh YH, Schacht V, Hirakawa S, Detmar M, Oliver G (2002) Prox1 is a master control gene in the program specifying lymphatic endothelial cell fate. Dev Dyn 225: 351-357

10. Huntington GS, McClure CFW (1908) The anatomy and development of the jugular lymph sacs in the domestic cat (*Felis domestica*). Anat Rec 2: 1-18

11. Jan YN, Jan LY (1998) Asymmetric cell division. Nature 392: 775-778

12. Kaiserling E (2003) Metastasis of malignant tumors. In: Földi M, Földi E, Kubik S (eds) Textbook of lymphology. Urban and Fischer, München, Jena, Germany, pp. 455-465

13. Kampmeier OF (1912) The value of the injection method in the study of the lymphatic development. Anat Rec 6: 223-233

14. Karkkainen MJ, Haiko P, Sainio K, Partanen J, Taipale J, Petrova TV, Jeltsch M, Jackson DG, Talikka M, Rauvala H, Betsholtz C, Alitalo K (2004) Vascular endothelial growth factor C is required for sprouting of the first lymphatic vessels from embryonic veins. Nat Immunol 5: 74-80

15. Lauria R, Perrone F, Carlomagno C, De Laurentiis M, Pettinato G, Panico L, Petrelle G, Bianco R, De Placido S (1995) The prognostic value of lymphatic and blood vessel invasion in operable breast cancer. Cancer 15: 1772-1778

16. Lee AKC, DeLellis RA, Silverman ML, Heatley GJ, Wolfe HJ (1990) Prognostic significance of peritumoral lymphatic and blood vessel invasion in node-negative carcinoma of the breast. J Clin Oncol 8: 1457-1465

17. Leu AJ, Berk DA, Lymboussaki A, Alitalo K, Jain RK (2000) Absence of Functional Lymphatics within a Murine Sarcoma: A Molecular and Functional Evaluation. Cancer Res 60: 4324-4327

18. Macchiarini P, Dulmet E, De Montpreville V (1995) Prognostic significance of peri-tumoural blood and lymphatic vessel invasion by tumour cells in T4 non-small cell lung cancer following induction therapy. Surg Oncol 4: 91-99

19. Maehara Y, Oshiro T, Baba H, Ohno S, Kohnoe S, Sugimachi K (1995) Lymphatic invasion and potential for tumor growth and metastasis in patients with gastric cancer. Surgery 117: 380-385

20. Ny A, Koch M, Schneider M, Neven E, Tong RT, Maity S, Fischer C, Plaisance S, Lambrechts D, Heligon C, Terclavers S, Ciesiolka M, Kalin R, Man WY, Senn I, Wyns S, Lupu F, Brandli A, Vleminckx K, Collen D, Dewerchin M, Conway EM, Moons L, Jain RK, Carmeliet, P (2005) A genetic Xenopus laevis tadpole model to study lymphangiogenesis. Nat Med 11: 998-1004

21. Oh S-J, Jeltsch MM, Birkenhäger R, McCarthy JEG, Weich HA, Christ B, Alitalo K, Wilting J (1997) VEGF and VEGF-C: specific induction of angiogenesis and lymphangiogenesis in the differentiated avian chorioallantoic membrane. Dev Biol 188: 96-109

22. Oliver G, Harvey N (2002) A stepwise model of the development of lymphatic vasculature. Ann N Y Acad Sci 979: 159-165

23. Oliver G, Sosa-Pineda B, Geisendorf S, Spana EP, Doe CQ, Gruss P (1993) Prox 1, a prospero-related homeobox gene expressed during mouse development. Mech Dev 44: 3-16

24. Papoutsi M, Siemeister G, Weindel K, Tomarev S, Kurz H, Schächtele C, Martiny-Baron G, Christ B, Marmé D, Wilting J (2000) Active interaction of human A375 melanoma cells with the lymphatics in vivo. Histochem Cell Biol 114: 373-385

25. Papoutsi M, Tomarev SI, Eichmann A, Pröls F, Christ B, Wilting J (2001) Endogenous origin of the lymphatics in the avian chorioallantoic membrane. Dev Dyn 222: 238-251

26. Pardanaud L, Altmann C, Kitos P, Dieterlen-Liévre F, Buck CA (1987) Vasculogenesis in the early quail blastodisc as studied with a monoclonal antibody recognizing endothelial cells. Development 100: 339-349

27. Pepper MS, Tille JC, Nisato R, Skobe M (2003) Lymphangiogenesis and tumor metastasis. Cell Tissue Res 314: 167-177

28. Petrova TV, Makinen T, Makela TP, Saarela J, Virtanen I, Ferrell RE, Finegold DN, Kerjaschki D, Yla-Herttuala S, Alitalo K (2002) Lymphatic endothelial reprogramming of vascular endothelial cells by the Prox-1 homeobox transcription factor. EMBO J 21: 4593-4599

29. Sabin FR (1902) On the origin of the lymphatic system from the veins and the development of the lymph hearts and thoracic duct in the pig. Amer J Anat 1: 367-389

30. Sabin FR (1909) The lymphatic system in human embryos, with a consideration of the morphology of the system as a whole. Am J Anat 9: 43-91

31. Schneider M, Othman-Hassan K, Christ B, Wilting J (1999) Lymphangioblast in the developing avian wing bud. Dev Dyn 216: 311-319

32. Tanigawa N, Kanazawa T, Satomura K, Hikasa Y, Hashida M, Muranishi S, Sezaki H (1981) Experimental study on lymphatic vascular changes in the development of cancer. Lymphology 4: 149-154

33. Weidner N (1995) Intratumoral microvessel density as a prognostic factor in cancer. Am J Pathol 147: 9-19

34. Wigle JT, Oliver, G (1999) Prox1 function is required for the development of the murine lymphatic system. Cell 98: 769-778

35. Wigle JT, Harvey N, Detmar M, Lagutina I, Grosveld G, Gunn MD, Jackson DG, Oliver G (2002) An essential role for Prox1 in the induction of the lymphatic endothelial cell phenotype. Embo J 21: 1505-1513

36. Wilting J, Becker J (2006) Two endothelial cell lines derived from the somite. Anat Embryol 211 Suppl 7: 57-63

37. Wilting J, Birkenhäger R, Eichmann A, Kurz H, Martiny-Baron G, Marmé D, McCarthy JE, Christ B, Weich HA (1996) VEGF$_{121}$ induces proliferation of vascular endothelial cells and expression of *flk-1* without affecting lymphatic vessels of the chorioallantoic membrane. Dev Biol 176: 76-85

38. Wilting J, Papoutsi M, Othman-Hassan K, Rodriguez-Niedenführ M, Pröls F, Tomarev SI, Eichmann A (2001) Development of the avian lymphatic system. Microsc Res Tech 55: 81-91

39. Wilting J, Hawighorst T, Hecht M, Christ B, Papoutsi M (2005) Development of lymphatic vessels: Tumour lymphangiogenesis and lymphatic invasion. Curr Med Chem 12: 3043-3053

40. Wilting J, Aref Y, Huang R, Tomarev SI, Schweigerer L, Christ B, Valasek P, Papoutsi M (2006) Dual origin of avian lymphatics. Dev Biol 292: 165-173

41. Yaniv K, Isogai S, Castranova D, Dye L, Hitomi J, Weinstein BM (2006) Live imaging of lymphatic development in the zebrafish. Nat Med 12: 711-716

42. Zeidman I, Copeland B, Waren S (1955) Experimental studies on the spread of cancer in the lymphatic system. II. Absence of the lymphatic supply in carcinoma. Cancer 8: 123-127

3. LYMPHATIC ORIGIN FROM EMBRYONIC STEM CELLS

MICHAEL DICTOR[1], SOFIA MEBRAHTU[1], MANUEL SELG[2], ZERINA LOKMIC[2], AND LYDIA SOROKIN[2]

Departments of [1]Pathology and [2]Experimental Pathology, Lund University Hospital, Sölvegatan 25, SE 22185 Lund, Sweden

INTRODUCTION

Lymph circulation is unidirectional and commences in the tissue within highly permeable but blind-ended capillaries composed of a single layer of endothelial cells. These capillaries (lymphatic initiators) are characterized by loosely arranged, overlapping endothelial cells, few intercellular tight junctions and occasional fragments of basement membrane, which account for lymphatic permeability to fluid, macromolecules, pathogens, immune cells, and metastatic tumor cells. The lymphatic vessels are anchored to the surrounding extracellular matrix via anchoring filaments arising from the endothelial cells. As the lymphatic capillaries coalesce into larger collecting ducts, they acquire smooth muscle cells outside of the endothelial layer and start to structurally resemble veins. The larger, collecting vessel has valves to prevent the retrograde flow of lymph, a continuous basement membrane, a muscle layer, and an adventitial layer anchoring it to the surrounding tissue (18).

Research into the lymphatic system has been hindered by the lack of lymphatic markers to clearly identify lymphatic vessels and has been consequently overshadowed by the intense research into the development of blood and the blood vascular system and the search for the common vascular and haematopoietic stem cell giving rise to both. With the identification of lymphatic vessel-specific markers such as the vascular endothelial growth factor receptor 3 (VEGFR-3), the hyaluronan receptor LYVE-1, transcription factor Prox1 (prospero-related homeobox 1) and podoplanin (4), lymphatic research has undergone a revival and promises to delineate molecular mechanisms governing the lymphatic development, maturation and remodeling.

DEVELOPMENT OF LYMPHATIC VESSELS IN THE EMBRYO

The early embryonic blood vessels express CD31, MECA-32 (7), CD34, VE-cadherin, the hyaluronan receptor LYVE-1, and vascular endothelial growth factor receptor 3 (VEGFR-3, Fms-like tyrosine kinase 4, Flt-4), a receptor for VEGF-C (8) and VEGF-D (1). The lymphatic system develops from venous endothelium starting at embryonic day 9–10.5 when a polarized subset of CD31+ endothelial cells in axial veins expresses the Prox1 transcription factor (17). At this point expression of VEGFR-3 (up to E12.5) and LYVE-1 in the mouse shifts to lymphatic endothelium in which CD31 becomes downregulated (9, 17). Lymphatics express also VE-cadherin but not MECA-32 (12). By budding and sprouting these initial lymphatics eventually form the entire lymphatic network (Fig. 1) (29). On E10.5–11.5 mesenchymal cell VEGF-C induces

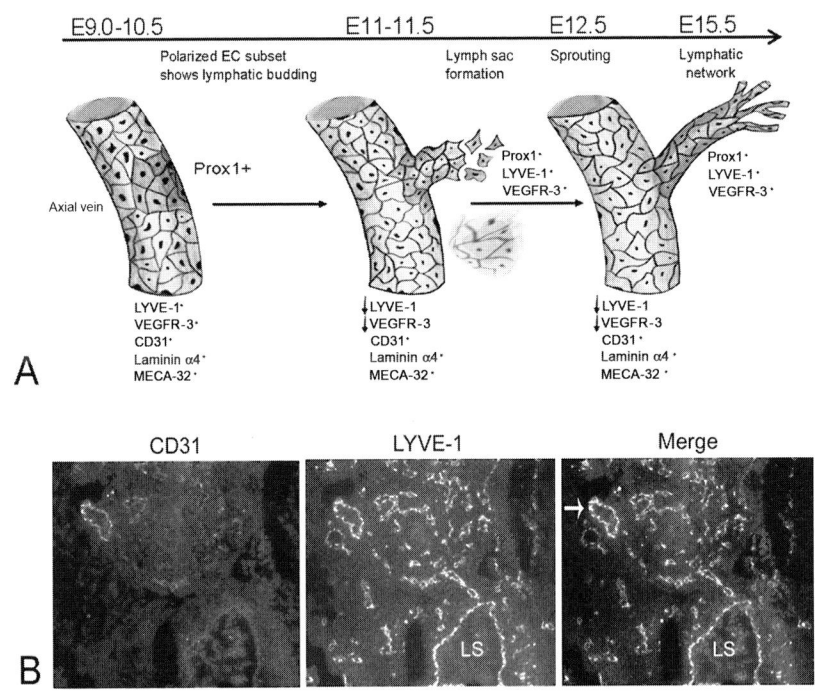

Figure 1. (**a**) Schematic of lymphatic development in mammalian embryogenesis with changes in expression patterns of cell surface molecules as the Prox1 transcription factor commits some venous cells to the lymphatic lineage. (**b**) Nuchal sections of mouse embryo at E10 show vessels brightly stained with LYVE-1 and a single vein intensely stained with CD31. This vein also expressed LYVE-1 in the merged photomicrograph (*arrow*). LS, lymph sac

lymphatic budding (17). Targeted gene inactivation of either Prox1 or VEGF-C prevents lymphatic development (29).

Following the commitment of the venous endothelial cell to lymphatic lineage under the direction of Prox1, other factors may play a role in the sprouting development of the lymphatic vessels, including basic fibroblast growth factor (bFGF) and hepatocyte growth factor (HGF), although their role is not clearly defined. EphrinB2, a transmembrane ligand, has been implicated in the formation and remodeling of the primary lymphoid vascular plexus (15).

The embryonic development of the smaller lymphatic vessels may be partly under control of neuropilin-2, a nonreceptor tyrosine kinase (30), while the absence of podoplanin, a membrane transport protein expressed by the lymphatic endothelium, results in structural and functional abnormalities of cutaneous and intestinal lymphatic vessels, depending on the mouse genetic background (23).

In addition to budding and sprouting, the lymphatic vessels undergo maturation and differentiation, a process thought to be similar to that described in blood vessels. Similar to blood vessel development, the maturation of the lymphatic vessel is signaled by the presence of the smooth muscle cell. FOXC2, a forkhead transcription factor, appears to play a role in recruitment of smooth muscle cells to the lymphatic endothelium during the process of remodeling and maturation (20).

Angiopoietin-2 (Ang-2), a ligand for Tie-2 receptor (14) is usually restricted to remodeling blood vessels during physiological angiogenesis. However, knocking out this gene leads to formation of chylous ascites, subcutaneous edema, disorganized and leaky lymphatic vessels, defects in the postnatal remodeling in the retina, and death of Ang-2 null mice within 2 weeks of birth (5). It is currently unknown if Ang-2 regulatory mechanisms are active in the lymphatic embryoid body cultures.

EMBRYOID BODY LYMPHANGIOGENESIS

Embryoid bodies (EB) are derived from differentiating murine embryonic stem cells and have been used to study early blood vessel formation, including the timing of relevant gene expression, which mimics the sequence of events in vivo (28). EB develop CD31$^+$ (pseudo)vessels early and the vessels survive for weeks. EB generated from hanging drops have a complex stereotypical though asymmetric development with a central core that may cavitate after proliferating cells have migrated down to the glass surface and spread out in a multilayer on the bottom of the well. Eccentrically opposed to the core and its vessels are collections of rhythmically contracting striated muscle cells. In and around the core wall is a plexiform vascular network, which is noted as early as day 5 post trypsinization. A number of multicellular "anchors" extend from the raised core (which flattens over time), some of which contain rare islands of endothelium in their center and may insert into small CD31$^+$ vascular foci in the spreading multilayer (Fig. 2).

Recent in vitro studies have shown that several major features of the in vivo lymphangiogenesis model can be replicated in differentiating murine embryonic

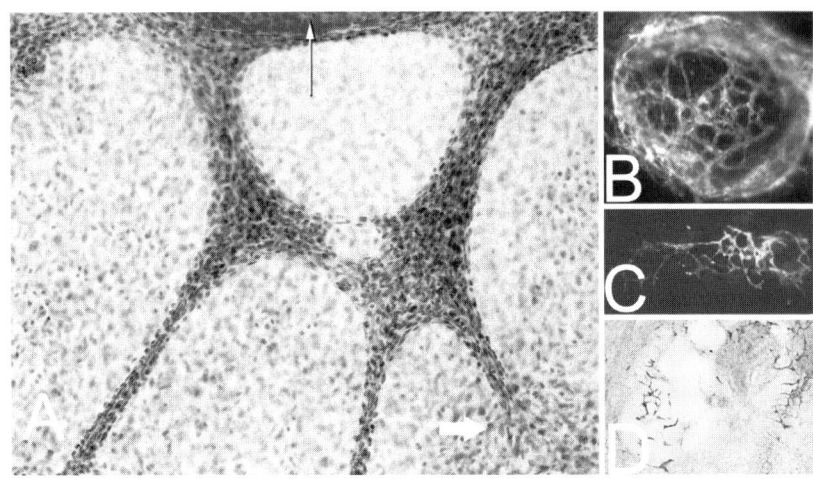

Figure 2. (a) H & E-stained EB at day 7 with cellular core (*thin arrow* at rim) giving rise to multiple "anchors" inserting in the multilayer on the chamber floor, the rightmost one anchored over a subsurface blood vessel plexus (*thick arrow*). **(b)** The core immunostained for CD31. **(c)** The subsurface plexus similarly stained. **(d)** A low power photograph of lymphatics within a single EB at day 6 (d. 5 + 1) stained with immunoperoxidase using anti-LYVE-1

stem cells (11, 12) and this has been partly confirmed in our own laboratory. Table 1 summarizes findings and highlights technical aspects which may account for the different results produced by various laboratories. While there is general agreement as to the anatomic and immunophenotypical features of lymphatic tubes relative to blood vascular tubes, there is less concordance as to the timing of events and the effects of VEGF isoforms on the developing lymphatics.

Our results are in agreement with Kreuger et al. (11) concerning the close proximity of LYVE-1$^+$/CD31$^-$ lymphatics to LYVE-1$^-$/CD31$^+$ blood vessels, which is consistent with the origin of lymphatics in veins. This close spatial relation can be appreciated in the three-dimensional effect of the deconvoluted image in Fig. 3. Co-expression of Prox1, podoplanin, and LYVE-1 has confirmed the lymphatic nature of LYVE-1$^+$/CD31$^-$/MECA-32$^-$ structures. VE-cadherin is present in postnatal vessels of both types and this was also confirmed in our EB. The lymphatic vascular tubes were usually parallel to or contiguous with CD31$^+$ vessels in the vicinity of the core but were also found scattered in smaller numbers within the multilayer unassociated with blood vessel structures.

Vessels staining for CD31 and MECA-32, especially large confluences, frequently contain aggregates of CD31$^+$/MECA-32$^-$ hematopoietic precursors, although we have found no such aggregates within lymphatic tubes.

Independent work in the three different laboratories has consistently identified a proportion of vessels in EB which co-expresses CD31 and LYVE-1. Using density slicing in which pixels are quantified at varying depths in EB we could verify a progressive decrease in double positives over time (Fig. 4), consistent both with the

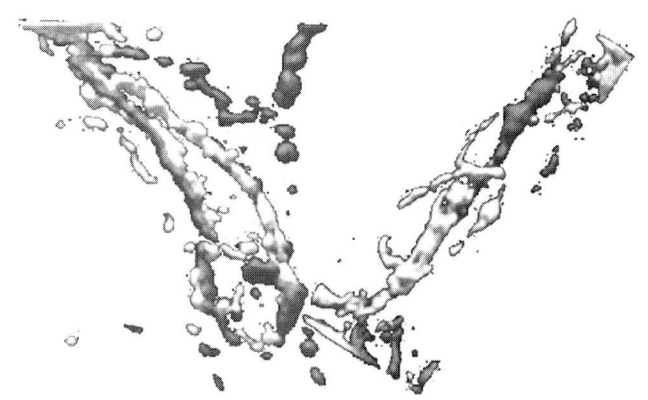

Figure 3. Deconvolution image of EB vessels stained with anti-CD31 (gray tone) and anti-LYVE-1 (light tone) depicts the intimate spatial relation, including focal contiguity, between blood vessels and lymphatics

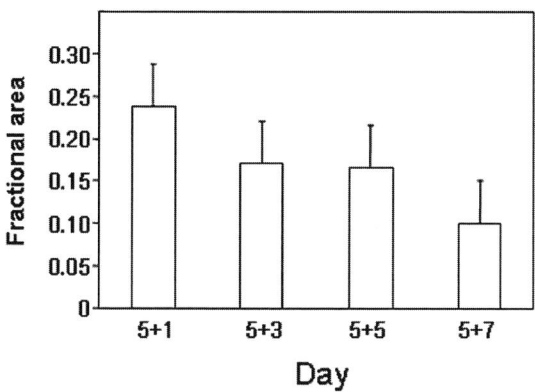

Figure 4. The time course of CD31/LYVE-1 double-positives by fractional EB area with each bar showing 5 days in hanging drop/suspension + x days in slide chambers (one S.D. at top of bar)

in vivo findings and the fact that the two vascular systems are derived from a common precursor cell at least one differentiation step after the hemangioblast in vasculogenesis. Liersch et al. (12) documented too that doubly positive vessels later began to express Prox1 which correlates with the observation that in embryogenesis Prox1 expression in the CD31[+]/LYVE-1[+] cardinal vein commits the endothelial cell to the lymphatic lineage.

Extracellular Matrix and Vessels in the Embryoid Body

The lymphangiogenic process can occur both in the presence and the absence of extracellular matrix, but neither of the above EB studies has examined whether differentiating lymphatic endothelial cells have the capacity to form their own matrix. Extracellular matrix appears also to follow in vivo patterns relative to vascular structures. As a constituent of basement membranes, laminin α4 chain is produced by embryonic blood vessel endothelium (6, 21, 24) but is barely detectable in lymphatics (13, 19, 27). We found that the α4 chain was strongly expressed by CD31⁺ EB vessels and it was correspondingly absent in the embryoid body lymphatics (Fig. 5). During embryogenesis, blood vessels produce the laminin α5 chain only in larger vessels and it first appears in the basement membranes of blood capillaries in postnatal life (26). As expected, we are unable to detect laminin α5 in the immature vessels of either lineage in the embryoid body.

To date, no comparative study has been made that examines if lymphatic vessels are structurally or functionally different when grown in three-dimensional matrix or not, or if growth regulation is affected by the type and quantity of matrix support.

We found LYVE-1⁺/CD31⁻/MECA-32⁻ lymphatic tubes as early as one day after seeding EB, i.e., 5 days post-trypsinization. In marked contrast, Kreuger et al. (11) did not identify complex lymphatic structures in cultures until day 12. Moreover, both Kreuger et al. and Liersch et al. reported continued lymphatic viability at 21 days and beyond, while lymphatics in our system unfailingly began to regress on day 10, regardless of supplementation with VEGF isoforms. The roots of these discrepancies may lie in the different technical approaches to EB culturing (Table 1) and suggests that comparative studies may reveal other factors critical for lymphatic growth.

Growth Factors in the Maintenance of Lymphatic Vessels

Importantly, for correlation with in vivo VEGF-C knockout data, in our laboratory, lymphatics fail to grow and form tubes if VEGFR-3 signaling is blocked by competitive inhibition with recombinant VEGFR-3/Fc (#743-R3, R&D, 3 μg/ml) or

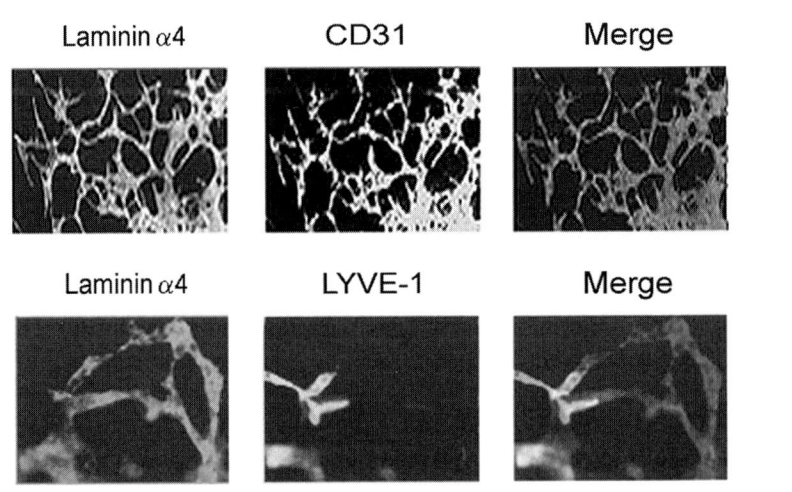

Figure 5. Double staining at day 6 for laminin α4 (originally red) and vascular membrane markers (green) indicates coexpression of laminin with CD31 but not LYVE-1

Table 1. EB lymphatic culture conditions, regulation and fate in three studies

Study	EB culture before trypsinisation	EB initiation & no./well	Medium for suspension culture	Supporting matrix	Onset of lymphatic growth (day)	VEGF-A effect	VEGF-C effect	VEGF-D effect	Lymphatic survival (days)	Origin of lymphatics	CD31+/ LYVE1+ cells	Serum deprivation effect
Liersch et al. (12)	Mitotically inactivated primary mouse fibroblasts in DMEM + 15% FBS, 1 M HEPES, 100 nM sodium pyruvate, 0.12% monothioglycerol, 1,000 IU/ml⁻¹ LIF	Single cell suspension; ref [23]; no. of wells not specified	Ref. (23)	None specified	18	D.14:5% FBS + 20 ng / ml⁻¹, (4 and 7 days) or 15% FBS + 20 ng/ml⁻¹, (d.4 & 7); *Increase*	D.14:5% FBS + 200 ng / ml or 15% FBS + 200 ng/ml⁻¹, (d.4 & 7); *Increase*	Not done	>27	From blood vessels formed in EB, not affected by bFGF	Yes	Not done
Kreuger et al. (11)	Mitotically arrested mouse embryonic fibroblasts + DMEM-Glutamax, 15% FBS, 25 mmol / L⁻¹ HEPES, pH 7.4, 1.2 mmol / L⁻¹ sodium pyruvate, 0.12% monothioglycerol, 1,000 IU/ml⁻¹ LIF; passaged every 48 h	1,200 cells into hanging drop + 30/ml⁻¹ VEGF-A: 8–10 EB/well	D. 0–4: DMEM-Glutamax, 15% FBS, 25 mmol L⁻¹ HEPES, pH 7.4, 1.2 mmol L⁻¹ sodium pyruvate, 0.12% monothioglycerol, 1,000 IU/ml⁻¹ LIF; From day 4: Ham's F12 medium + 5 mmol L⁻¹ NaOH, 20 mmol L⁻¹ HEPES, 0.225% NaHCO3, 1% Glutamax-1	D.4: 3D collagen I gel (1.5 mg/ml⁻¹)	12	15% FBS + 30 mg/ml *No effect*	30 ng/ml; *Increase,* synergistic effect with 30 ng/ml⁻¹ VEGF-A	Not done	24	From blood vessels formed in EB + de novo formation, headed by a tip cell	Yes	Not done

(Continued)

Table 1. EB lymphatic culture conditions, regulation and fate in three studies—cont'd

Study	EB culture before trypsinisation	EB initiation & no./well	Medium for suspension culture	Supporting matrix	Onset of lymphatic growth (day)	VEGF-A effect	VEGF-C effect	VEGF-D effect	Lymphatic survival (days)	Origin of lymphatics	CD31+/ LYVE1+ cells	Serum deprivation effect
Present data	Mitotically inactivated primary mouse fibroblasts in DMEM + 15% FBS, 1 M HEPES, 100 nM sodium pyruvate, 1,000 IU/ml⁻¹ LIF	600 cells/2d hanging drop culture in DMEM + 20% FBS, β-ME, 1× nonessential amino acids; 1 EB/well	D.5: DMEM + 20% FBS	None	<5	Not done	5% FBS + 100 ng/ml⁻¹, starting with hanging drop; *No effect*	5% FBS + 300 ng/ml⁻¹ starting with hanging drop; *No effect*	Up to d.11 then regress	From blood vessels formed in the EB + de novo formation	Yes, with progressive decline	Lymphatic regression

if EB are cultured in serum deprivation (5% FBS), while the viability of the CD31$^+$ blood vessels is unaffected. Similarly, lymphangiogenesis is blocked in mice expressing soluble VEGFR-3 (16) or lacking the receptor (10).

Because EB vessels are highly asymmetric and grow with varying robustness in individual EB, area measurements of selected fields such as reported by both groups is semiquantitative with an element of subjectivity, as implied by Kreuger et al. (11). Our own subjective evaluation (involving four independent observers) of lymphatics in whole EB showed no difference between controls and EB supplemented with VEGF-C and/or VEGF-D. On the other hand, Liersch et al. (12) found that VEGF-A and VEGF-C each promoted lymphatic development, whereas VEGF-A alone did not promote lymphangiogenesis according to Kreuger et al. (11). The latter group did, however, find increased lymphatics with VEGF-C and even more so with combined VEGF-C and VEGF-A. Furthermore, bFGF-2, hepatocyte growth factor and (Kreuger group only) hypoxia had no effect on the development of lymphatic vessels in the EB. Neither group of authors report lymphatic regression.

The above inconsistencies notwithstanding, the time-dependent regression of serum-supplemented lymphatic vessels, the stunting of lymphatic development in serum-depleted medium, and the failure of the growth factors VEGF-C and VEGF-D to reverse these events, in addition to the inhibition of lymphatic development caused by inactivation of VEGFR-3 signaling suggest that in addition to VEGFR-3 ligand binding, at least two other factors or endothelial cell interactions are necessary for the early survival of lymphatics rather than simply their continued proliferation. In addition to addressing these issues, the model can also be utilized to examine if the developed vessels are recruiting supporting cells (such as smooth muscle) from the cells constituting the embryonic body, which signals are involved in this process, and to what degree the process of lymphatic maturation is similar to that of the well-described vascular remodeling (22).

CONCLUSION

Lymphatic development in EB replicates lymphangiogenesis in vivo and is initiated by the transcription factor Prox1. The timing and fate of EB lymphatics appear to be strongly influenced by culture conditions such as supplementation with extracellular matrix proteins acting in concert with growth factors and possibly other supplements. Cells co-expressing lymphatic and blood vessel markers decline over time, consistent with differentiation toward the lymphatic lineage. In addition, competitive blockage of signaling through VEGFR-3 causes failure of lymphatic development, which corroborates the in vivo effect of abrogating the ligand VEGF-C.

We suggest that EB may be used to test the effect of heterologous gain-of-function genes, gene knockouts, biological modifiers, and co-cultured cancer cells on endothelial development. Advantages over in vivo models include shortened experiment times, reduced costs, and the availability of unlimited quantities of pluripotent stem cells without ethical implications. In addition, problems with embryonic lethality due to gene modifications may be avoided, while still allowing analysis of gene function, particularly if robust quantitative methods are applied. Differentiating embryonic stem cells with loss of one or both alleles for angiopoietin-2 or FOXC2 would, for example, offer potential models for comparison with in vivo data.

METHODS

Embryoid Body Cultures

For in vitro immunophenotypical analysis after growth factor supplementation, wild-type R1 ES maintained undifferentiated on both mouse fibroblast feeders and in leukemia inhibitory factor were trypsinized and then grown 2 days in DMEM containing 20% FCS, β-mercaptoethanol (β-ME), and nonessential amino acids (NEA) in hanging drops (600 cells per drop), as previously described (3). Nascent EB were then suspended for 3 days in medium, prior to seeding on day 5 one EB per chamber on eight-chamber slides (Lab-Tek). EB growing in 20% FCS were supplemented from day 1 with 100 ng ml^{-1} recombinant human vascular endothelial growth factor C (VEGF-C, #752-VC-025, R&D Systems, England), 300 ng ml^{-1} recombinant mouse VEGF-D (#469-VD-025, R&D), or recombinant mouse chimeric VEGFR-3/Fc (#743-R3, R&D) at a final concentration of 3 μg ml^{-1}. These supplements were replenished daily in suspension culture and with fresh medium (125 μl) every day after seeding. Other hanging-drop EB started in 20% FCS were grown in 5% FCS from day 3 onward at which time a similar regimen of supplements was begun in order to more precisely determine the effect of growth factors on lymphatic development in the face of serum depletion. Control slides with either serum concentration received no supplementary growth factors throughout the culture period. EB were grown up to 10 days (denoted as day 5 + x) in chamber prior to fixation in cold methanol and immunostaining. The effects of VEGF-C, VEGF-D, and competitive binding of VEGFR-3 ligand were assessed on day 5 + 2.

Production of Anti-LYVE-1

Polyclonal rabbit antimouse LYVE-1 antiserum was raised against the 212-aa putative extracellular domain of mouse LYVE-1, essentially as described previously (2). The protein was expressed in NIH 293 cells for immunization of rabbits by subcutaneous injection. The resultant antiserum displayed properties similar to those already described. Specific intense immunofluorescence staining was noted on lymphatic cell membranes (and some macrophages) in all lymphatic-bearing tissues tested, including skin, lymph node, and bowel but not brain or kidney. Similarly, rat monoclonal antimouse LYVE-1 was produced as previously described (25).

Antibodies

In addition to rabbit anti–LYVE-1 antibody, primary antibodies for endothelial markers included monoclonal rat antimouse CD31, anti-CD34 (both 1:100, BD Pharmingen, USA), and goat antimouse VEGFR-3 (1:100, R&D Systems, USA). For basement membrane proteins, polyclonal rabbit antisera were used against mouse laminin chains $\alpha 4$ (21) and $\alpha 5$ (26) in double stains with anti–CD31 or rat monoclonal anti–LYVE-1 in clones 24C5 (1:200). Secondary antibodies included adsorbed Cy3-(or Texas red) conjugated goat antirat and goat antirabbit-FITC (all 1:200, Jackson Labs, USA).

Stained slides were viewed in a Zeiss Axioplan 2 fluorescence microscope controlled by the Open Lab software package and equipped with single bandpass filters appropriate for the above fluorochromes.

Density Slicing of EB

The ratio of double stained LYVE-1/CD31 areas to single stained areas in entire EB was determined by density slicing on days 6, 8, 10, and 12 (5 + 1, 5 +3, 5 + 5 and 5 + 7) using the appropriate software module. Selection criteria included the intensity of colorized red and green channels, and yellow in the merged images, corresponding to vessel structures.

APPENDIX

EF medium for fibroblast feeder cells: DMEM high glucose with Na-pyruvate and 2 mM L-glutamine or Glutamax (Gibco), 10% fetal bovine serum (FBS, Gibco).

ES medium for ES cells: DMEM high glucose, Na-pyruvate (Gibco) and Glutamax or 2 mM L-glutamine, 15–20% heat-inactivated FBS, β-mercaptoethanol 0.1 mM, 3.5 μl per 500 ml medium, 100 × nonessential amino acids (NEA, Gibco), 5 ml per 500 ml medium, LIF (leukemia inhibitory factor) 1,000 U ml^{-1} (ESGRO from Chemicon, #ESG1107). LIF concentrate should be dissolved in 10 ml DMEM + 20% FBS, aliquoted 0.5 ml × 20 and is then stable at 4°C. Use 0.5 ml LIF per 500 ml medium.

EB medium for embryoid bodies: As ES medium above but with 5–20% FBS and *no* LIF.

Undifferentiated ES can be cryopreserved after trypsinizing in trypsin/EDTA for 15 min at 37°C and then aliquoting in ice-cold DMEM with 15–20% FBS and 10% dimethylsulfoxide and storage at −80°C.

ACKNOWLEDGMENTS

The authors are indebted to Prof. Reinhard Fässler for introducing us to embryonic stem cell techniques. Gunnel Roos provided expert help in sectioning and staining. This work was supported by grants from the LU-ALF Fund through the Lund University Medical Faculty (L.S. and M.D.), the Deutsche Forschungsgellschaft (So285/5-1 and So285/5-2), the Alfred Österlund Foundation, the Knut and Alice Wallenberg Foundation (KAW 2002.0056), and the Swedish Research Council (L.S.) and Stiftelsen Forskning utan djurförsök (M.D.).

REFERENCES

1. Achen MG, Jeltsch M, Kukk E, Makinen T, Vitali A, Wilks AF, Alitalo K, Stacker SA (1998) Vascular endothelial growth factor D (VEGF-D) is a ligand for the tyrosine kinases VEGF receptor 2 (Flk1) and VEGF receptor 3 (Flt4). Proc Natl Acad Sci U S A 95:548-553
2. Banerji S, Ni J, Wang SX, Clasper S, Su J, Tammi R, Jones M, Jackson DG (1999) LYVE-1, a new homologue of the CD44 glycoprotein, is a lymph-specific receptor for hyaluronan. J Cell Biol 144:789-801

3. Bloch W, Forsberg E, Lentini S, Brakebusch C, Martin K, Krell HW, Weidle UH, Addicks K, Fassler R (1997) Beta 1 integrin is essential for teratoma growth and angiogenesis. J Cell Biol 139:265-278

4. Breiteneder-Geleff S, Soleiman A, Kowalski H, Horvat R, Amann G, Kriehuber E, Diem K, Weninger W, Tschachler E, Alitalo K, Kerjaschki D (1999) Angiosarcomas express mixed endothelial phenotypes of blood and lymphatic capillaries: podoplanin as a specific marker for lymphatic endothelium. Am J Pathol 154:385-394

5. Gale NW, Thurston G, Hackett SF, Renard R, Wang Q, McClain J, Martin C, Witte C, Witte MH, Jackson D, Suri C, Campochiaro PA, Wiegand SJ, Yancopoulos GD (2002) Angiopoietin-2 is required for post-natal angiogenesis and lymphatic patterning, and only the latter role is rescued by Angiopoietin-1. Dev Cell 3:411-423

6. Hallmann R, Horn N, Selg M, Wendler O, Pausch F, Sorokin LM (2005) Expression and function of laminins in the embryonic and mature vasculature. Physiol Rev 85:979-1000

7. Hallmann R, Mayer DN, Berg EL, Broermann R, Butcher EC (1995) Novel mouse endothelial cell surface marker is suppressed during differentiation of the blood brain barrier. Dev Dyn 202:325-332

8. Joukov V, Pajusola K, Kaipainen A, Chilov D, Lahtinen I, Kukk E, Saksela O, Kalkkinen N, Alitalo K (1996) A novel vascular endothelial growth factor, VEGF-C, is a ligand for the Flt4 (VEGFR-3) and KDR (VEGFR-2) receptor tyrosine kinases. Embo J 15:1751

9. Kaipainen A, Korhonen J, Mustonen T, van Hinsbergh VW, Fang GH, Dumont D, Breitman M, Alitalo K (1995) Expression of the fms-like tyrosine kinase 4 gene becomes restricted to lymphatic endothelium during development. Proc Natl Acad Sci U S A 92:3566-3570

10. Karkkainen MJ, Haiko P, Sainio K, Partanen J, Taipale J, Petrova TV, Jeltsch M, Jackson DG, Talikka M, Rauvala H, Betsholtz C, Alitalo K (2004) Vascular endothelial growth factor C is required for sprouting of the first lymphatic vessels from embryonic veins. Nat Immunol 5:74-80

11. Kreuger J, Nilsson I, Kerjaschki D, Petrova T, Alitalo K, Claesson-Welsh L (2006) Early lymph vessel development from embryonic stem cells. Arterioscler Thromb Vasc Biol 26:1073-1078

12. Liersch R, Nay F, Lu L, Detmar M (2006) Induction of lymphatic endothelial cell differentiation in embryoid bodies. Blood 107:1214-1216

13. Maatta M, Liakka A, Salo S, Tasanen K, Bruckner-Tuderman L, Autio-Harmainen H (2004) Differential expression of basement membrane components in lymphatic tissues. J Histochem Cytochem 52:1073-1081

14. Maisonpierre PC, Suri C, Jones PF, Bartunkova S, Wiegand SJ, Radziejewski C, Compton D, McClain J, Aldrich TH, Papadopoulos N, Daly TJ, Davis S, Sato TN, Yancopoulos GD (1997) Angiopoietin-2, a natural antagonist for Tie2 that disrupts in vivo angiogenesis. Science 277:55-60

15. Makinen T, Adams RH, Bailey J, Lu Q, Ziemiecki A, Alitalo K, Klein R, Wilkinson GA (2005) PDZ interaction site in ephrinB2 is required for the remodeling of lymphatic vasculature. Genes Dev 19:397-410

16. Makinen T, Jussila L, Veikkola T, Karpanen T, Kettunen MI, Pulkkanen KJ, Kauppinen R, Jackson DG, Kubo H, Nishikawa S, Yla-Herttuala S, Alitalo K (2001) Inhibition of lymphangiogenesis with resulting lymphedema in transgenic mice expressing soluble VEGF receptor-3. Nat Med 7:199-205.

17. Oliver G (2004) Lymphatic vasculature development. Nat Rev Immunol 4:35-45

18. Oliver G, Alitalo K (2005) The lymphatic vasculature: recent progress and paradigms. Annu Rev Cell Dev Biol 21:457-483

19. Petajaniemi N, Korhonen M, Kortesmaa J, Tryggvason K, Sekiguchi K, Fujiwara H, Sorokin L, Thornell LE, Wondimu Z, Assefa D, Patarroyo M, Virtanen I (2002) Localization of laminin alpha4-chain in developing and adult human tissues. J Histochem Cytochem 50:1113-1130

20. Petrova TV, Karpanen T, Norrmen C, Mellor R, Tamakoshi T, Finegold D, Ferrell R, Kerjaschki D, Mortimer P, Yla-Herttuala S, Miura N, Alitalo K (2004) Defective valves and abnormal mural cell recruitment underlie lymphatic vascular failure in lymphedema distichiasis. Nat Med 10:974-981

21. Ringelmann B, Roder C, Hallmann R, Maley M, Davies M, Grounds M, Sorokin L (1999) Expression of laminin alpha1, alpha2, alpha4, and alpha5 chains, fibronectin, and tenascin-C in skeletal muscle of dystrophic 129ReJ dy/dy mice. Exp Cell Res 246:165-182

22. Risau W (1997) Mechanisms of angiogenesis. Nature 386:671-674

23. Schacht V, Ramirez MI, Hong YK, Hirakawa S, Feng D, Harvey N, Williams M, Dvorak AM, Dvorak HF, Oliver G, Detmar M (2003) T1alpha/podoplanin deficiency disrupts normal lymphatic vasculature formation and causes lymphedema. Embo J 22:3546-3556

24. Sixt M, Engelhardt B, Pausch F, Hallmann R, Wendler O, Sorokin LM (2001) Endothelial cell laminin isoforms, laminins 8 and 10, play decisive roles in T cell recruitment across the blood-brain barrier in experimental autoimmune encephalomyelitis. J Cell Biol 153:933-946

25. Sorokin LM, Conzelmann S, Ekblom P, Battaglia C, Aumailley M, Timpl R (1992) Monoclonal antibodies against laminin A chain fragment E3 and their effects on binding to cells and proteoglycan and on kidney development. Exp Cell Res 201:137-144

26. Sorokin LM, Pausch F, Frieser M, Kroger S, Ohage E, Deutzmann R (1997) Developmental regulation of the laminin alpha5 chain suggests a role in epithelial and endothelial cell maturation. Dev Biol 189:285-300

27. Thyboll J, Kortesmaa J, Cao R, Soininen R, Wang L, Iivanainen A, Sorokin L, Risling M, Cao Y, Tryggvason K (2002) Deletion of the laminin alpha4 chain leads to impaired microvessel maturation. Mol Cell Biol 22:1194-1202

28. Vittet D, Prandini MH, Berthier R, Schweitzer A, Martin-Sisteron H, Uzan G, Dejana E (1996) Embryonic stem cells differentiate in vitro to endothelial cells through successive maturation steps. Blood 88:3424-3431

29. Wigle JT, Oliver G (1999) Prox1 function is required for the development of the murine lymphatic system. Cell 98:769-778

30. Yuan L, Moyon D, Pardanaud L, Breant C, Karkkainen MJ, Alitalo K, Eichmann A (2002) Abnormal lymphatic vessel development in neuropilin 2 mutant mice. Development 129:4797-4806

4. LYMPHATIC MARKERS, TUMOUR LYMPHANGIOGENESIS AND LYMPH NODE METASTASIS

DAVID G. JACKSON, B.A. (Mod.) Ph.D.

MRC Human Immunology Unit and University of Oxford, Oxford UK

INTRODUCTION

Many of the most common human cancers disseminate from the site of primary tumour growth to distant tissues via the vessels and organs of the lymphatic system. In melanomas, cancers of the breast and colorectum, and in head and neck squamous cell carcinomas, early metastasis to lymph nodes is a common clinical finding, and one that is associated with poorer prognosis. Treatments to specifically block dissemination through the lymphatic network could in theory provide an independent therapy for some cancers, or at least an adjunct to existing chemotherapy. However, such a rational basis for the design of treatments is currently hindered by our poor understanding of the fundamental biology of lymphatics, and in particular lymphatic endothelial cell (LEC) biology.

Evidence derived largely from animal models indicates that most if not all lymphatic vessels originate by sprouting from fetal blood vessels during early embryogenesis, confirming predictions from early in the last century (1) (see (2) for review). However, it has only recently become possible to distinguish between the two vasculatures at the level of microscopy, thanks to the identification of new, lineage-specific lymphatic endothelial markers such as the sialylated mucoprotein podoplanin, the chemokine scavenging receptor D6 and the hyaluronan receptor LYVE-1. These new tools are now enabling researchers to identify lymphatic vessels in pathological tissue specimens; they are also facilitating the isolation of lymphatic vessel endothelial cells from such sources for characterization and phenotypic analysis. It can be anticipated that the results flowing from such studies will inform us about the molecular mechanisms underlying normal lymphatic function as well as how these functions may be subverted in lymphedema and cancer. This chapter outlines the current state of the art for lymphatic markers, some critical issues in relation to their use in studies of tumour lymphangiogenesis and lymph node metastasis, and some novel research that is revealing how tumour lymphatics may differ from their "normal" tissue counterparts.

LYMPHATIC MARKERS – THE MAJOR PLAYERS

Studies on tumour lymphangiogenesis rely upon the ability of the investigator to visualize the often small and indistinct lymphatic capillaries within and around the tumour so that they can be quantitated, and their density recorded and correlated with various clinical parameters such as invasion or nodal involvement, or assessed against prognosis or long term survival. All this requires the availability of markers that not only distinguish between lymphatic vessels and other non-endothelial structures such as epithelia, fibroblasts and inflammatory cells, but also distinguish lymphatic vessels from blood vessels (3). Basic research during the last decade has identified a small number of such molecules, mainly through serendipity. Although these new tools have greatly simplified the study of lymphangiogenesis, it should still be appreciated that no individual marker is entirely specific for lymphatic endothelium and due care and attention must always be exercised in order to avoid under- or overestimating lymph vessel density as this could lead to misinterpretation of its significance (see below).

Amongst the limited number of cell surface receptors, extracellular matrix proteins and transcription factors that show differential expression in lymph and hemovascular endothelial cells, those that have received most use as lymphatic markers are VEGFR3, PROX-1, podoplanin, D6 and LYVE-1 (see Table 1). Although other molecules such as the chemokine CCL21 (*slc*, secondary lymphoid chemokine) and to a lesser extent the non-signalling VEGFR-like receptor neuropilin 2 (*nrp2*) show selective expression in lymphatic endothelium (4, 5) they have received more limited use as markers to date, and are mentioned only in passing here.

Table 1. Features of the main lymphatic endothelial markers in current usage

VEGFR-3	Tyrosine kinase receptor for VEGF-C/VEGF-D
Prox-1	Homeobox domain transcription factor
Podoplanin (T1α/Aggrus/E11/PA2.26)	Cell surface sialylated glycoprotein
D6	Endocytic 7TM receptor for inflammatory β chemokines
LYVE-1	Link superfamily glycoprotein receptor for hyaluronan
CCL 21 (secondary lymphoid chemokine)	Chemoattractant for DC in lymph vessels and nodes
Neuropilin-2	Co-receptor for VEGFs and ligand for semaphorins involved in axonal guidance

Vascular endothelial growth factor receptor 3 (VEGFR3), the fms-like tyrosine kinase receptor (aka flt4) that binds the lymphangiogenic growth factors VEGF-C and VEGF-D (6, 7) is expressed on venous endothelia early in development, prior to the sprouting of the first lymph buds (8, 9). Thereafter, the expression of VEGFR3 shuts down on most adult hemovascular structures but is retained rather selectively on lymphatic endothelium (10). This pattern of expression is reflected in the finding that deletion of the gene for VEGFR3 leads to early embryonic death, due to catastrophic defects in cardiovascular development (11). While VEGFR3 was the first receptor to be employed as a true lymphatic marker (12) due to its key involvement in adult tumour lymphangiogenesis (8, 13-17) it has come to light subsequently that the molecule is present also in fenestrated capillaries of spleen, bone marrow and hepatic sinus and in kidney glomeruli. More importantly for cancer studies, re-expression of VEGFR3 has been observed in the endothelium of blood capillaries in breast and vascular tumours (18, 19), and this has restricted its use as a lymphatic marker in neoplasia. Nevertheless, antibodies to VEGFR3 are still used widely in studies of physiological lymphangiogenesis (20) and are available commercially from several sources.

The transcription factor PROX-1, (Drosophila prospero related homeobox gene) like VEGFR3, is also expressed early during embryonic lymphangiogenesis (2), where it marks sprouting of the first lymph buds from the cardinal vein during mouse embryogenesis (21, 22). Interestingly, PROX-1 appears to maintain differentiation of lymphatic endothelium in adult tissue and its expression is regarded as synonymous with the lymphatic endothelial phenotype (23). For example, transfection of blood vessel endothelial cells with PROX-1 cDNA is sufficient to induce differentiation towards an overtly lymphatic endothelial phenotype in vitro (22). In practical terms, PROX-1 is distinct from other markers insofar as it is localized within the nucleus rather than at the cell surface. Hence, it is normally used in combination with surface markers such as the pan-endothelial antigen CD31, or the lymphatic endothelial markers LYVE-1 or podoplanin, so as to allow visualization of the cell body (see eg. (24, 25)). As regards non-endothelial tissue expression, PROX-1 is detected within cells of a number of different tissues including the liver, pancreas, heart and nervous system (26). Commercial antibodies to PROX-1 have recently become available.

Originally identified as the T1a/Aggrus/PA2.26/E11 protein on airway epithelia (27), fibroblasts, keratinocytes (28) osteoblasts/osteocytes (29), and renal tubular epithelial cells respectively (30), the protein now known as podoplanin in humans is a small (162 residue) highly glycosylated transmembrane sialomucoprotein expressed at high levels on most lymphatic vessel endothelia (31). The precise function of podoplanin is unclear. However, mice with a targeted deletion of the podoplanin gene were shown recently to have either impaired lymphatic function and lymphedema (32) or lung defects (33) according to genetic background. This might imply that the role of podoplanin is largely structural, although other functions such as chemokine sequestration/presentation (34) and the promotion of platelet aggregation have been reported - the latter involving tandem repeats of a platelet-activation-like domain (PLAG) present within the N-terminal region of the ectodomain (35). Podoplanin interacts with the actin cytoskeleton via conserved motifs within the cytoplasmic tail that bind ERM proteins (Ezrin, Radixin, Moesin) – molecules that link the cell surface to the contractile fibres that control cell shape and polarity. Moreover, podoplanin has been shown recently to induce the formation of filopodia in cells via Rho-mediated remodelling of the actin cytoskeleton (36); curiously this latter function has been observed in tumour cells, rather than normal endothelia. How these roles in tumour invasion and metastasis might translate to the function of podoplanin in lymphatic endothelium is still unclear. Antibodies to podoplanin, including the commonly used mouse D2-40 mAb that has been validated recently with recombinant human podoplanin Fc are commercially available (37).

The orphan chemokine receptor D6 belongs to the family of 7TM spanning receptors (38, 39), and functions in the uptake and degradation of inflammatory C-C chemokines (38, 40, 41). Failure to fulfill this function in D6 gene knockout mice was recently shown to delay the resolution of inflammation in a mouse model of contact dermatitis (42, 43). Available evidence indicates that the D6 molecule is expressed rather exclusively in lymphatic endothelium in addition to a subset of vascular tumours, but not in blood vascular endothelium (44). At the time of writing, there is no commercial supplier of antibodies to D6 and these reagents are available only through academic collaborations.

Finally, LYVE-1, the primary lymphatic endothelial receptor for hyaluronan (an abundant extracellular mucopolysaccharide that is metabolized in the lymphatic system) has been shown to be a specific marker for lymphatic endothelium in a wide variety of different tissues, and to distinguish lymphatic from blood vascular endothelium in numerous human tumours (45). LYVE-1 is also expressed in a subset of tissue macrophages (46), including those which infiltrate tumours, as well as in liver and spleen sinus endothelium and airway epithelium (45, 47, 48). Despite these other locations, the marker is probably the most specific, reliable and robust for pathology and basic research applications. As regards biological function, the considerable structural similarity between LYVE-1 and the related leukocyte inflammatory homing receptor CD44 (both are members of the Link protein superfamily) suggests a potential role for LYVE-1 in lymphatic trafficking (45, 49-51). Confounding such predictions however, LYVE-1-/- mice display no obvious phenotype in terms of lymphatic development, fluid uptake or cell trafficking through afferent lymphatics (52). Preliminary studies on primary tumour growth and metastasis in LYVE-1-/- mice indicate these processes are also unaltered in the absence of the receptor (52). Hence it may be that the true function of LYVE-1 is manifest only under specific pathological conditions. Antibodies to LYVE-1 generated against both synthetic peptide epitopes and the recombinant receptor ectodomain are available from a variety of commercial sources (see below for further discussion).

LYMPHATIC MARKERS – METHODOLOGICAL CONSIDERATIONS

While each of the aforementioned markers has been instrumental in published studies of tumour lymphangiogenesis, it is important to re-iterate that none is absolutely specific in detecting the vasculature. As outlined above, LYVE-1 marks liver and spleen sinusoidal endothelium, whereas podoplanin and PROX-1 are expressed in several non-vascular sites including epithelium and connective tissue. In addition, the elevated expression of podoplanin has been reported within tumour cells of numerous cancers including skin, larynx, cervix, lung and breast where it is concentrated at the invading margin and contributes to metastasis in the absence of epithelial-mesenchymal transition (36). Indeed podoplanin/T1a (also known as Aggrus) was independently identified as a marker of type I alveolar lining epithelium in the lung (27). Curiously, several lymphatic markers including LYVE-1 and VEGFR3 also stain certain types of macrophage. Hence it should be clear that reliance on any single molecule for estimation of tumour lymph vessel density is unwise and may lead to errors due to mis-identification.

A less obvious pitfall is that some lymphatic markers may exhibit downmodulation either during lymphangiogenesis or in response to conditions such as inflammation that persist within the environment of certain tumours. If overlooked, this phenomenon could lead to significant underestimation of vessel numbers and incorrect interpretation of data. To date, the best documented examples of marker downregulation relate to LYVE-1. Our own studies, for example, have demonstrated that LYVE-1 is rapidly downregulated within lymphatic endothelial cells in response to inflammation in vitro, most notably after exposure to cytokines such as TNF α and IL-1 (Johnson, L.A. Clasper, S. and Jackson, D.G. submitted for publication). Release of these cytokines by tumour infiltrating leukocytes could well promote LYVE-1 downregulation in vivo. Although we have not confirmed an association with inflammation, we have observed LYVE-1[low] and LYVE-1[negative] lymphatics in human squamous cell carcinoma lesions assessed by immunohistochemical staining. Other reports have documented the reduced expression of LYVE-1 in lymphatics within breast cancer primary tumours and those close to their secondary metastases (53-55). Furthermore, in a recent study of human pancreatic endocrine carcinomas (56), of some 39 cases that contained podoplanin-positive intratumoural lymphatic vessels, only 13 stained positive for LYVE-1. Further research will be needed to assess how widespread is the phenomenon of marker loss, and what mechanisms are involved.

Finally, there is the potential complication that some marker preparations may have different reactivity towards their targets, depending upon the commercial source of the antibody. For example, not all commercial LYVE-1 antibodies are directed to the same epitope and some are generated against recombinant antigen expressed in non-human cell lines. Such differences may yet explain some of the apparent anomalies observed in tumour studies. Based upon the many considerations outlined in the foregoing paragraphs, one international consortium has gone so far as to recommend the preferential use of the podoplanin mAb D2-40 for estimation of lymphatic vessel density in tumour studies (57). In light of the current uncertainties regarding the reasons for apparent marker instability, and the many non-lymphatic structures that stain with D2-40 we would caution the recommendation of any single marker at this time but suggest instead that estimations be verified using two different markers. Further clarification on this issue is warranted and should be forthcoming in the near future.

TUMOUR LYMPHANGIOGENESIS AND ITS RELATIONSHIP TO METASTASIS

One of the key questions currently being addressed using lymphatic markers is whether the spread of tumours via the lymphatics involves formation and invasion of new lymphatics (tumour lymphangiogenesis) or the co-option of normal lymphatic vessels [see Fig 1 and (51) for separate review]. Knowledge in this area could have immediate prognostic value in identifying those patients whose tumours are likely to relapse and hence would require more aggressive chemotherapy. In the longer term, there is also scope for tumour lymphangiogenesis, like tumour hemangiogenesis, to be a target for drug therapy.

Seminal studies in mice using LYVE-1 and VEGFR3 as markers have established that the artificial induction of lymphangiogenesis in xenotransplanted human tumours can

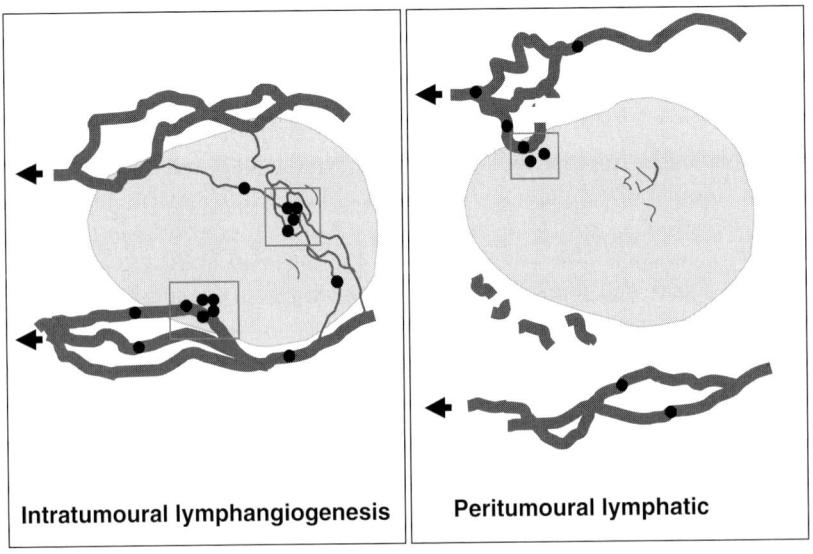

| Intratumoural lymphangiogenesis | Peritumoural lymphatic |

Figure 1. Two alternative models to explain the patterns of lymphatic vessel growth observed around metastatic human tumours. In the cartoon depicting intratumoural lymphangiogenesis (eg melanoma, head and neck squamous cell carcinoma, see text) lymphangiogenesis in and around the tumour provides conduits for the invasion and dissemination of metastatic tumour cells to lymph nodes. In the cartoon depicting peritumoural lymphangiogenesis, the tumour experiences only growth of local pre-existing lymphatics. The additional possibility included is that either new or pre-existing lymphatic vessel growth does occur, but the vessels are subsequently destroyed. Primary tumours are in each case colored light grey, lymphatic vessels dark grey, points where tumours might exit to lymph are boxed and tumour cells are shown as black circles.

be sufficient to promote lymph node metastasis in immunocompromised animals (58, 59). In these and other similar studies, overexpression of the lymphangiogenic growth factors either VEGF-C or VEGF-D generally induced potent lymphatic vessel recruitment and proliferation throughout the tumour i.e., both intra- and peritumourally. Notably however, in the case of pancreatic islet tumours grown in RIP-TAg transgenic animals, vessel enlargement rather than new vessel development appeared to accompany metastasis and no intratumoural lymphangiogenesis was apparent (60). Nonetheless, these findings sowed the seeds of a dogma that lymphangiogenesis was the key event for lymph node metastasis, and that intratumoural lymphatics were the likely conduit.

Subsequent to these mouse experiments, there have been numerous studies carried out on lymphangiogenesis in human cancers using LYVE-1, VEGFR3 and the more recently identified podoplanin molecule as markers. These have sought mostly to quantify lymphatic vessel density in and around tumours in patient groups, relating the values to the levels of lymphangiogenic growth factors such as VEGF-C and VEGF-D, and in some cases to clinicopathological characteristics including vessel invasion (by tumour), nodal involvement and long-term survival. In general the results have failed to reveal a straightforward association between the levels of lymphangiogenic growth factor and the density of tumour lymphatics, although an association with metastasis seems clear. Secondly, they have shown that lymphangiogenesis and the pattern of lymphatic vessel growth differ among cancer types; in some cases new vessels are clearly visible whereas in others there is only an enlargement or even an apparent reduction of existing vessels (Table 2). For example, in cancers of the head and neck, in melanomas, and in pancreatic ductal and thyroid papillary carcinomas (61-67), proliferating lymphatic vessels have been detected within the body of the tumour mass as well as in the surrounding stroma using LYVE-1 immunohistochemistry. In some cases the intratumoural LVD correlated with nodal metastasis as well as poor prognosis (68). A similar pattern of intratumoural lymphangiogenesis has also been found in a separate study of head and neck squamous carcinomas by Kyzas et al (69) using podoplanin as marker, and this was reported to correlate with lymphatic invasion, early nodal metastasis (ie at time of diagnosis) and poor prognosis.

In other tumours such as breast, cervical, prostate and colorectal carcinoma, proliferation of lymphatic vessels is apparent only in the peritumoural regions (70-78). Indeed in the case of prostate cancer, evidence suggests that lymphatic vessel density decreases during malignant transformation. For example, one recent study reported a higher LVD in patients with benign prostatic hypertrophy than in prostate carcinoma but no correlation between LVD and tumour stage (74). Furthermore, the virtual absence of lymphatic vessels within tumours of breast carcinoma assessed using LYVE-1 immunohistochemistry (71) and colorectal carcinoma using transmission electron microscopy (79) have led to suggestions that these vessels may undergo destruction, possibly by infiltrating inflammatory cells (79). Nevertheless, in recent studies of colorectal cancer high lymphatic microvessel density and in some cases positive lymphatic vessel invasion scored using podoplanin (D2-40) were negatively associated with overall survival (p = 0.0011 and p = 0.0118, respectively) and with liver and lymph node involvement (80, 81).

Table 2. Patterns of lymphatic vessel growth in human cancers

Cancer type	Lymph vessel pattern		Lymph vessel proliferation	Association with metastasis or disease-free survival
	Intratumoral	Peritumoral a **		
Head and neck Squamous Ca.	Yes	Yes	Ki67 +ve Intratumoral	Intratumoral/peritumoral LVD with nodal metastasis (61, 64, 69)
Melanoma	Yes	Yes	Ki67/PCNA +ve	Intratumoral + peritumoral LVD with nodal metastasis + long-term survival (62, 66, 67)
Thyroid papillary	Yes	N.D.	N.D.	Intratumoral LVD with nodal metastasis (65)
Pancreatic	Yes	N.D.	N.D.	Intratumoral LVD with liver metastasis (56, 63)
Breast Ca.	V. rarely	Yes	No/N.D.	Peritumoral LVD with axillary node metastasis + poor survival (70, 71, 75)
Prostate Ca.	No	No	N.D.	Peritumoral LVD with tumour stage. Association with metastasis unclear (73, 74)
Cervical	No	Yes	N.D.	Peritumoral LVD with vessel invasion and nodal metastasis? (78)
Colorectal	V. rarely	Yes	Ki67 +ve	Peritumoral LVD with nodal metastasis in one case (76) No significant association in another case (77)

**Increased relative to normal

How are we to interpret these disparate findings ? It seems likely to us that tumours genuinely differ from one another in how they manipulate the lymphatics for dissemination. In the more rare examples such as melanoma and head and neck carcinoma, newly dividing lymphatics may form within the tumour body (Figure 1) due either to initial growth of these cancers in an area of extensive lymphatic supply (i.e. the subcutaneous site) or to particular growth characteristics/chemotactic properties of the tumours themselves. However, the suggestion that these intratumoural lymphatics act as conduits for tumour metastasis has aroused great controversy (82). Many within the field cite the results of lymphangiography as proof that intratumoural lymphatics are "nonfunctional" due to the large compressive force exerted by the surrounding tumour mass (83-85). Of course the failure to drain fluorescent dyes need not necessarily equate with a failure to traffic tumour cells; a resolution to this contentious issue is probably still far away. Nevertheless, the absence of a mechanistic explanation for metastasis does not preclude the fact that lymphangiogenesis may yet have prognostic value.

It appears likely that most tumours compress and exclude lymphatic vessels rather than promoting their proliferation and branching. In these cases one would expect that only pre-existing lymphatics and newly enlarged or dividing lymphatics at the periphery of the tumour would contribute to nodal metastasis (Figure 1). Indeed it has been argued that such peritumoural lymphatics, which are functional by the criteria of fluid flow and dye uptake, enhance invasion by tumour simply by promoting increased lymph circulation (86). The promotion of metastasis may also be due as much to the capacity of new lymphatics to chemoattract tumour cells as the capacity of the tumour to promote lymphangiogenesis (87). Other features emerging from recent research include the role of tumour-derived factors in preparing the vasculature and architecture of draining lymph nodes for subsequent metastasis ("Seed and Soil" theory (88, 89)) and the realization that many other proteins besides VEGF-C and VEGF-D, such as VEGF-A, platelet derived growth factor (PDGF), fibroblast growth factor (FGF), insulin-like growth factor (IGF) and hepatocyte growth factor (HGF) are also mitogenic for lymphatic endothelium and may play separate roles in the metastatic process (89-93). Further studies of different human cancers will be required to clarify the importance of these phenomena.

One final possibility is that lymphatics are altered biochemically by their close proximity to tumour cells and acquire properties that render them more accessible to invasion by tumour cells. Such a possibility might even explain the discrepancy in the literature between lymphangiogenic growth factor levels, lymphatic vessel density and lymph node metastasis that has been noted in many clinical studies. Put simply, the quality of tumour lymphatics rather than their quantity may turn out to be the key factor in terms of dissemination.

TUMOUR LYMPHATICS – DO THEY DIFFER FROM NORMAL TISSUE LYMPHATICS ?

As intimated in the previous section, the propensity for nodal metastasis that is characteristic of certain tumour types might be explained at least in part, if such tumours induced particular changes to the architecture or function of lymphatics, be they pre-existing local lymphatics or new lymphatics, that were advantageous for invasion. The precedent for such a notion comes from parallel studies of tumour blood vessel endothelium that have identified a number of tumour-specific endothelial markers or "TEMs" (94-96), and more recent studies using *in vivo* screening of phage peptide libraries that have indicated the existence of tumour-specific target receptors in lymphatic endothelium (97). Recently, we explored the phenomenon in a mouse tumour model by comparing the RNA profile of primary lymphatic endothelial cells (LEC) isolated from the vasculature of subcutaneous tumour and normal tissue in animals transplanted with the lymph node metastasizing T-241/VEGF-C fibrosarcoma (Clasper et al. submitted for publication). Curiously, we found significant differences in expression of some 800 genes that coded for a variety of proteins including components of endothelial junctions, sub-endothelial matrix and vessel growth/patterning. These differences were also observed by immunohistochemical staining of vessels within T-241 tumours using appropriate antibodies. Overall, the phenotype of tumour LEC suggested increased expression of certain receptors associated with functions such as intercellular junction formation and cell trafficking and an apparent loosening/re-modelling of the sub-endothelial matrix. Although it might have been anticipated that these changes would derive from autocrine effects of VEGF-C which is overexpressed by the T-241 cells themselves, this did not appear to be the case. Rather, they appeared to reflect some more complex influence of the tumour/host environment. Moreover, a recent study into the expression profile of normal primary human LEC found only modest changes were induced by VEGF-C treatment (98), and these were distinct from the ones detected in the mouse tumour study. The implication from these findings are that tumour lymphatic vessels, much like tumour blood vessels, have a distinct transcriptional fingerprint. The studies are only in their infancy, and further work will be required to determine whether such a fingerprint is common to all tumour types, or whether it is associated with those displaying a particular pattern of lymphangiogenesis or capacity for lymph node metastasis. Regardless, they will surely have major implications for prognosis, and perhaps even therapy.

ACKNOWLEDGEMENTS

I would like to thank the MRC and Cancer Research UK for generously funding the research outlined in this chapter.

REFERENCES

1. Sabin, FR, (1902) The lymphatic system in human embryos, with consideration of the morphology of the system as a whole. Am. J. Pathol. 1: 367-389.
2. Oliver, G, (2004) Lymphatic vasculature development. Nat. Rev. Immunol. 4: 35-45.
3. Jackson, DG, (2001) New molecular markers for the study of tumour lymphangiogenesis. Anticancer Res. 21: 4279-4283.
4. Sallusto, F, Schaerli, P, Loetscher, P, Schaniel, C, Lenig, D, Mackay, CR, Qin, S, and Lanzavecchia, A, (1998) Rapid and co-ordinated switch in chemokine receptor expression during dendritic cell maturation. Eur. J. Immunol. 28: 2760-2769.
5. Yuan, L, Moyon, D, Pardanaud, L, Breant, C, Karkkainen, MJ, Alitalo, K, and Eichmann, A, (2002) Abnormal lymphatic vessel development in neuropilin 2 mutant mice. Development. 129: 4797-4806.

6. Joukov, V, Pajusola, K, Kaipainen, A, Chilov, D, Lahtinen, I, Kukk, E, Saksela, O, Kalkkinen, N, and Alitalo, K, (1996) A novel vascular endothelial growth factor, VEGF-C, is a ligand for the Flt4 (VEGFR-3) and KDR (VEGFR-2) receptor tyrosine kinases. EMBO. J. 15: 290-298.

7. Makinen, T, Veikkola, T, Mustjoki, S, Karpanen, T, Catimel, B, Nice, EC, Wise, L, Mercer, A, Kowalski, H, Kerjaschki, D, Stacker, SA, Achen, MG, and Alitalo, K, (2001) Isolated lymphatic endothelial cells transduce growth, survival and migratory signals via the VEGF-C/D receptor VEGFR-3. EMBO. J. 20: 4726-4773.

8. Kukk, E, Lymboussaki, A, Taira, S, Kaipainen, A, Jeltsch, M, Joukov, V, and Alitalo, K, (1996) VEGF-C receptor binding and pattern of expression with VEGFR-3 suggests a role in lymphatic vascular development. Development. 122: 3829-3837.

9. Karkkainen, MJ, Haiko, P, Sainio, K, Partanen, J, Taipale, J, Petrova, TV, Jeltsch, M, Jackson, DG, Talikka, M, Rauvala, H, Betsholtz, C, and Alitalo, K, (2004) Vascular endothelial growth factor C is required for sprouting of the first lymphatic vessels from embryonic veins. Nat Immunol. 5: 74-80.

10. Kaipainen, A, Korhonen, J, Mustonen, T, van Hinsbergh, VW, Fang, GH, Dumont, D, Breitman, M, and Alitalo, K, (1995) Expression of the fms-like tyrosine kinase 4 gene becomes restricted to lymphatic endothelium during development. Proc Natl Acad Sci U S A. 92: 3566-3570.

11. Dumont, DJ, Jussila, L, Taipale, J, Lymboussaki, A, Mustonen, T, Pajusola, K, Breitman, M, and Alitalo, K, (1998) Cardiovascular failure in mouse embryos deficient in VEGF receptor-3. Science. 282: 946-949.

12. Lymboussaki, A, Partanen, TA, Olofsson, B, Thomas-Crusells, J, Fletcher, CDM, de Waal, RMW, Kaipainen, A, and Alitalo, K, (1998) Expression of the vascular endothelial growth factor C receptor VEGFR-3 in lymphatic endothelium of the skin and in vascular tumors. Am. J. Pathol. 153: 395-403.

13. Jeltsch, M, Kaipanen, A, Joukov, V, Meng, X, Lakso, M, Rauvala, H, Swartz, M, Fukumura, D, Jain, RK, and Alitalo, K, (1997) Hyperplasia of lymphatic vessels in VEGF-C transgenic mice. Science. 276: 1423-1425.

14. Kubo, H, Fujiwara, T, Jussila, L, Hashi, H, Ogawa, M, Shimizu, K, Awane, M, Sakai, Y, Takabayashi, A, Alitalo, K, Yamaoka, Y, and Nishikawa, SI, (2000) Involvement of vascular endothelial growth factor receptor-3 in maintenance of integrity of endothelial cell lining during tumor angiogenesis. Blood. 96: 546-553.

15. Veikkola, T, Jussila, L, Makinen, T, Karpanen, T, Jeltsch, M, Petrova, TV, Kubo, H, Thurston, G, McDonald, DM, Achen, MG, Stacker, SA, and Alitalo, K, (2001) Signalling via vascular endothelial growth factor receptor-3 is sufficient for lymphangiogenesis in transgenic mice. EMBO. J. 20: 1223-1231.

16. He, Y, Kozaki, K, Karpanen, T, Koshikawa, K, Yla-Herttuala, S, Takahashi, T, and Alitalo, K, (2002) Suppression of tumor lymphangiogenesis and lymph node metastasis by blocking vascular endothelial growth factor receptor 3 signaling. J. Natl. Cancer Inst. 94: 819-825.

17. He, Y, Karpanen, T, and Alitalo, K, (2004) Role of lymphangiogenic factors in tumor metastasis. Biochim Biophys Acta. 1654: 3-12.

18. Valtola, R, Salven, P, Heikkila, P, Taipale, J, Joensuu, H, Rehn, M, Pihlajaniemi, T, Weich, H, deWaal, R, and Alitalo, K, (1999) VEGFR-3 and its ligand VEGF-C are associated with angiogenesis in breast cancer. Am. J. Pathol. 154: 1381-1390.

19. Partanen, TA, Alitalo, K, and Miettinen, M, (1999) Lack of lymphatic vascular specificity of vascular endothelial growth factor receptor 3 in 185 vascular tumors. Cancer. 86: 2406-2412.

20. Saharinen, P, Tammela, T, Karkkainen, MJ, and Alitalo, K, (2004) Lymphatic vasculature: development, molecular regulation and role in tumor metastasis and inflammation. Trends Immunol. 25: 387-395.

21. Wigle, JT and Oliver, G, (1999) Prox-1 function is required for the development of the murine lymphatic system. Cell. 98: 769-778.

22. Hong, YK, Harvey, N, Noh, YH, Schacht, V, Hirakawa, S, Detmar, M, and Oliver, G, (2002) Prox1 is a master control gene in the program specifying lymphatic endothelial cell fate. Dev Dyn. 225: 351-357.

23. Wigle, JT, Harvey, N, Detmar, M, Lagutina, I, Grosveld, G, Gunn, MD, Jackson, DG, and Oliver, G, (2002) An essential role for Prox1 in the induction of the lymphatic endothelial cell phenotype. Embo J. 21: 1505-1513.

24. Agarwal, B, Saxena, R, Morimiya, A, Mehrotra, S, and Badve, S, (2005) Lymphangiogenesis does not occur in breast cancer. Am J Surg Pathol. 29: 1449-1455.

25. Johnson, LA, Clasper, S, Holt, A, Lalor, P, Baban, D, and Jackson, DG, (2006) An inflammation-induced mechanism for leukocyte transmigration of lymphatic endothelium. J. Exp. Med. 203: 2763-2777.

26. Stacker, SA, Achen, MG, Jussila, L, Baldwin, ME, and Alitalo, K, (2002) Lymphangiogenesis and cancer metastasis. Nat. Rev Cancer. 2: 573-583.

27. Dobbs, LG, Williams, MC, and Gonzalez, R, (1988) Monoclonal antibodies specific to apical surfaces of rat alveolar type I cells bind to surfaces of cultured, but not freshly isolated, type II cells. Biochim. Biophys. Acta. 970: 146-156.

28. Gandarillas, A, Scholl, FG, Benito, N, Gamallo, C, and Quintanilla, M, (1997) Induction of PA2.26, a cell-surface antigen expressed by active fibroblasts, in mouse epidermal keratinocytes during carcinogenesis. Mol. Carcinog. 20: 10-18.

29. Wetterwald, A, Hoffstetter, W, Cecchini, MG, Lanske, B, Wagner, C, Fleisch, H, and Atkinson, M, (1996) Characterization and cloning of the E11 antigen, a marker expressed by rat osteoblasts and osteocytes. Bone. 18: 125-132.

30. Breiteneder-Geleff, S, Matsui, K, Soleiman, A, Meraner, P, Poczewski, H, Kalt, R, Schaffner, G, and Kerjaschki, D, (1997) Podoplanin, novel 43-kd membrane protein of glomerular epithelial cells, is down-regulated in puromycin nephrosis. Am J Pathol. 151: 1141-1152.

31. Breiteneder-Geleff, S, Soleiman, A, Horvat, R, Amann, G, Kowalski, H, and Kerjaschki, D, (1999) [Podoplanin—a specific marker for lymphatic endothelium expressed in angiosarcoma]. Verh Dtsch Ges Pathol. 83: 270-275.

32. Schacht, V, Ramirez, MI, Hong, YK, Hirakawa, S, Feng, D, Harvey, N, Williams, M, Dvorak, AM, Dvorak, HF, Oliver, G, and Detmar, M, (2003) T1 alpha/podoplanin deficiency disrupts normal lymphatic vasculature formation and causes lymphedema. EMBO. J. 22: 3546-3556.

33. Ramirez, MI, Millien, G, Hinds, A, Cao, Y, Seldin, DC, and Williams, MC, (2003) T1alpha, a lung type I cell differentiation gene, is required for normal lung cell proliferation and alveolus formation at birth. Dev. Biol. 256: 61-72.

34. Kerjaschki, D, Regele, HM, Moosberger, I, Nagy-Bojarski, K, Watschinger, B, Soleiman, A, Birner, P, Krieger, S, Hovorka, A, Silberhumer, G, Laakkonen, P, Petrova, T, Langer, B, and Raab, I, (2004) Lymphatic neoangiogenesis in human kidney transplants is associated with immunologically active lymphocytic infiltrates. J Am Soc Nephrol. 15: 603-612.

35. Kaneko, M, Kato, Y, Kunita, A, Fujita, N, Tsuruo, T, and Osawa, M, (2004) Functional sialylated O-glycan to platelet aggregation on Aggrus (T1alpha/Podoplanin) molecules expressed in Chinese hamster ovary cells. J Biol Chem. 279: 38838-38843.

36. Wicki, A, Lehembre, F, Wick, N, Hantusch, B, Kerjaschki, D, and Christofori, G, (2006) Tumor invasion in the absence of epithelial-mesenchymal transition: podoplanin-mediated remodeling of the actin cytoskeleton. Cancer Cell. 9: 261-272.

37. Schacht, V, Dadras, SS, Johnson, LA, Jackson, DG, Hong, YK, and Detmar, M, (2005) Up-regulation of the lymphatic marker podoplanin, a mucin-type transmembrane glycoprotein, in human squamous cell carcinomas and germ cell tumors. Am J Pathol. 166: 913-921.

38. Nibbs, RJ, Wylie, SM, Yang, J, Landau, NR, and Graham, GJ, (1997) Cloning and characterization of a novel promiscuous human beta-chemokine receptor D6. J Biol Chem. 272: 32078-32083.

39. Nibbs, RJ, Wylie, SM, Pragnell, IB, and Graham, GJ, (1997) Cloning and characterization of a novel murine beta chemokine receptor, D6. Comparison to three other related macrophage inflammatory protein-1alpha receptors, CCR-1, CCR-3, and CCR-5. J Biol Chem. 272: 12495-12504.

40. Fra, AM, Locati, M, Otero, K, Sironi, M, Signorelli, P, Massardi, ML, Gobbi, M, Vecchi, A, Sozzani, S, and Mantovani, A, (2003) Cutting Edge: scavenging of inflammatory CC chemokines by the prmiscuous putatively silent chemokine receptor D6. J. Immunol. 170: 2279-2282.

41. Weber, M, Blair, E, Simpson, CV, O'Hara, M, Blackburn, PE, Rot, A, Graham, GJ, and Nibbs, RJ, (2004) The chemokine receptor D6 constitutively traffics to and from the cell surface to internalize and degrade chemokines. Mol Biol Cell. 15: 2492-2508.

42. Jamieson, T, Cook, DN, Nibbs, RJ, Rot, A, Nixon, C, McLean, P, Alcami, A, Lira, SA, Wiekowski, M, and Graham, GJ, (2005) The chemokine receptor D6 limits the inflammatory response in vivo. Nat Immunol. 6: 403-411.

43. Martinez de la Torre, Y, Locati, M, Buracchi, C, Dupor, J, Cook, DN, Bonecchi, R, Nebuloni, M, Rukavina, D, Vago, L, Vecchi, A, Lira, SA, and Mantovani, A, (2005) Increased inflammation in mice deficient for the chemokine decoy receptor D6. Eur. J. Immunol. 35: 1342-1346.

44. Nibbs, RJB, (2001) The b-chemokine receptorD6 is expressed by lymphatic endotheliumand a subset of vascular tumours. Am. J. Pathol. 158: 867-877.

45. Banerji, S, Ni, J, Wang, SX, Clasper, S, Su, J, Tammi, R, Jones, M, and Jackson, DG, (1999) LYVE-1, a new homologue of the CD44 glycoprotein, is a lymph-specific receptor for hyaluronan. J Cell Biol. 144: 789-801.

46. Maruyama, K, Ii, M, Cursiefen, C, Jackson, DG, Keino, H, Tomita, M, Van Rooijen, N, Takenaka, H, D'Amore, PA, Stein-Streilein, J, Losordo, DW, and Streilein, JW, (2005) Inflammation-induced lymphangiogenesis in the cornea arises from CD11b-positive macrophages. J Clin Invest. 115: 2363-2372.

47. Prevo, R, Banerji, S, Ferguson, DJ, Clasper, S, and Jackson, DG, (2001) Mouse LYVE-1 is an endocytic receptor for hyaluronan in lymphatic endothelium. J Biol Chem. 276: 19420-19430.

48. Carreira, CM, Nasser, SM, di Tomaso, E, Padera, TP, Boucher, Y, Tomarev, SI, and Jain, RK, (2001) LYVE-1 is not restricted to the lymph vessels : expression in normal liver blood sinusoids and down-regulation in human liver cancer and cirrhosis. Cancer Res. 61: 8079-8084.

49. Jackson, DG, (2003) The lymphatics revisited: new perspectives from the hyaluronan receptor LYVE-1. Trends Cardiovasc Med. 13: 1-7.

50. Jackson, DG, (2004) The lymphatic endothelial hyaluronan receptor LYVE-1. Glycoforum. www.glycoforum.gr.jp/science/hyaluronan/HA28/HA28E.html.
51. Jackson, DG, (2004) Biology of the lymphatic marker LYVE-1 and applications in research into lymphatic trafficking and lymphangiogenesis. APMIS. 112: 526-538.
52. Gale, NW, Prevo, R, Espinosa-Fematt, J, Ferguson, DJ, Dominguez, MG, Yancopoulos, GD, Thurston, G, and Jackson, DG, (2007) Normal lymphatic development and function in mice deficient for the lymphatic hyaluronan receptor LYVE-1. Mol. Cell. Biol. 27: 595-604.
53. Stessels, F, Van den Eynden, G, Van der Auwera, I, Salgado, R, Van den Heuvel, E, Harris, AL, Jackson, DG, Colpaert, CG, van Marck, EA, Dirix, LY, and Vermeulen, PB, (2004) Breast adenocarcinoma liver metastases, in contrast to colorectal cancer liver metastases, display a non-angiogenic growth pattern that preserves the stroma and lacks hypoxia. Br J Cancer. 90: 1429-1436.
54. Van der Auwera, I, Van den Eynden, GG, Colpaert, CG, Van Laere, SJ, van Dam, P, Van Marck, EA, Dirix, LY, and Vermeulen, PB, (2005) Tumor lymphangiogenesis in inflammatory breast carcinoma: a histomorphometric study. Clin Cancer Res. 11: 7637-7642.
55. Van den Eynden, GG, Van der Auwera, I, Van Laere, SJ, Huygelen, V, V Colpaert, CG, Van Dam, P, Dirix, LY, Vermeulen, PB, and Van Marck, EA, (2006) Induction of lymphangiogenesis in and around axillary lymph node metastases of patients with breast cancer. Br. J. Cancer. 95: 1362-1366.
56. Rubbia-Brandt, L, Terris, B, Giostra, E, Dousset, B, Morel, P, and Pepper, MS, (2004) Lymphatic vessel density and vascular endothelial growth factor-C expression correlate with malignant behavior in human pancreatic endocrine tumors. Clin Cancer Res. 10: 6919-6928.
57. Van der Auwera, I, Cao, Y, Tille, JC, Pepper, MS, Jackson, DG, Fox, SB, Harris, AL, Dirix, LY, and Vermeulen, PB, (2006) First International consensus on the methodology of lymphangiogenesis quantification in solid human tumours. Br. J. Cancer. 1-15.
58. Skobe, M, Hawighorst, T, Jackson, DG, Prevo, R, Janes, L, Velasco, P, Riccardi, L, Alitalo, K, Claffey, K, and Detmar, M, (2001) Induction of tumor lymphangiogenesis by VEGF-C promotes breast cancer metastasis. Nat Med. 7: 192-198.
59. Stacker, SA, Caesar, C, Baldwin, ME, Thornton, GE, Williams, RA, Prevo, R, Jackson, DG, Nishikawa, S, Kubo, H, and Achen, MG, (2001) VEGF-D promotes the metastatic spread of tumor cells via the lymphatics. Nat Med. 7: 186-191.
60. Mandriota, SJ, Jussila, L, Jeltsch, M, Compagni, A, Baetens, D, Prevo, R, Banerji, S, Huarte, J, Montesano, R, Jackson, DG, Orci, L, Alitalo, K, Christofori, G, and Pepper, MS, (2001) Vascular endothelial growth factor-C-mediated lymphangiogenesis promotes tumour metastasis. Embo J. 20: 672-682.
61. Beasley, NJ, Prevo, R, Banerji, S, Leek, RD, Moore, J, van Trappen, P, Cox, G, Harris, AL, and Jackson, DG, (2002) Intratumoral lymphangiogenesis and lymph node metastasis in head and neck cancer. Cancer Res. 62: 1315-1320.
62. Dadras, SS, Paul, T, Bertoncini, J, Brown, LF, Muzikansky, A, Jackson, DG, Ellwanger, U, Garbe, C, Mihm, MC, and Detmar, M, (2003) Tumor lymphangiogenesis: a novel prognostic indicator for cutaneous melanoma metastasis and survival. Am J Pathol. 162: 1951-1960.
63. Von Marschall, Z, Scholz, A, Stacker, S, Achen, M, Jackson, DG, Alves, F, Schirner, M, Haberey, M, Thierauch, K-H, Wiedenmann, B, and Rosewicz, S, (2005) Vascular endothelial growth factor-D induces lymphangiogenesis and lymphatic metastasis in human pancreatic cancer. 27: 669-679.
64. Maula, SM, Luukkaa, M, Grenman, R, Jackson, D, Jalkanen, S, and Ristamaki, R, (2003) Intratumoral lymphatics are essential for the metastatic spread and prognosis in squamous cell carcinomas of the head and neck region. Cancer Res. 63: 1920-1926.
65. Hall, FT, Freeman, JL, Asa, SL, Jackson, DG, and Beasley, NJ, (2003) Intratumoral lymphatics and lymph node metastases in papillary thyroid carcinoma. Arch Otolaryngol Head Neck Surg. 129: 716-719.
66. Shields, JD, Borsetti, M, Rigby, H, Harper, SJ, Mortimer, PS, Levick, JR, Orlando, A, and Bates, DO, (2004) Lymphatic density and metastatic spread in human malignant melanoma. Br J Cancer. 90: 693-700.
67. Straume, O, Jackson, DG, and Akslen, LA, (2003) Independent prognostic impact of lymphatic vessel density and presence of low-grade lymphangiogenesis in cutaneous melanoma. Clin Cancer Res. 9: 250-256.
68. Audet, N, Beaasley, NJ, MacMillan, C, Jackson, DG, Gullane, PJ, and Kamel-Reid, S, (2005) Lymphatic vessel density, nodal metastases, and prognosis in patients with head and neck cancer. Arch. Otolaryngol. Head Neck Surg. 131: 1065-1070.
69. Kyzas, PA, Geleff, S, Batistatou, A, Agnantis, NJ, and Stefanou, D, (2005) Evidence for lymphangiogenesis and its prognostic implications in head and neck squamous cell carcinoma. J Pathol. 206: 170-177.
70. Bono, P, Wasenius, V, Lundin, J, Jackson, DG, and Joensuu, H, (2004) High peritumoral LYVE-1 positive lymphatic vessel numbers are associated with axillary lymph node metastases and poor outcome in early breast cancer. Clin Cancer Res. 10: 7144-7149.

71. Williams, CS, Leek, RD, Robson, AM, Banerji, S, Prevo, R, Harris, AL, and Jackson, DG, (2003) Absence of lymphangiogenesis and intratumoural lymph vessels in human metastatic breast cancer. J Pathol. 200: 195-206.

72. Van Trappen, PO, Steele, D, Lowe, DG, Baithun, S, Beasley, N, Thiele, W, Weich, H, Krishnan, J, Shepherd, JH, Pepper, MS, Jackson, DG, Sleeman, JP, and Jacobs, IJ, (2003) Expression of vascular endothelial growth factor (VEGF)-C and VEGF-D, and their receptor VEGFR-3, during different stages of cervical carcinogenesis. J Pathol. 201: 544-554.

73. Trojan, L, Michel, MS, Rensch, F, Jackson, DG, Alken, P, and Grobholz, R, (2004) Lymph and blood vessel architecture in benign and malignant prostatic tissue: lack of lymphangiogenesis in prostate carcinoma assessed with novel lymphatic marker lymphatic vessel endothelial hyaluronan receptor (LYVE-1). J Urol. 172: 103-107.

74. Trojan, L, Rensch, F, Voss, M, Grobholz, R, Weiss, C, Jackson, DG, Alken, P, and Michel, MS, (2006) The role of the lymphatic system and its specific growth factor, vascular endothelial growth factor C, for lymphogenic metastasis in prostate cancer. BJU Int. 98: 903-906.

75. Schoppmann, SF, Birner, P, Studer, P, and Breiteneder-Geleff, S, (2001) Lymphatic microvessel density and lymphovascular invasion assessed by anti-podoplanin immunostaining in human breast cancer. Anticancer Res. 21: 2351-2355.

76. Liang, P, Hong, JW, Ubukata, H, Liu, HR, Watanabe, Y, Katano, M, Motohashi, G, Kasuga, T, Nakada, I, and Tabuchi, T, (2006) Increased density and diameter of lymphatic microvessels correlate with lymph node metastasis in early stage invasive colorectal carcinoma. Virchows Arch. 448: 570-575.

77. Omachi, T, Kawai, Y, Mizuno, R, Nomiyama, T, Miyagawa, S, Ohhashi, T, and Nakayama, J, (2006) Immunohistochemical demonstration of proliferating lymphatic vessels in colorectal carcinoma and its clinicopathological significance. Cancer Lett. 246: 167-172.

78. Birner, P, Schindl, M, Obermair, A, Breitenecker, G, Kowalski, H, and Oberhuber, G, (2001) Lymphatic microvessel density as a novel prognostic factor in early-stage invasive cervical cancer. Int J Cancer. 95: 29-33.

79. Sacchi, G, Weber, E, Agliano, M, Lorenzoni, P, Rossi, A, Caruso, AM, Vernillo, R, Gerli, R, and Lorenzi, M, (2003) Lymphatic vessels in colorectal cancer and their relation with inflammatory infiltrate. Dis Colon Rectum. 46: 40-47.

80. Matsumoto, K, Nakayama, Y, Inoue, Y, Minagawa, N, Katsuki, T, Shibao, K, Tsurudome, Y, Hirata, K, Nagata, N, and Itoh, H, (2007) Lymphatic microvessel density is an independent prognostic factor in colorectal cancer. Dis Colon Rectum. 50: 308-314.

81. Saad, RS, Kordunsky, L, Liu, YL, Denning, KL, Kandil, HA, and Silverman, JF, (2006) Lymphatic microvessel density as prognostic marker in colorectal cancer. Mod. Pathol. 19: 1317-1323.

82. Jain, RK and Fenton, BT, (2002) Intratumoral lymphatic vessels: a case of mistaken identity or malfunction ? J. Natl. Cancer Inst. 94: 417-421.

83. Leu, AJ, Berk, DA, Lymboussaki, A, Alitalo, K, and Jain, RK, (2000) Absence of functional lymphatics within a murine sarcoma: a molecular and functional evaluation. Cancer Res. 60: 4324-4327.

84. Padera, TP, Kadambi, A, Di Tomaso, E, Mouta Carreira, C, Brown, EB, Bpucher, Y, Choi, NC, Mathisen, D, Wain, J, Mark, EJ, Munn, LL, and Jain, RK, (2002) Lymphatic metastasis in the absence of functional intratumor lymphatics. Science 296:1883-1886.

85. Padera, T. P., Stoll, BR, Tooredman, JB, Capen, D, Di Tomaso, E, and Jain, RK, (2004) Pathology: Cancer cells compress intratumour vessels. Nature. 427: 695.

86. Hoshida, T, Isaka, N, Hagendoorn, J, Di Tomaso, E, Chen, Y-L, Pytowski, B, Fukumura, D, Padera, TP, and Jain, RK, (2006) Imaging steps of lymphatic metastasis reveals that vascular endothelial growth factor-c increases metastasis by increasing delivery of cancer cells to lymph nodes: therapeutic implications. Cancer Res. 66: 8065-8075.

87. Shields, J, Emmett, MS, Dunn, DBA, Joory, KD, Sage, LM, Rigby, H, Mortimer, PS, Orlando, A, Levick, JR, and Bates, DO, (2006) Chemokine - mediated migration of melanoma cells towards lymphatics - a mechanism contributing to metastasis. Oncogene. epubl. 27 November 2006.

88. Qian, CN, Berghuis, B, Tsarfaty, G, Bruch, M, Kort, EJ, Ditlev, J, Tsarfaty, I, Hudson, E, Jackson, DG, Petillo, D, Chen, J, Resau, JH, and Teh, BT, (2006) Preparing the soil: the primary tumor induces vasculature reorganization in the sentinel lymph node before the arrival of metastatic cancer cells. Cancer Res. 66: 10365-10376.

89. Hirakawa, S, Kodama, M, Kunstfeld, R, Kajiya, K, Brown, LF, and Detmar, M, (2005) VEGF-A induces tumor and sentinel lymph node lymphangiogenesis and promotes lymphatic metastasis. J. Exp. Med. 201: 1089-1099.

90. Cao, R, Bjorndahl, MA, Religa, P, Clasper, S, Garvin, S, Galter, D, Meister, B, Ikomi, F, Tritsaris, K, Dissing, S, Ohhashi, T, Jackson, DG, and Cao, Y, (2004) PDGF-BB induces intratumoral lymphangiogenesis and promotes lymphatic metastasis. Cancer Cell. 6: 333-345.

91. Kajiya, K, Hirakawa, S, Ma, B, Drinnenberg, I, and Detmar, M, (2005) Hepatocyte growth factor promotes lymphatic vessel formation and function. EMBO. J. 24: 2885-2895.
92. Bjorndahl, M, Cao, R, Nissen, LJ, Clasper, S, Johnson, LA, Xue, Y, Zhou, Z, Jackson, D, Hansen, AJ, and Cao, Y, (2005) Insulin-like growth factors 1 and 2 induce lymphangiogenesis in vivo. Proc Natl Acad Sci U S A. 102: 15593-15598.
93. Tammela, T, Petrova, TV, and Alitalo, K, (2005) Molecular lymphangiogenesis: new players. Trends Cell Biol. 15: 434-441.
94. St Croix, B, Rago, C, Velculescu, V, Traverso, G, Romans, KE, Montgomery, E, Lal, A, Riggins, GJ, Lengauer, C, Vogelstein, B, and Kinzler, KW, (2000) Genes expressed in human tumor endothelium. Science. 289: 1197-1202.
95. Carson-Walter, EB, Watkins, DN, Nanda, A, Vogelstein, B, Kinzler, K, and St Croix, B, (2001) Cell surface tumor endothelial markers are conserved in mice and humans. Cancer Res. 61: 6649-6655.
96. Nanda, A and St Croix, B, (2004) Tumor endothelial markers: new targets for cancer therapy. Curr Opin Oncol. 16: 44-49.
97. Zhang, L, Giraudo, E, Hoffman, JA, Hanahan, D, and Ruoslahti, E, (2006) Lymphatic zip codes in premalignant lesions and tumors. Cancer Res. 66: 5696-5706.
98. Yong, C, Bridenbaugh, EA, Zawieja, D, and Swartz, MA, (2005) Microarray analysis of VEGF-C responsive genes in human lymphatic endothelial cells. Lymphatic Res. Biol. 3: 183-207.

5. ANATOMY OF THE HUMAN LYMPHATIC SYSTEM

MAURO ANDRADE AND ALFREDO JACOMO

Department of Surgery, University of Sao Paulo, Brazil

INTRODUCTION

The lymphatic system transports lymph from interstitial space in different organs toward the base of the neck. Its pathway begins after resorption from initial lymphatics and lymph transport to progressively larger vessels (lymphatic collectors and trunks), finally reaching the confluence of the internal jugular and subclavian veins as lymphatic and thoracic ducts, respectively, at the right and left venous angles.

Even though important physiopathological and therapeutical issues may exist due to the close anatomical, embryological, and functional relationship of blood and lymphatic vessels, there are some marked differences between the two systems (1).

In that sense, unlike blood vessels, the lymphatic system cannot be considered as a real circulatory system. While blood circulates in a closed circle pumped by the heart, both in systemic and pulmonary circulation, lymph flow is unidirectional from peripheral tissues to blood and is considered to be an open semicircular system.

The lymphatic system is ubiquitous and exists in all tissues where blood vessels are also found, placenta being an exception. Cornea does not contain lymphatics (10). For a long time, the existence of lymphatics in the central nervous system has been a subject of discussion among anatomists. However, liquor is now considered as the neuroaxis lymph and it has a clear relationship with cervical lymphatic pathways.

Study of lymphatics has always been troublesome for the anatomists due to the small caliber of the lymphatic vessels and their transparent content. After the initial observation of the chylous vessels by Aselli in 1627, methods were developed to observe the lymph vessels. In the seventeenth century, mercurial injections were employed and Gerota's solution, idealized at the end of the nineteenth century, is still in use today with some modifications (3, 6–9).

GENERAL ORGANIZATION OF THE LYMPHATIC SYSTEM

The fluid originated from capillary filtration flows preferentially through the tissue channels, the "microcirculatory highway" of the interstitium. After absorption of the interstitial fluid by the initial lymphatics, lymph is transported through progressively larger and structurally more complex vessels until its final destination into the blood system. All along the way, compact chains of capsulated lymphocytes, the lymph nodes, filter the lymph and are responsible for another essential role of the system: the immune response (14).

According to Kubik, lymphatic vessels can be classified in a crescent order of size and complexity in lymph capillaries, precollectors, collectors, and trunks. The first two are denominated initial lymphatics (12).

The structure of lymph capillaries, whose prime function is absorption of fluid and macromolecules, differs from blood capillaries in some essential features: their format resembles glove fingers, they have incomplete basal membrane, and are larger than the correspondent blood capillary vessels (1). Their endothelial cells have a small number of open junctions, not found in blood vessels (except for sinusoidal capillaries and injured vessels). In some areas, adjacent endothelial cells partially overlap, creating a point of entry for interstitial fluid and at the same time acting as an antireflux mechanism. Anchoring filaments are a unique anatomical feature presented by lymph capillaries; these structures are extensions of the endothelial cells and originate on the outer surface of the intercellular contact area between two adjacent cells. Their adhesions to interstitial elastic and collagen fibers open the intercellular space when interstitial volume increases and are a major feature of lymph absorption.

Collector vessels and trunks present structure similar to veins, even though their three layers – intimae, media, and adventitia – are thinner and have a less evident separation than those observed in the venous system. They have semilunar valves, more numerous and histologically similar to the vein valves, formed by folds of endothelium, smooth muscle, and connective tissue. There is also a valve at the lymphatic confluence at the jugulosubclavian junction, thus avoiding blood reflux to the major lymphatic ducts (10).

The lymphatic system, according to its topography, can be divided into three systems: superficial, deep, and visceral. The superficial system drains skin and subcutaneous tissue whereas the deep lymphatic system is responsible for the subfascial tissue drainage. The visceral system can also be considered a part of the deep system. Perforating vessels cross the fascia and connect the superficial and deep systems. Some authors consider another group of vessels: the communicating vessels, which communicate areas drained by different bundles. Lymphatic collectors of the limbs, both superficial and deep, accompany neighboring vessels (2), the drained volume through the superficial system being far more important to the lymphatic drainage of the extremities.

Lymph nodes consist in an agglomerate of lymphoid tissue surrounded by a capsule of dense connective tissue and some smooth muscle fibers and their inner framework is formed by trabeculae, extensions of the inner aspect of the capsule that limit lymph follicles. After reaching the lymph node, lymph flows through its subcapsular space and is filtered in the network formed by the trabecular and medullar sinuses. Lymph nodes are arranged as chains found in reasonably constant areas of the body and contain a variable number of nodes; the total number of lymph nodes in humans is estimated to be around 600–700 (13). The shape of the lymph nodes is usually spherical or round, and can vary considerably in size, and may reach a normal diameter of up to 1 in. Structurally, they have a small depression called the hilus and an opposite convex surface. Efferent lymph vessels and nodal arteries and veins are found in the hilus whereas afferent lymph vessels reach the lymph node in many points along its convex surface. Afferent lymph vessels are generally smaller and more numerous than the efferent vessels (14).

The same as in lymph vessels, lymph node groups, or chains can be classified according to their location as superficial, when they are embedded into the subcutaneous tissue, or deep, situated under the muscular fascia or inside abdominal or thoracic cavities (2).

FORMATION OF THE MAIN LYMPHATIC TRUNKS AND DUCTS

There are 11 lymphatic trunks: gastrointestinal, lumbar, bronchomediastinal, subclavian, jugular, and descending intercostals (10). All, except for the gastrointestinal trunk, are paired.

Lumbar trunks are formed by the union of lymphatic vessels, which drain the following regions: lower limbs, urogenital system, anatomical structures irrigated by the inferior mesenteric artery, and the infraumbilical portion of the abdominal wall.

Efferent lymph vessels from celiac and superior mesenteric lymph nodes originate the gastrointestinal trunk.

The right and left bronchomediastinal trunks are responsible for the transport of lymph coming from the deep layer of the superior and anterior areas of the abdomen and thorax, the anterior portion of the diaphragm, lungs, heart, and visceral aspect of the right lobe of the liver.

The subclavian trunks are formed by lymphatic collectors draining the upper limbs, supraumbilical area of the abdominal wall, and anterior thoracic wall.

Lymph from the head, face, inner structures of the neck, and posterior cervical region drain toward the jugular trunks.

The descending intercostal trunks collect the lymph originated at the deep posterior thoracic region, corresponding to the last five intercostal spaces.

There are two lymphatic ducts: the right lymphatic duct and the thoracic duct. The first is formed by the confluence of the right jugular trunk, right subclavian trunk, and right bronchomediastinal trunk; generally, this duct empties into the right jugulosubclavian confluence.

The thoracic duct is originated from the descending intercostal trunks, the right and left lumbar trunks, and the gastrointestinal trunk. Cisterna chyli is an ampular dilatation frequently observed where those trunks meet and is located between the azygous vein and aorta at the level of L2 to D12. Just after its origin, the thoracic duct runs cranially through the aortic hiatus of the diaphragm, to the right of the median sagittal plane, and around D5 level it turns to the left side, crossing the posterior aspect of the thoracic esophagus. At the base of the neck, it reaches the left jugulosubclavian junction and near its terminal portion receives the left jugular, left subclavian, and left bronchomediastinal trunks.

Therefore, according to the lymphatic drainage, the body can be divided into four quadrants and all but the upper right quadrant are drained by the thoracic duct.

ANATOMY OF THE LYMPHATICS OF THE UPPER LIMBS

The lymphatic drainage of the superior limbs has two components: a superficial drainage and a less important one, the deep lymphatic system. Both systems anastomose and most of the upper limb lymph has a common final destination: the axillary lymph nodes. The superficial lymphatic system has ten bundles (Figs. 1 and 2), each one of them with one to many lymphatic collectors. Anastomoses between bundles are frequent.

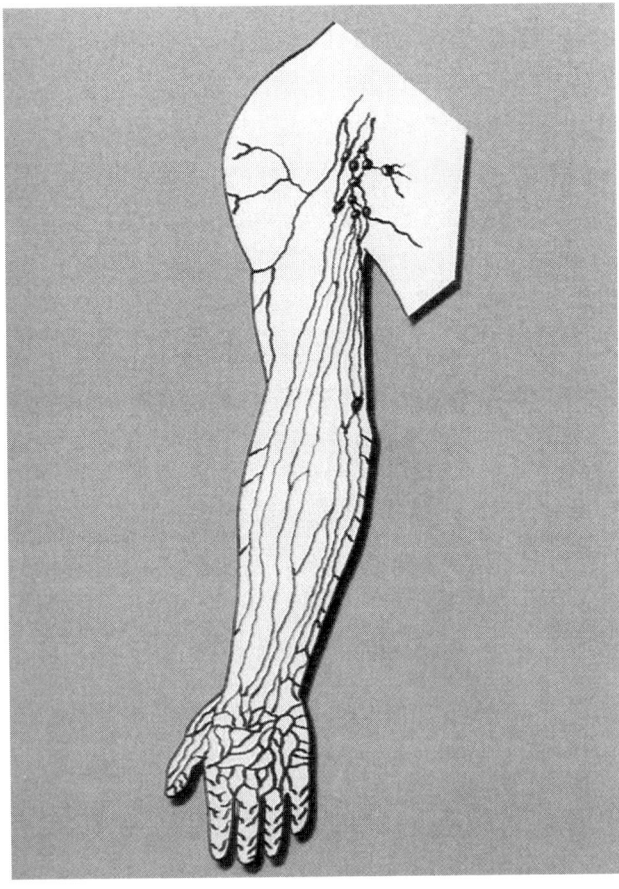

Figure 1. Anterior view of the upper limb. Schematic distribution of the superficial bundles of the forearm and arm. Observe the epitroclear lymph node

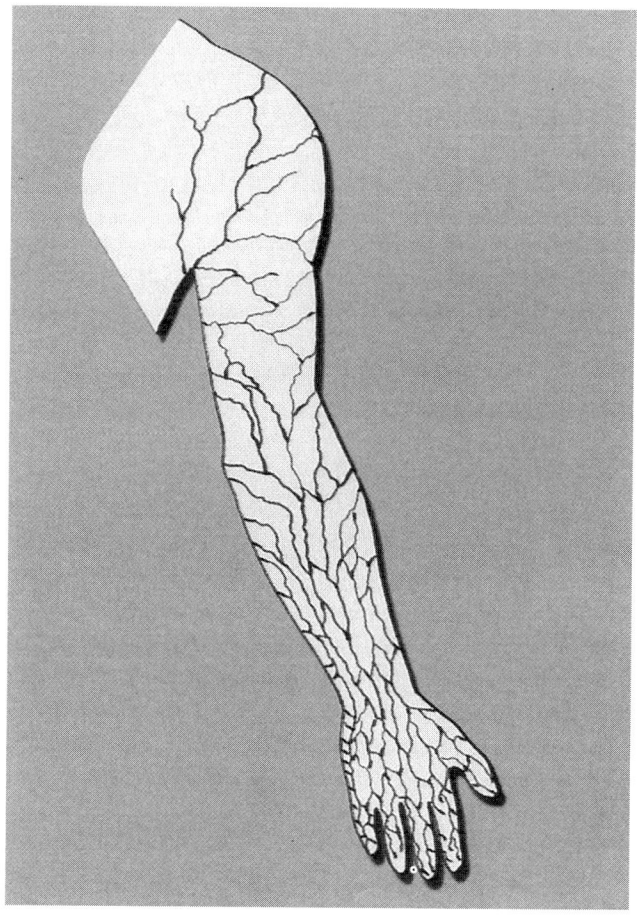

Figure 2. Posterior view of the superficial lymphatic bundles of the upper limb

Didactically, the bundles can be divided into six proximal bundles in the arm and four distal in the forearm and hand. The proximal bundles are further subdivided into three anterior and three posterior bundles (4).

Anterior bundles are, according to their drainage area, cephalic, basilic (Fig. 3), and prebicipital; and the posterior ones are posteromedial, posterior, and posterolateral.

The four bundles that drain the distal regions are divided into two anterior (anterior radial and anterior ulnar) and two posterior (posterior radial and posterior ulnar).

The deep lymphatic drainage of the upper arms has six bundles: two proximal in the arm and four distal. The proximal bundles are denominated brachial (Fig. 4) and deep brachial due to their anatomical relation witsh the homonymous arteries.

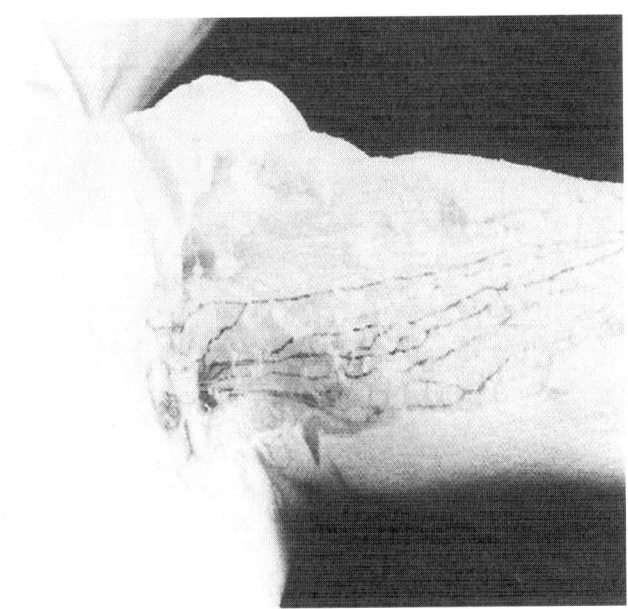

Figure 3. Basilic bundle observed after intradermal injection of Gerota's mass in the anterior aspect of the forearm. Impregnation of lymph nodes of the anterior and lateral lymph node groups of the axilla

The four distal comprise three anterior bundles: deep radial, deep ulnar, and anterior interosseal (Fig. 5), and one posterior: posterior interosseal (6–9) (Fig. 6).

Derivative pathways are lymph collectors that do not reach the expected drainage site at the root of the limbs. For the upper limbs, two different derivative pathways can be identified. They are the cephalic and the posterior bundles that run to the supraclavicular nodes and posterior scapular nodes, respectively. These derivative pathways are one of the possible explanations of why lymphedema does not always develop after axillary resection and radiation for breast cancer treatment (4).

Lymph nodes of the upper limbs can also be classified as superficial and deep (4). Superficial lymph nodes are found in the arm (Fig. 1) accompanying the basilic vein, called epitroclear lymph nodes, and in the deltoideopectoral sulcus, called deltoideopectoral lymph nodes. Deep lymph nodes (Figs. 4–6) are located in the arm and in the forearm. Arm lymph nodes are found close to the vessels and are so denominated brachial and deep brachial lymph nodes. In the forearm, there are anterior lymph nodes (radial, ulnar, and anterior interosseal) and a posterior one (posterior interosseal) (6–9).

Lymph nodes in the axilla (Figs. 7–9) are organized as lymph centers or chains and receive lymph from the following regions: upper limb, supraumbilical area up to the clavicle, and dorsal region (10). These chains are classified according to their location in:

1. *Anterior group (also pectoral or external mammary or lateral thoracic)*. Located at the inferior border of the pectoralis major muscle and related with the lateral thoracic artery. This chain receives lymph from most of the breast and supraumbilical region.

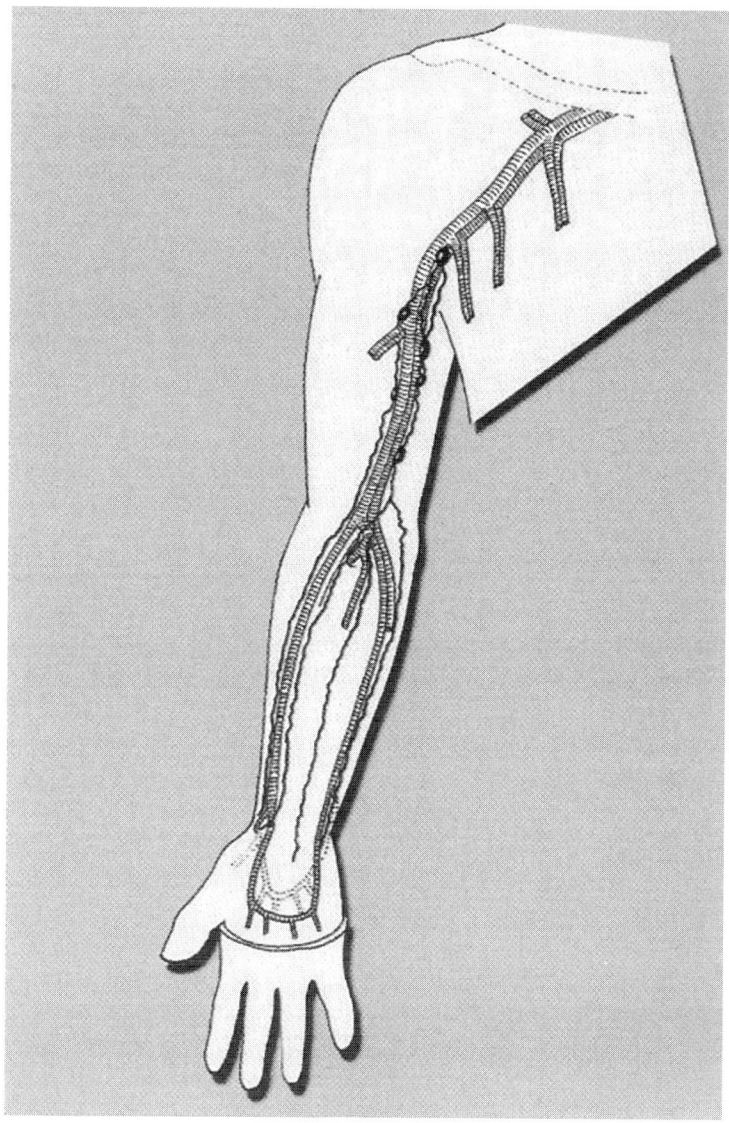

Figure 4. Schematic anterior view of the deep bundles and lymph nodes of the arm and their relationship with the arteries

2. *Posterior group (also subscapular).* Situated anterior to the subscapular muscle, all along the subscapular vessels and receives lymph from the dorsum.
3. *Lateral group (or axillary).* This chain accompanies the axillary vessels, situated anterior, posterior, superior, and inferior to them and drains lymph from the upper limb, except the lymph that flows through derivative pathways.

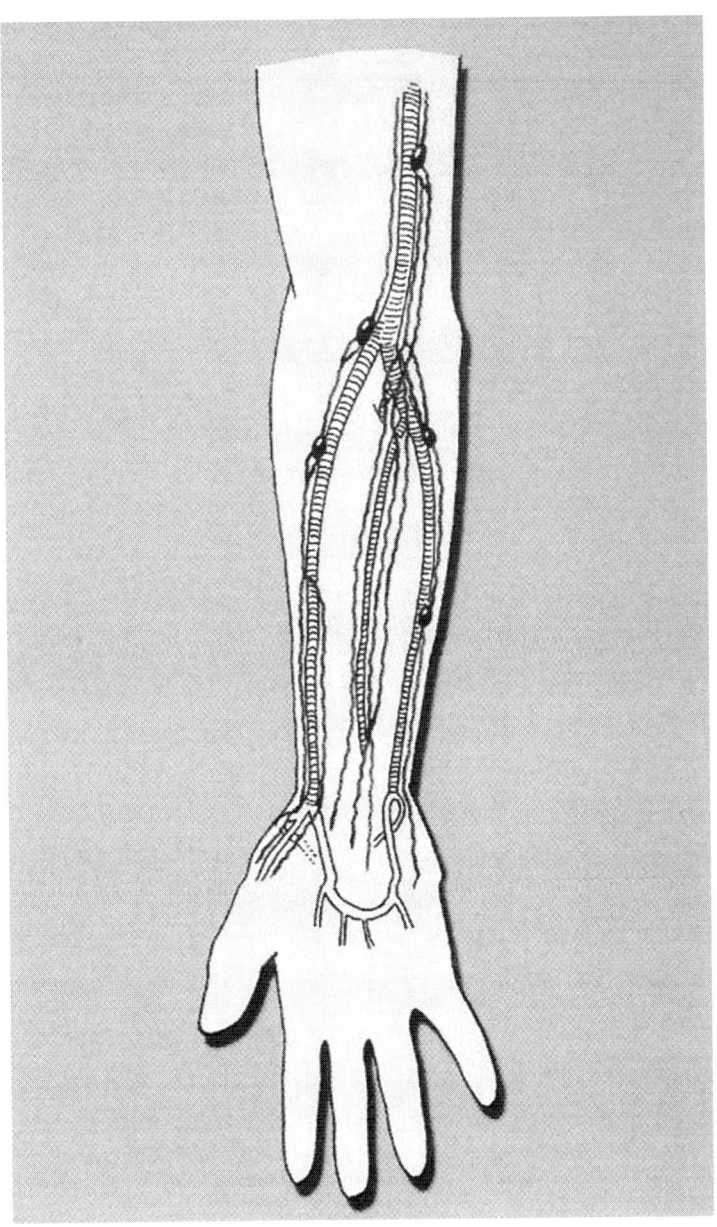

Figure 5. Anterior view of the deep bundles and lymph nodes of the forearm

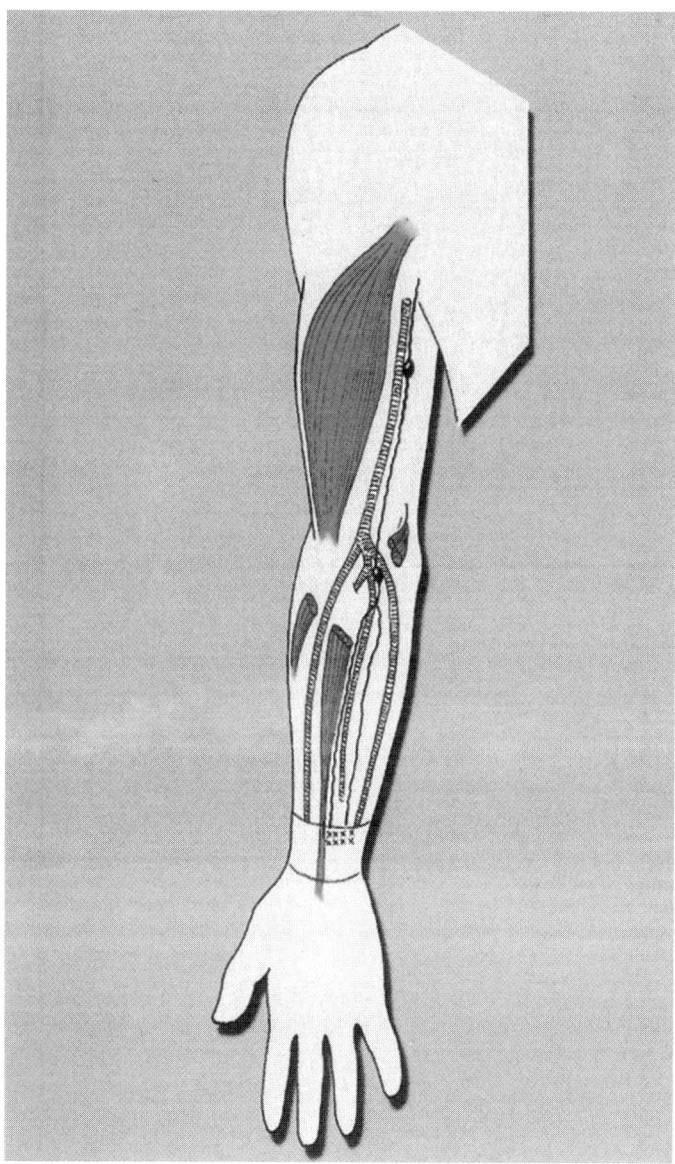

Figure 6. Anterior view of the deep bundles and lymph nodes of the arm, medial and posterior to the biceps muscle

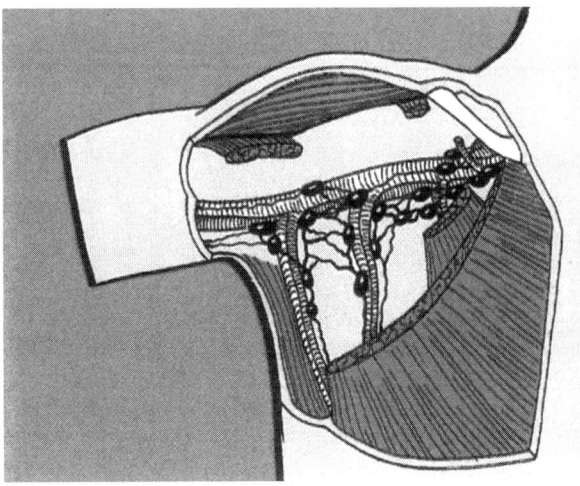

Figure 7. Lymph nodes of the axilla. The anterior group is related to the lateral thoracic artery and is followed by the lateral and posterior chains. The intermediate group receives afferent vessels from the previous groups. Medial or apical chain is located medial to the minor pectoralis muscle

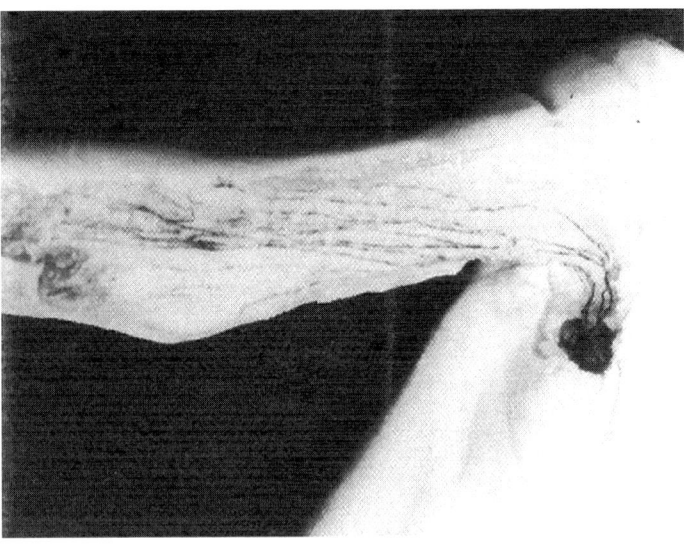

Figure 8. Basilic bundle and lateral lymph nodes of the axilla after injection in the hand

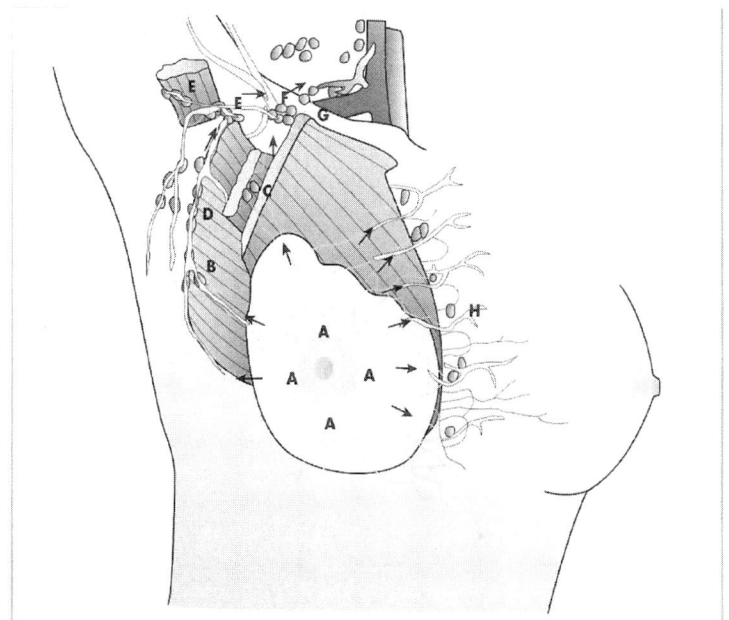

Figure 9. Lymphatic drainage of the breast to the lymph nodes of the axilla and internal mammary chain

4. *Intermediate group (or central).* This is also located following the axillary vessels but is immediately medial to the previous group, receiving lymph from efferent vessels of the lateral chain.
5. *Medial group (or apical).* This last group is situated medial to the pectoralis minor muscle, receives efferent vessels from the intermediate group and from this group, efferent vessels form the subclavian trunk that flows to the lymphatic duct on the right side and thoracic duct on the left.

ANATOMY OF THE LYMPHATICS OF THE LOWER LIMBS

The lymphatic drainage of the lower limbs also consists of two different systems: the deep and the superficial system (2).

The superficial system has six different bundles (11) (Figs. 10–12), two distal in the foot and in the leg, named according to the main vein they follow: great saphenous bundle (or ventromedial) and lesser saphenous (or posterolateral) bundle. The other four proximal bundles are located in the thigh and are subsequently divided in two anterior and two posterior bundles. The anterior bundles are the anteromedial of the thigh (or ventromedial or great saphenous bundle) and anterolateral of the thigh. The posterior bundles of the thigh are denominated posteromedial and posterolateral.

The great saphenous bundle of the leg extends upward and continues as the anteromedial bundle of the thigh. These lymphatic vessels converge posterior to the medial condilum of the femur to reach the thigh. The great saphenous bundle of

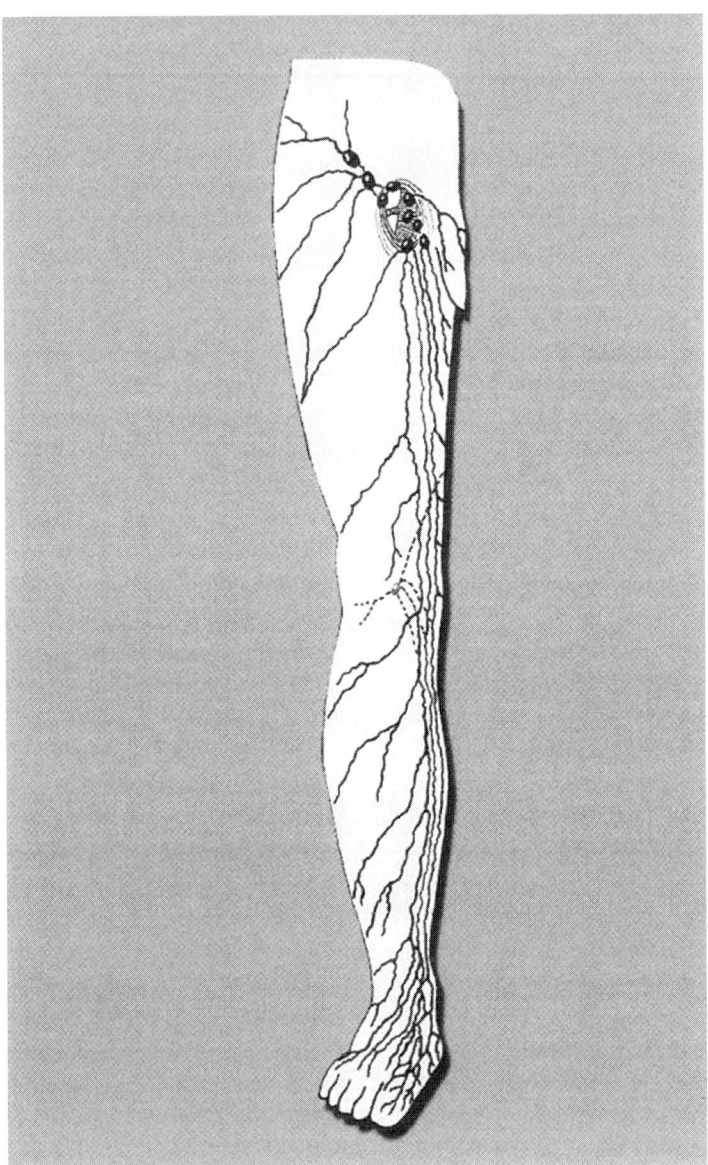

Figure 10. Anterior view of the lower limb. Schematic distribution of the superficial bundles of the leg and thigh. Observe that the accessory saphenous bundle is restricted to the thigh

the leg receives anastomotic vessels from the lesser saphenous bundle. The antero-lateral bundle of the thigh, also called the accessory saphenous bundle, originates in the thigh so there is no direct connection between this bundle and the lymphatics of the leg (5) (Fig. 10). It is also important to notice the close relationship between the great saphenous vein and the accompanying lymphatic bundle, especially in the

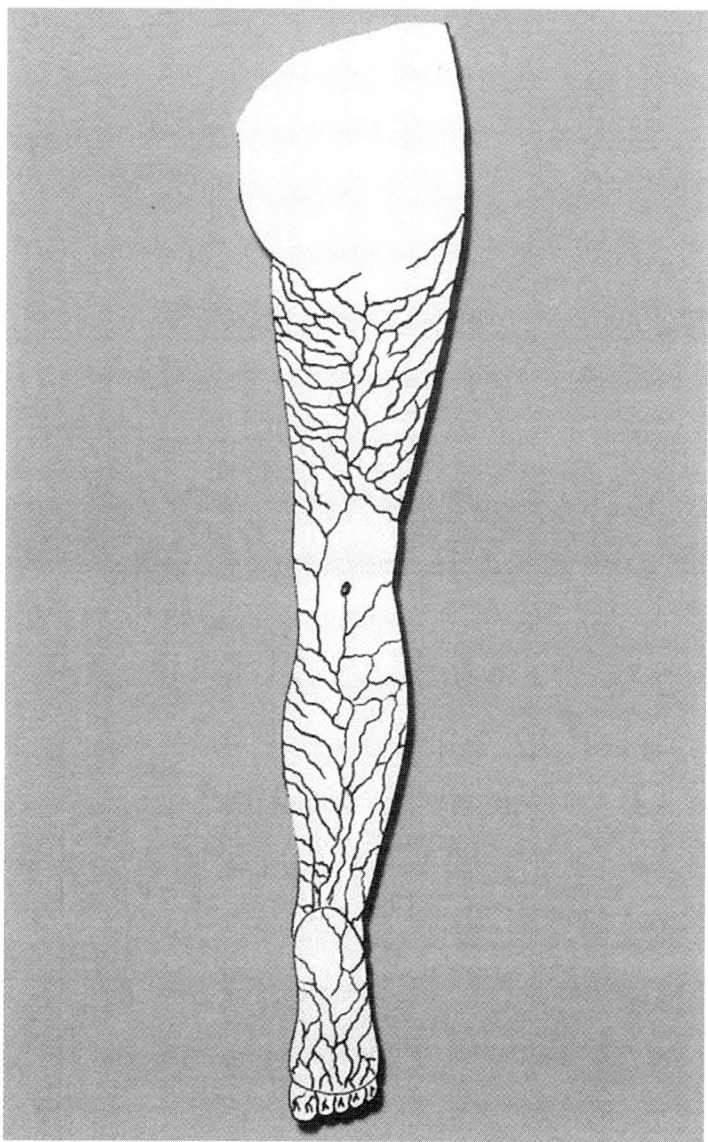

Figure 11. Posterior view of the lower limb. Observe the superficial popliteal lymph node

knee area, which makes the latter susceptible to trauma in operations for saphenous harvest to aortocoronary bypass and some surgical procedures for varicose veins (2).

The deep lymphatic drainage of the lower limb has five lymphatic bundles, being three distal (leg and foot) and two proximal in the thigh.

The deep lymphatic bundles of the foot and leg are divided in one anterior (Fig. 13) and two posterior (Fig. 14). The anterior bundle is named anteromedial

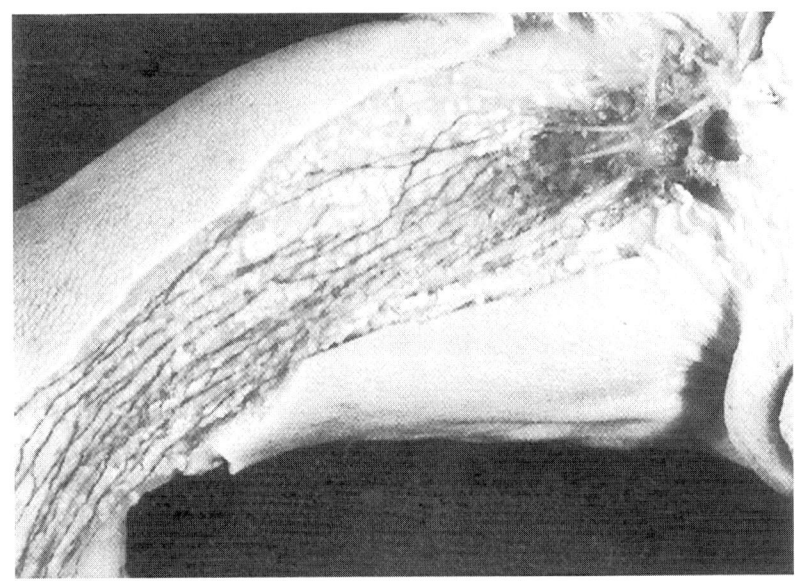

Figure 12. Superficial inguinal lymph nodes and their relationship with the branches of the great saphenous vein after injection in the foot

bundle or anterior tibial and the posterior ones are called posteromedial or posterior tibial, and the last one posterolateral or fibular bundle.

In the thigh, the deep lymphatic bundles accompany the femoral artery and the deep femoral artery (Fig. 15) and drain into the deep inguinal lymph nodes (6–9).

Lower limbs also have deep and superficial lymph nodes (3). Superficial lymph nodes are found in the subcutaneous of the inguinal (Figs. 13 and 15) and popliteal regions (Fig. 14). Inguinal lymph nodes are related to the superficial regional veins: great saphenous, accessory lateral saphenous, superficial circumflex iliac, superficial epigastric, and external pudenda.

The superficial inguinal lymph nodes are named according to their anatomical relationship with the neighboring vein (Fig. 16). There are six superficial nodal chains: three of them are located inferiorly and contain one single node (great saphenous, lateral accessory saphenous, and intersaphenous) and the remaining three are cranial to the saphenofemoral junction, and usually multinodal (superficial circumflex iliac, superficial epigastric, and external pudenda).

Usually, the lymphatic drainage of the lower limbs reaches the inferior inguinal lymph nodes (great saphenous, lateral accessory saphenous, and intersaphenous), while superior ones receive lymph from infraumbilical abdominal area, gluteus, external genitalia, and part of the uterus. The major labia of pudendum have both homolateral and contralateral drainage (6–9) (Figs. 16 and 17).

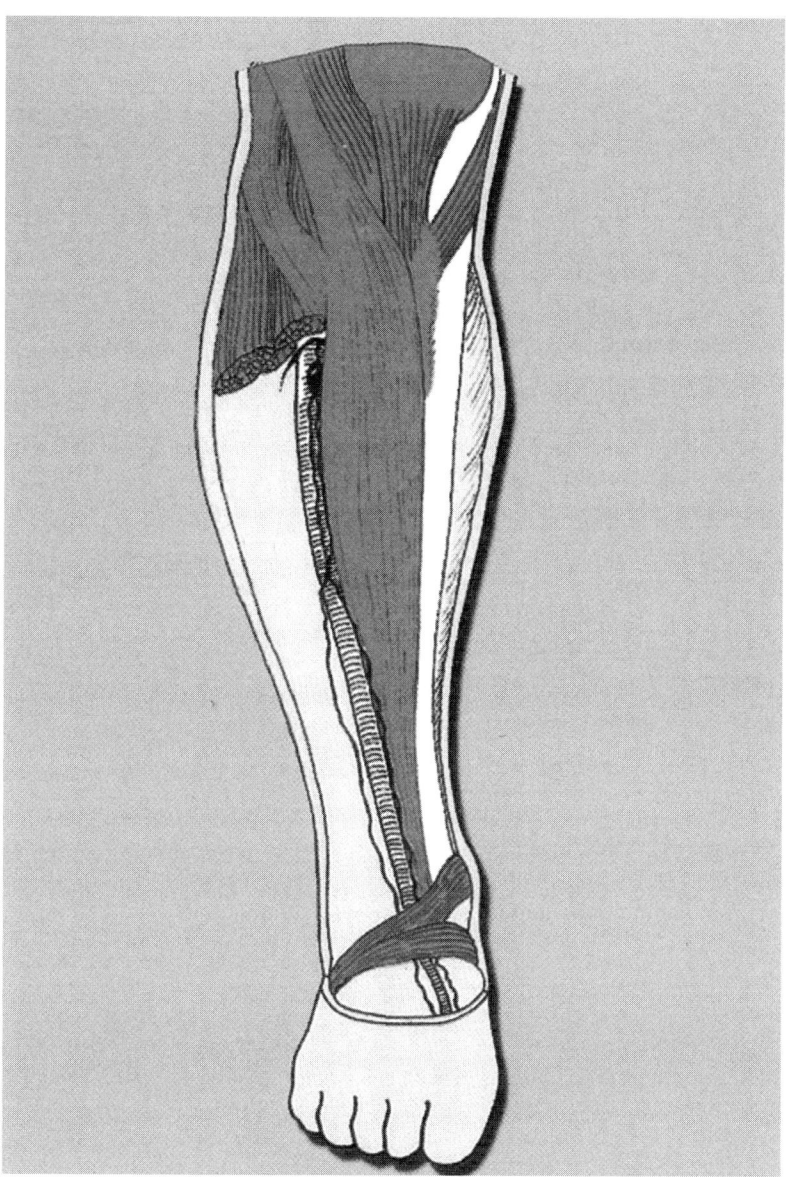

Figure 13. View of the anterior deep bundle and lymph node of the leg

Superficial inguinal lymph nodes, mainly the inferior nodes, can be severed during great saphenous vein stripping and dissections of the inguinal area, due to their relationship with saphenofemoral junction, which may lead to lymphatic blockage and edema of the lower limb.

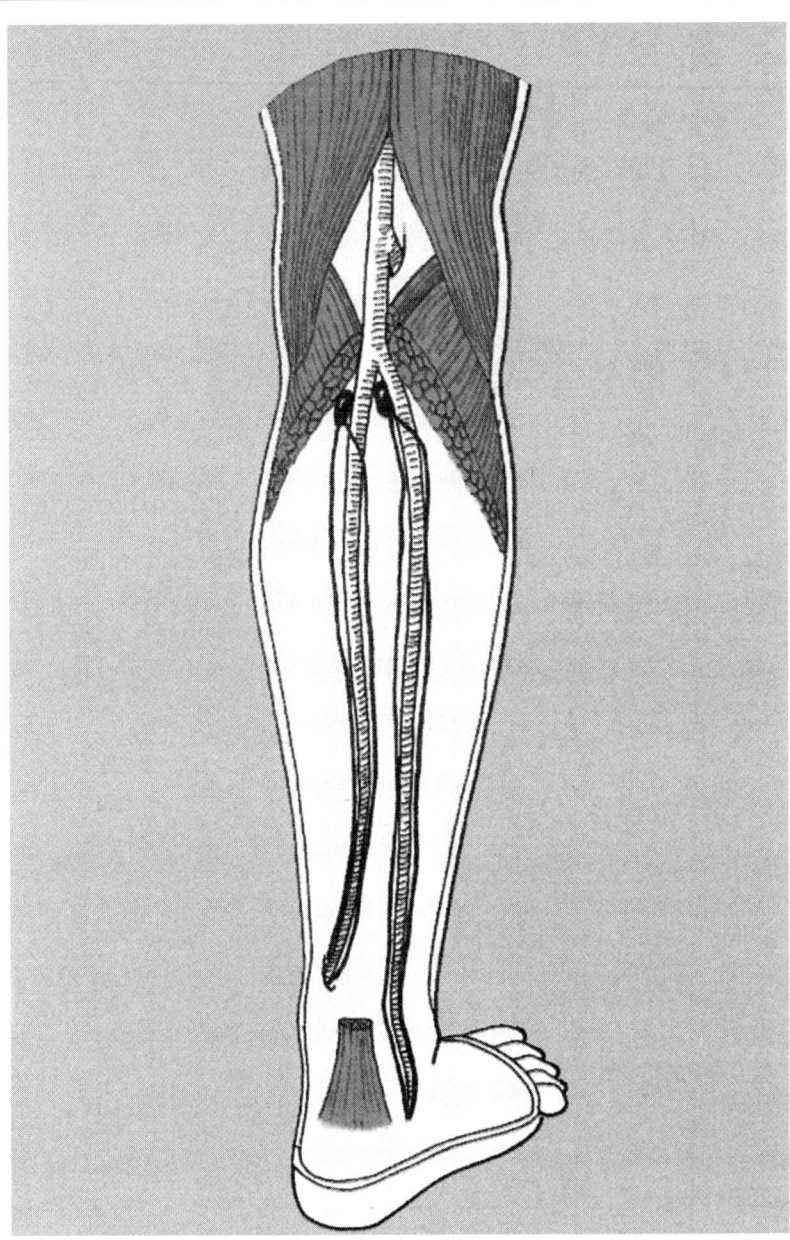

Figure 14. View of the posterior deep bundles of the leg accompanying the posterior tibial and fibular arteries

In the popliteal region, the superficial popliteal node is commonly unique and receives lymph from the posterolateral bundle of the leg (Fig. 18).

Concerning deep lymph nodes, they are located in the leg, popliteal, and inguinal regions.

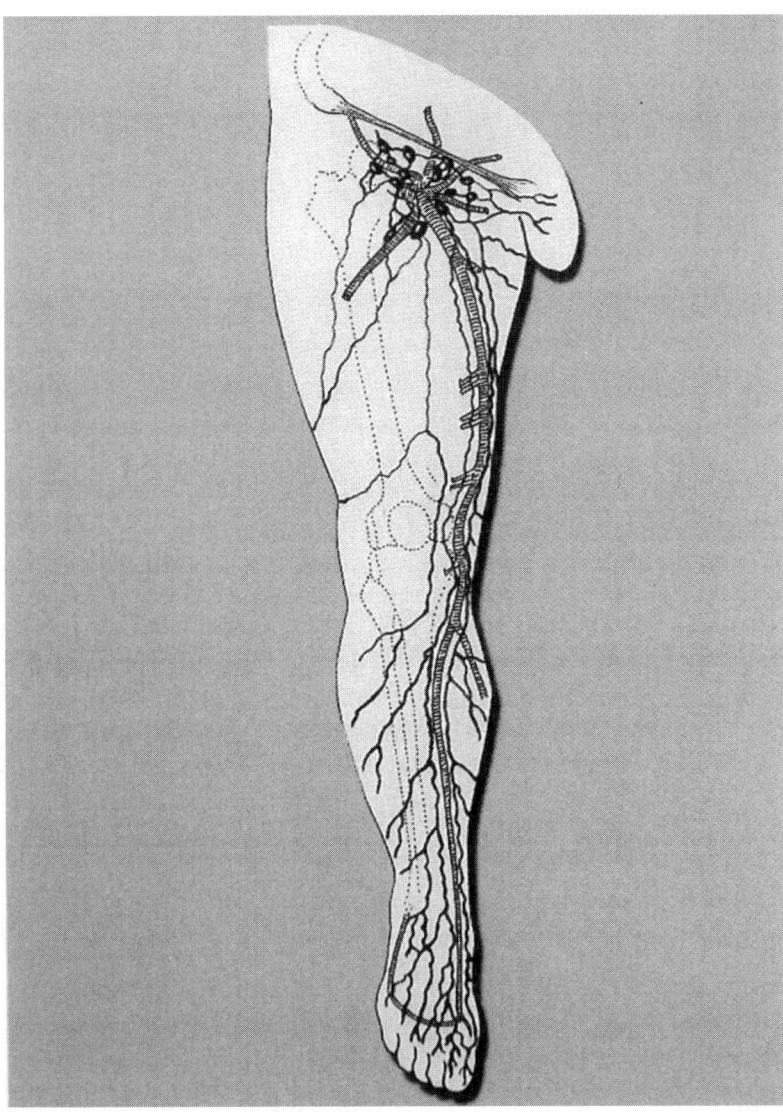

Figure 15. Superficial inguinal lymph nodes and superficial bundles of the lower limb and their relationship with the great saphenous vein

Deep leg lymph nodes are usually situated near to the origin of the arteries, thus anterior tibial, posterior tibial, and fibular, and they receive lymph from the leg and foot (11). Deep popliteal chain (Fig. 19) usually contains ten lymph nodes and has the following distribution, according to their position regarding the popliteal vessels: one is anterior to the popliteal artery (anterior popliteal or prearterial); the nine lymph nodes remaining are related to the popliteal vein. Of those, three are

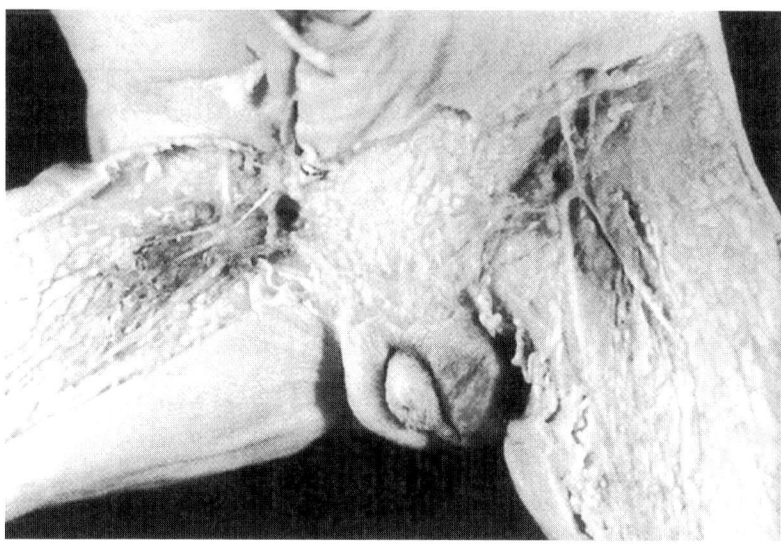

Figure 16. Superficial inguinal lymph nodes after injection in both feet and left major labium with masses of different colors. Lymphatic drainage of the genital area injected goes to both inguinal areas

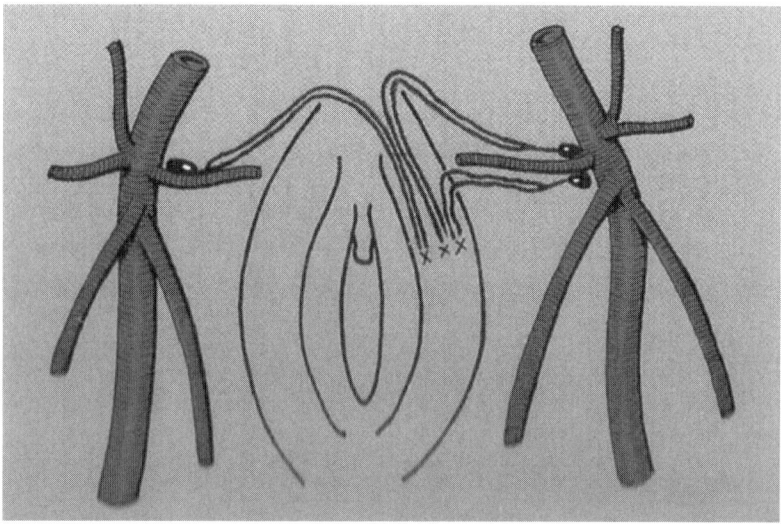

Figure 17. Schematic distribution of the lymphatic drainage of the major labia of the pudendum

situated lateral to the vein and three are medial. They have the denomination of superior, median, and inferior in each side, considering their location related to the joint. The three deep posterior lymph nodes (retropopliteal) receive their denomination according to their position cranial or caudal to the lesser saphenous popliteal

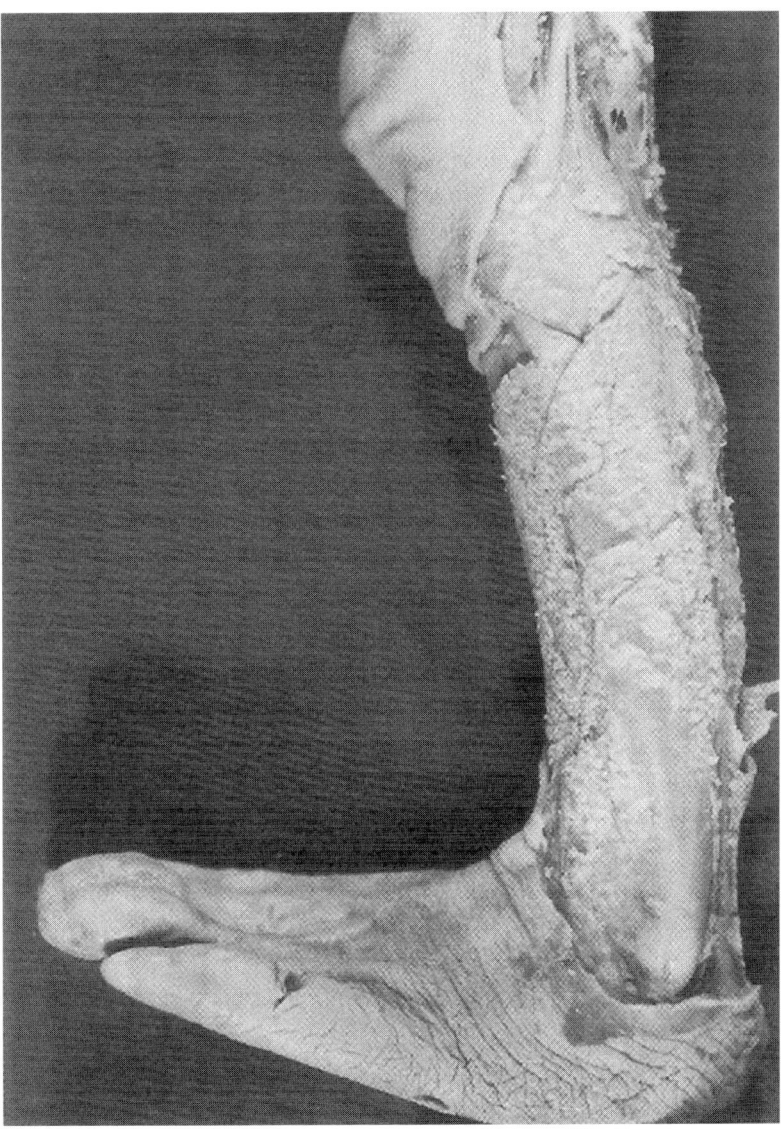

Figure 18. Superficial popliteal lymph node and posterolateral bundle of the leg after injection in the lateral aspect of the foot

junction as two suprasaphenous and one infrasaphenous (2, 3, 11). This entire group drains lymph from subfascial portions of the leg and foot and can also receive lymph from the superficial area through perforator vessels.

Deep inguinal lymph nodes are located medial to the femoral vein and deep to saphenous femoral junction. There are fewer nodes as compared to the superficial chain and one of them, always present, lays near to the lacunar ligament and is called

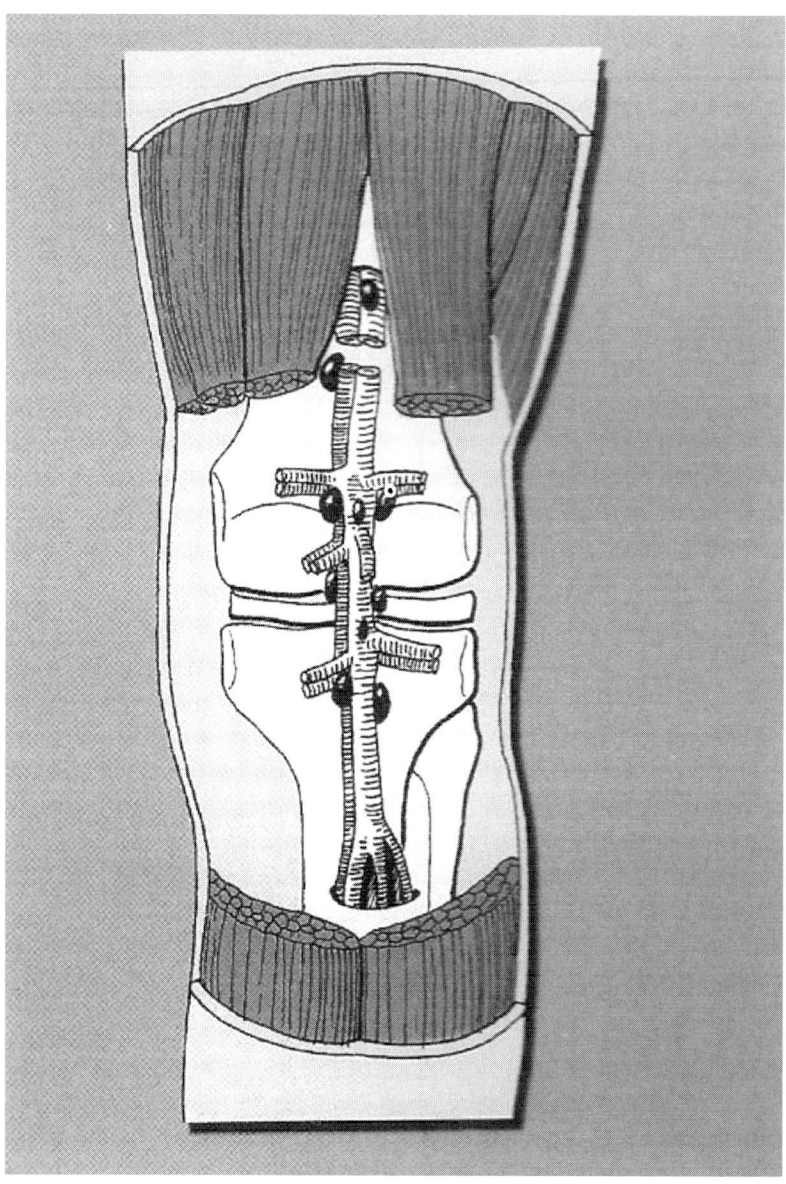

Figure 19. Deep popliteal lymph nodes and their relationship with the popliteal vessels

Cloquet's lymph node (2, 3). This chain receives lymph from efferent vessels that accompany the femoral artery and also from the superficial area.

After the inguinal lymph nodes, lymph of the lower limbs reaches external iliac and common iliac lymph nodes. Subsequently, it passes through lumbar aortic lymph nodes that form the lumbar trunks and finally drain into the thoracic duct.

ANATOMY OF THE LYMPHATICS OF THE PELVIS

Pelvic lymph nodes receive their denomination according to their topographic relationship to the iliac vessels as external, internal, and common iliac lymph nodal chains (10).

The external iliac chain, which follows inguinal lymph nodes, is subdivided into lateral, intermediate, and medial. The lateral lymph nodes are located at the lateral aspect of the external iliac artery and are superficial to the psoas muscle. The intermediate chain is found between the artery and the vein, and its more cranial lymph node is found near the common iliac artery bifurcation and is closely related to the ureter.

Medial external iliac lymph nodes are found medial to the external iliac vein and near the obturator nerve. Its more caudal node has a close relationship with Cloquet's node (2, 3).

The internal iliac chain lies near to the internal iliac artery and its branches and has parietal and visceral lymph nodes.

The parietal nodes are superior and inferior gluteal, lateral sacral, and obturators. The visceral are lateral, anterior and posterior vesical, rectal, and uterine. As visceral internal iliac lymph nodes are closely related to the pelvic organs, they are usually the first to be reached by lymphatic metastasis.

The common iliac lymph chain is located along the homonymous artery, and medial, lateral, and intermediate lymph nodes can also be identified. The medial one is the most cranial of them and sometimes is included in the subaortic lymph nodes group.

Thorough comprehension of lymphatic vessels and nodes of the pelvis, particularly those of the uterus, is very important due to the incidence of uterine carcinoma.

Thus, the fundus and upper part of the uterine body drain through lymphatic vessels of the round ligament to the superficial inguinal lymph nodes. Laterally, on the superior region of the broad ligament, its lymphatic drainage follows that of the uterine tube and ovary, accompanying the ovarian vessels to the lumbar aortic chain. On the other hand, the lymphatic drainage of the inferior portion of the uterine body and neck goes mainly to the pelvic lymph nodes, external, internal, and even common. Because of this massive spread of the cervical lymph drainage, complete removal of pelvic lymph nodes is sometimes required for the treatment of cervical carcinoma.

ANATOMY OF THE LYMPHATICS OF THE ABDOMEN

Lymph node chains of the abdominal cavity are retroperitoneal and are divided into aortoceliac and aortolumbar, respectively, superior and inferior to the left renal vessels. The first will form the gastrointestinal trunk and the latter the lumbar trunks (10).

The celiac aortic lymph nodes have three different chains:

1. Left aortoceliac, located between the lateral aspect of the aorta and the left diaphragmatic pillar

2. Right aortoceliac, between the right side of the aorta and the right diaphragmatic pillar
3. Anterior aortoceliac, near the superior mesenteric artery origin

These three chains receive lymph from the spleen, pancreas, abdominal esophagus, liver, gallbladder, stomach, small intestine, cecum, ascending colon, and proximal two-thirds of the transverse colon. Also, some vessels from the left colic flexure and distal third of the transverse colon drain to this chain.

Aortolumbar lymph nodes are divided into three groups: preaortic, left aortic or left lateral aortic, and right aortic. Some authors describe a posterior aortic chain, which we believe does not exist because aortic pulse against the vertebra could damage them.

The preaortic chain is located anterior to the abdominal aorta and its lymph nodes are around the inferior mesenteric artery origin up to the inferior aspect of the left renal artery. This chain receives efferent lymph vessels from the left colic flexure, distal third of the transverse colon, descending colon, sigmoid and most of the rectum. Therefore, the distal part of the transverse colon and the left flexure have double lymphatic drainage.

The left aortic chain is located between the lateral aspect of the aorta and the psoas muscle. This chain collects lymph from the kidney, suprarenal gland, left common iliac chain, testicle or ovary, uterine tube, left superior portion of the uterus, and deep layer of the abdominal wall.

The right aortic chain is divided into precaval, interaortocaval, laterocaval, and retrocaval. The precaval group is represented by lymph nodes situated from the origin of the inferior cava vein until the inferior border of the right renal vessels. The interaortocaval group is found between the inferior cava vein and abdominal aorta until the inferior border of the left renal vessels. The laterocaval group is situated to the right of the vein and the retrocaval group is found posterior to the cava, anterior to the psoas muscle. These four lymph nodal groups receive the lymphatic drainage from the kidney, suprarenal gland, testicle or ovary, uterine tube, superior and lateral portion of the uterus, deep layer of the abdominal wall, and right common iliac chain.

The aortolumbar chains join at the median line and the main efferent lymph vessels from either side form two lumbar trunks that join with the gastrointestinal trunk to form the thoracic duct.

ANATOMY OF THE LYMPHATICS OF THE HEAD AND NECK

The lymphatic drainage from the head is made through four pathways (10):

1. *Anterior or facial vessels*. It receives the drainage from the frontal area and anterior portion of the face, except for the chin and inferior lip (that drain to the submental lymph nodes) and subsequently drains to the submandibular lymph nodes.
2. *Parotideal*. It receives the lymphatic drainage from the lateral aspect of the face, including the eyelid, flowing to parotideal lymph nodes.

3. *Retroauricular.* It receives lymph from the parietal and temporal areas and drains to the mastoid or retroauricular lymph nodes.
4. *Occipital.* It receives lymph from the occipital region and drains to the occipital lymph nodes.

Superficial cervical lymph nodes are distributed along the external jugular vein, superficial to the sternocleidomastoid muscle, and their efferent vessels reach the deep cervical lymph nodes.

Deep cervical lymph nodes accompany the internal jugular vein, beneath the sternocleidomastoid muscle; some of these lymph nodes run posteriorly together with the accessory nerve and others run downward along with the subclavian vessels.

One lymph node located deep to the posterior body of the digastric muscle is denominated jugulodigastric and another, located superiorly to the tendon of the omohyoid muscle, is called juguloomohyoid.

Efferent lymph vessels from submental, submandibular, parotideal, retromandibular, and occipital reach the deep cervical lymph nodes (jugulodigastric), located cranial to the internal jugular vein. The jugular trunk is formed by lymphatic vessels coming from deep cervical lymph nodes and flows to the thoracic duct on the right and to the thoracic duct on the left (10, 14).

REFERENCES

1. Andrade MFC, Jacomo AL (2000) Sistema linfático dos membros inferiores. In: Petroianu A (ed) Anatomia cirúrgica. Guanabara-Koogan, Rio de Janeiro, pp. 726-728
2. Andrade MFC, Buchpiegel CA, De Luccia N (2000) Lymph absorption and transport in acute deep venous thrombosis of the lower limbs. Lymphology 33(Supp): 95-8
3. Caplan I (1978) The lymphatic system of the big toe. Folia Angiol 26:241 245
4. Caplan I, Ciucci JL (1995) Drenaje linfático superficial del miembro superior. Linfologia 1:33-36
5. Jacomo AL, Caplan I (1991) Estudio e investigación del drenaje linfático cutaneo antero-externo de la region tibial anterior. I Congreso de la sociedad de ciencias morfologicas de La Plata, La Plata, Argentina
6. Jacomo AL, Rodrigues Jr, Figueira LNT (1993) Estudo da drenagem linfática do musculo vasto lateral da coxa, no homem. Acta Ortop Bras 1(1):12-14
7. Jacomo AL, Rodrigues Jr, Figueira LNT (1993) Estudo da drenagem linfática do músculo pronador quadrado. Acta Ortop Bras 1(2):60-62
8. Jacomo AL, Rodrigues Jr AJ, Figueira LNT (1993) Drenagem linfática cutânea – modelo de estudo anatômico. Rev Bras Angiol Cir Vasc 9(3):53
9. Jacomo AL, Rodrigues Jr AJ, Figueira LNT (1993) Estudo da drenagem linfática cutânea dos lábios maiores do pudendo. XVI Congresso Brasileiro de Anatomia, VII Congresso Luso-Brasileiro de Anatomia, São Paulo
10. Jacomo AL, Rodrigues Jr AJ (1995) Anatomia clínica do sistema linfático. In: Vogelfang D (ed) Linfologia básica, Ícone, São Paulo, pp 19-34
11. Jacomo AL, Rodrigues Jr AJ, Figueira LNT (1994) Drenagem linfática superficial da pele da região plantar. Acta Ortop Bras 2:35-37
12. Kubik S (1998) Atlas of the lymphatics of the lower limbs. Servier, Paris
13. Kubik S (2003) Anatomy of the lymphatic system. In: Foldi, Foldi, Kubik (ed) Textbook of Lymphology. Urban & Fischer, Munchen
14. Rouvière H (1981) Anatomie des lymphatiques de l'Homme. Masson, Paris

6. SPECT–CT FUSION IMAGING RADIONUCLIDE LYMPHOSCINTIGRAPHY: POTENTIAL FOR LIMB LYMPHEDEMA ASSESSMENT AND SENTINEL NODE DETECTION IN BREAST CANCER

A. P. PECKING, M. WARTSKI, R. V. CLUZAN,
D. BELLET, AND J. L. ALBÉRINI

Centre René Huguenin, Saint-Cloud, France

INTRODUCTION

Radionuclide lymphoscintigraphy (RNL) has progressively superseded lymphangiography and may be considered as the most advanced method for the assessment of the limb lymphatic system (1, 2). As a safe, noninvasive, and physiological method, RNL is commonly used in lymphology for the evaluation of limb lymphedemas and in oncology for the detection of the sentinel node (SN) (3, 4). However, conventional planar imaging sometimes failed to preoperatively identify the exact localization of the detected lymph nodes (5). Since 2000 (6), hybrid cameras combining a dual head gamma camera with a low-dose radiograph tube mounted on the same gantry were developed, and image fusion has been successfully introduced in clinical practice. We report our experience of this new imaging method in lymphology and oncology, particularly for the SN detection in patients with breast cancer.

METHODS

Lymphoscintigraphic Protocol for Lower Limb Lymphedemas

– Injection: A small volume (<0.2 ml) of calibrated nanocolloids labeled with technetium 99m was used (GE Healthcare, Amersham, UK). The standard procedure involves a simultaneous bilateral subcutaneous injection performed into the first web space of each foot. This easy and reproducible protocol is dedicated to visualize the superficial lymphatic ducts and the corresponding lymph nodes.

- Imaging: All patients were asked to walk (10 min) and whole body detection was first performed 40 min after injection using a large and rectangular field of view camera (GE millennium VG Hawkeye). The lymphatic system is considered as normal when lymph node impregnation is obtained within 40 min with visualization of the superficial lymphatic channels running along the saphena magna. Different pathological situations can be observed: few or no lymph node impregnation in the pelvis 40 min after injection, radiolabeled colloid carried out through the superficial and/or the deep lymphatic system with visualization of popliteal nodes while the superficial femorounguinal nodes are not demonstrated, stasis of the isotopic material in certain areas (dermal back flow) and lymphatic blockades. Secondly, lymphoscintigraphic SPECT and anatomical CT data on selected areas were performed using a dual-modality integrated SPECT–CT imaging system (GE millennium VG Hawkeye). The hybrid camera was fitted with high-resolution, low-energy collimators and 360° SPECT images were acquired in a 128 × 128 matrix size (3° angle step, 20 s per frame). Because of the low level of activity in the limbs reconstruction was performed by filtered backprojection. Transaxial, sagittal, and coronal fusion images of the superimposed anatomical (CT) and functional (SPECT) were finally obtained.

Lymphoscintigraphic Protocol for SN Detection

- Injection: An average dose of 111 MBq (94–135) of calibrated nanocolloids labeled with technetium 99m (GE Healthcare, Amersham, UK) in 0.2 ml was injected in the peritumoral tissue at one site the afternoon before surgery.
- Imaging: Detection was performed around 18 h (16–20) postinjection, about 1 h before surgery using a hybrid camera fitted with a high-resolution and low-energy collimator (GE millennium VG Hawkeye). Images were obtained first in a planar projection (anterior and lateral view of the tumor side) and secondly on a SPECT–CT mode. 360° SPECT images were acquired in a 128 × 128 matrix size (3° angle step, 20 s per step) over the chest. Reconstruction was then performed with two iterations, each with ten subsets of ordered-subset expectation maximization. The CT data were used for attenuation correction and image fusion.

IMAGE INTERPRETATION

A two-sequence image analysis (planar scintigraphic images first and tomographic fusion images second) was separately performed by two senior nuclear medicine physicians either for lymphoscintigraphic images of the limbs or sentinel detection.

PATIENTS

Lower Limb Lymphedemas

One hundred and fifteen patients (age ranging 23–77 years) with symptoms of impaired lymphatic function or transient clinical lower limb lymphedema without venous disease at the venous evaluation were referred for a baseline RNL from

2003 to 2005. All patients were stage 0 or I according to the International Society of Lymphology clinical four stages classification:

Stage 0. No clinical sign and symptoms of impaired lymphatic function.

Stage I. Spontaneous, reversible, soft and doughy tissue swelling, pitting edema, extensive regression when the extremity is kept elevated, very little or no fibrous tissue, negative or borderline Stemmer sign.

Stage II. Spontaneous, irreversible, hard and no pitting edema, no regression with elevated positioning of the extremity, moderate to marked fibrosis, positive Stemmer sign.

Stage III. Lymphostatic elephantiasis, hard and no pitting edema, skin lesions, relapsing infections, no regression with elevated positioning of the extremity, pronounced fibrosis, positive Stemmer sign.

SN Detection

Thirty-four consecutive breast cancer patients, age ranging from 34 to 47 years, were referred for SN detection. Diagnosis was first obtained on core biopsies performed on 8 nonpalpable and 26 palpable lesions. Histological types were ductal carcinomas in 28 patients and lobular carcinomas in 6 patients. All were planed for conservative surgery and lymph node dissection.

RESULTS

Lower Limb Lymphedemas

Among the 29 patients classified as stage 0, four patients (13.8%) had a slow lymphatic progression in the superficial ducts, with a compensatory pathway to the deep lymphatic system through the popliteal nodes on planar images. This particular aspect was confirmed on SPECT–CT fusion images and is typically related to a superficial lymphatic functional insufficiency. A mild lymphostasis was detected on planar images in six of them (20.6%), while fusion imaging detected a lymphatic disturbance in 18 patients (62%). Only seven patients had a normal RNL either on planar or SPECT–CT detection and no explanations could be given to their clinical symptoms, mainly heaviness of the legs. All patients (86) classified stage I had an abnormal RNL. The planar detection demonstrated a unilateral superficial lymphatic insufficiency in 67 patients (74%) and a bilateral superficial lymphatic insufficiency in 11 patients (12.8%). Fused images have detected enlarged lymphatic vessels related to an intravascular lymphostasis in 21 out of these 78 cases. In eight cases, a lack of inguinal nodes was detected, either at the planar or the SPECT–CT imaging (Fig. 1).

SN Detection in Breast Cancer

On planar images gathering anterior and lateral projection, a SN was clearly detected in 21 patients (61.7%) and probably detected in nine others (26.4%). Planar detection was not able to demonstrate a SN in four cases. SPECT–CT clearly demonstrated a SN in 31 patients (91.1%) and particularly in a patient where the planar images failed to detect an intramammary SN close to the injection site. The

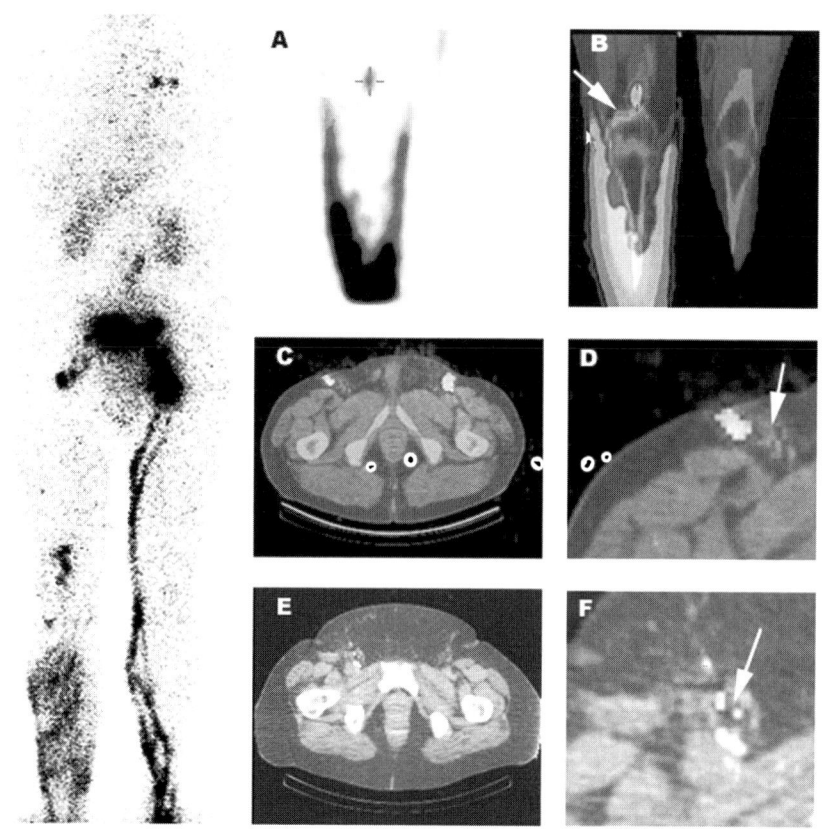

Figure 1. RNL in a patient with a transient right lower limb lymphedema classified as stage I. On the right, the whole body scan demonstrating scintigraphic patterns of distal lymphostasis and deep progression of the radiocolloid through the popliteal nodes related to a superficial lymphatic insufficiency. SPECT images on the legs (**a**) showing a transversal lymph duct (*arrow*) and the SPECT–CT fusion image at the same level (**b**) where the pathway to the deep system is clearly noticed (*arrow*). (**c–f**) are SPECT–CT fusion images at the groin level with a magnification on a nonfunctional inguinal lymph node (**d**, *arrow*) and on enlarged dilated lymphatic vessels in relation to an intravascular lymphostasis (**f**, *arrow*)

localization was more precise on SPECT–CT fusion images (31 patients) than on planar views (21 patients). When comparing SPECT to SPECT–CT images, SPECT–CT appeared to be more accurate in nine patients where SPECT alone was not precise enough (Fig. 2). Drainage to internal mammary lymph nodes was observed in four patients either on planar or SPECT–CT images.

DISCUSSION

There are no attempts to assess the limb lymphatic system with SPECT–CT. Fused images are bringing additional and useful information to the lymphologist. In stages 0 and I, the lymphatic disturbance can be demonstrated, particularly an intravascular

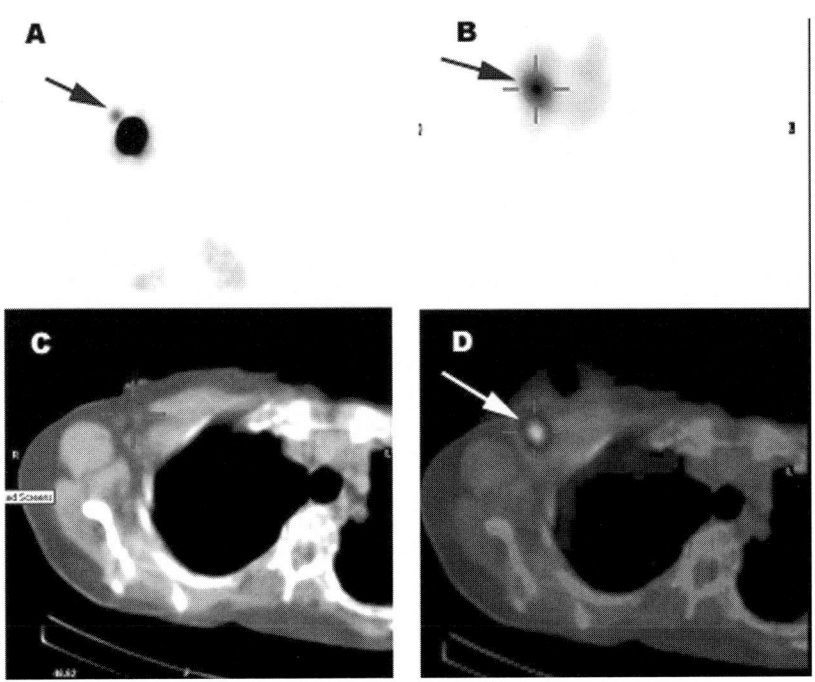

Figure 2. SN detection in a right breast cancer (T1N0M0). Planar image in (**a**) clearly demonstrates an axillary SN (*arrow*). The localization of this SN is not precise. SPECT image in (**b**) confirms the SN detection but the exact localization of the SN is only achieved on SPECT–CT fusion image in (**d**, *arrow*)

lymphostasis, while the lymphatic system seems nearly normal. In cases of superficial lymphatic insufficiency, fusion images can confirm a subfacial dermal backflow with a normal deep system. Hybrid imaging is also giving a precise location of a blockade, and may verify which lymph nodes are functional or not. For the clinician, this new imaging approach can be used to modify the treatment protocol, resulting in a well-adapted treatment. All of these patients with a swelling were treated with manual lymphatic drainage without bandaging and exercise. A good clinical response was observed in 86% of all stage 0 and in 67% of all stage I. The RNL data could be used as a helpful tool to have a better classification of the clinical low stages.

There is little literature dealing with SPECT–CT for SN mapping. Since 2003, attempts were carried out on melanoma patients (7, 8), head and neck squamous cell carcinoma (9), prostate cancer (10), cervical cancer (11), and bladder cancer (12), demonstrating promisingly more precise results. Lerman et al. (13) and Husarik and Steinert (14) have compared planar images to SPECT–CT in SN mapping of breast cancer. They found that SPECT–CT was a better method and was able to detect SN not detected on planar images, as well as unexpected sites of drainage. Husarik and Steinert demonstrated that integrated SPECT–CT was clearly superior to SPECT alone or planar images, especially with regard to exact anatomical localization of the SN. They also report that the high-anatomical accuracy of integrated SPECT–CT seems to facilitate the detection of the SN during minimal invasive surgery. The sensitivity and the specificity of RNL are higher, reducing false-negative SN and avoiding false-positive interpretation of hot spots in case of radioactive contamination. In our study we have injected all patients the afternoon before the surgery and the detection was made 1 hour before surgery. The results of the SPECT–CT are so anatomically precise that we can expect to perform a guided fine needle aspiration of the detected SN. It could be possible to detect the occurrence of tumor cells in this lymph node and then to modify the lymphatic dissection.

CONCLUSION

RNL is an evolving method, however planar or SPECT images remain a little bit esoteric. Using a hybrid camera to perform fusion lymphographic images, our results are more accurate and have a direct clinical impact on the therapeutic decision. Hybrid fusion images probably are a determinant of progress in clinical imaging.

REFERENCES

1. Pecking AP, Cluzan RV, Desprez-Curely JP, Guérin P.: (1986) Functional study of the limb lymphatic system. Phlebology 1,129-133
2. Pecking AP, Cluzan RV, Desprez-Curely JP, Guérin P.: (1986) Indirect lymphoscintigraphy in patients with limb edemas. Phlebology 1, 215-217
3. Monon DL, Wen DR, Wong JH, et al: (1992) Technical details of intraoperative lymphatic mapping for early Stage melanoma. Arch Surg 127:392-399
4. Krag DN, Weaver DL, Alex JC, et al: (1993) Surgical resection and radiolocalization of the sentinel lymph node in breast cancer using a gamma probe. Surg Oncol2:335-340
5. Hill AD, Tran KN, Akhursl T, et al: (1999) Lessons learned from 500 cases of lymphatic mapping for breast cancer. Ann Surg 229:528-535
6. Bocher M, Balan A, Krausz Y, et al: (2000) gamma camera mounted anatomical Xray tomography: technology, system characteristic and first images. Eur J Nucl med 27:619-627 2000
7. Kretschmer T, Altenvoerde G, Meller J, et al: (2003) Dynamic lymphoscintigraphy and image fusion of SPECT and pelvic CT-scans allow mapping of aberrant pelvic sentinel lymph nodes in mahgnam melanoma. Eur J Cancer 39:175-183
8. Even-Sapir E, Leonan H, Lievshitz G, et al: (2003) Lymphoscintigraphy for sentinel node mapping using a hybrid SPECT/CT system. J Nucl Med 44:1413-142
9. Wagner A, Schicho K, Glaser C, et al: (2004) SPECT–CT for topographic mapping of sentinel lymph nodes prior to gamma probe-guided biopsy in head and neck squamous cell carcinoma. J Craniomaxillofac Surg 32:343-349
10. Kizu H, Takayama T, Fukuda M, et al: (2005) Fusion of SPECT and multidetector CT images for accurate localization of pelvic sentinel lymph nodes in prostate cancer patients. J. Nucl Med Technol 33:78-82
11. Zhang WJ, Zheng R, Wu LY, et al: (2006) Clinical application of sentinel lymph node detection to early stage cervical cancer. Ai Zheng 25:224-228
12. Sherif A, Garske V, Torre Mde L, et al: (2006) Hybrid SPECT. CT: an additional technique for sentinel node detection of patients with invasive bladder cancer. Eur Urol 50:83-91
13. Lerman H, Metser U.l, Lievshitz G, et al: (2006) lymphoscintigraphic sentinel node identification in patients with breast cancer: the role of SPECT–CT Eur Nucl Med Mol Imaging 33:329-337
14. Husarik DB, Steinert HC. (2007) Single Photon Emission Tomography/Computed Tomography for sentinel node mapping in breast cancer. Semin Nucl Med. 37:29-33

7. SENTINEL NODE IDENTIFICATION USING RADIONUCLIDES IN MELANOMA AND BREAST CANCER

EDWIN C. GLASS

V.A. Greater Los Angeles Healthcare System, Los Angeles, California, USA
John Wayne Cancer Institute, Santa Monica, California, USA

INTRODUCTION

Background of Lymphatic Mapping

The metastatic spread of breast cancer to regional lymph nodes has been recognized for centuries (1), and the propensity of melanoma for lymphatic spread was documented in the nineteenth century (2). The basis for the sentinel node hypothesis is that tumors with a propensity for lymphatic invasion initially spread preferentially to nodes located on their draining lymphatic pathways. Hence these lymph nodes are the ones most likely to contain metastatic cells (3, 4), and they can be regarded as sentinel for the lymphatic spread of the cancer. Knowledge of the tumor status of these sentinel lymph nodes is now recognized as essential for staging and treating malignancies with a propensity for lymphatic invasion. Before discussing the mechanics and details of sentinel node localization, it is worthwhile to review relevant lymphatic physiology.

LYMPHATIC CONTENT AND FUNCTION

The lymphatic system plays important, interrelated roles in fluid homeostasis, removal of toxins, and immune function. The system is particularly well developed and extensive in the skin, oropharynx, and intestinal tract where potentially offending organisms and substances are ever present and abundant.

The distal ends of lymphatic channels are lined with clefts that can be forced open by external pressure from surrounding interstitial fluid, under the influences of oncotic and hydrostatic pressures. Cellular breakdown products, bacteria, proteins, and other materials gain entrance to the lymphatics through these clefts. Malignant cells can also enter through these clefts or by directly invading and penetrating the walls of lymphatic vessels. A continuous flow of interstitial fluid from these distal lymphatic origins carries materials to lymph nodes downstream.

Molecular expressions on many substances are recognized innately by macrophages, and the materials may be engulfed peripherally or in draining nodes by macrophages or dendritic cells. Examples include the mannose on cell walls of mycobacteria and other pathogens, lipotechoic acid in the cell walls of gram-positive bacteria, or lipopolysaccharides on the cell walls of gram-negative organisms (5). These substances can be suspended in lymph, can be bound to albumin, immunoglobulins, or other proteins, or can be engulfed within macrophages. Intact cancer cells may similarly be transported to draining lymph nodes, although presumably their rate of transit would be slower due to their relatively larger size.

Upon arrival to a lymph node, foreign substances and cells are further processed, in the matrix and sinuses of the node. Importantly, antigens can be processed and presented to B- and T-lymphocytes present in the node, to initiate adaptive immune responses that allow these antigens to be recognized subsequently by antibodies, lymphocytes, and macrophages.

IMAGING THE LYMPHATIC SYSTEM

Strategies for imaging the lymphatic system have been developed based on the functional and mechanical properties of the system outlined above. Substances with properties that allow uptake into, transport within, processing within, or binding in the lymphatic system can be employed for imaging the system, provided that they can be monitored or visualized. Hence fluorescent materials, radiolabeled compounds, or magnetic molecules have been employed to study the lymphatic system using wavelength controlled light sources, radiosensitive probes or cameras, or magnetic resonance imaging devices, respectively.

Examples of schemes employed for fluorescent lymphatic imaging include the use fluorescent proteins or dyes, and quantum dots that exhibit near-infrared fluorescence at invisible near-infrared frequencies (6). Some of the most widely employed tracking schemes have utilized radioactive reporter molecules, including radioactive colloidal materials and radiolabeled mannosyl compounds (7) that are bound to innately recognized mannose receptors. Iron ferrumoxtran is an example of a colloid material developed for imaging lymph nodes based on trapping of the iron-containing colloidal particles within lymph nodes, with external detection using magnetic resonance imaging devices (8) or magnetically sensitive probes.

DEFINITION OF A SENTINEL NODE

Notwithstanding the principles on which sentinel node detection is based, as discussed above, surgeons need a practical definition for routine clinical use. Many working definitions of a "sentinel" node have been proposed. Examples include the first lymph node to appear after injection of a tracer, the hottest node, all nodes with radioactive countrates exceeding a given background level, the nodes that are first encountered on all independent lymphatic drainage pathways, and other definitions. These disparate definitions are usually pragmatic in orientation, and are developed to provide surgeons with a practical means for the intraoperative determination of which lymph node or nodes to remove. At a more fundamental level however, the intent of sentinel node procedures is to identify, remove, and analyze the node or nodes that are most likely to contain metastatic cancer cells.

In practice, procedures are needed that will, in a period of minutes, to at most hours, define he most likely routes and locations for spread of cancer cells in lymphatic channels. The spread of malignant cells, however, evolves over many hours to months. Since many factors may influence the biological spread of cells, a relatively brief lymphatic mapping procedure using a foreign tracer substance may not always reproduce the path of spread of malignant cells from a primary tumor. Procedures for localizing sentinel nodes are therefore pragmatic, and their accuracy should be assiduously pursued, given that at best they can only approximate the complex process of cancer spread through lymphatics.

COLLOIDS IN LYMPHATICS

Among the various tools developed for lymphatic mapping for sentinel node localization, radiolabeled colloids have received the widest application, and have been in use for half a century (9, 10). Interstitially injected proteins and colloids are absorbed into, and migrate within, regional draining lymphatics. Early applications included mapping internal mammary lymph nodes in patients with breast cancer using subcostal injections (11), intralymphatic therapy (12), and radionuclide lymphangiography (13).

These initial techniques were extended to evaluation of specific tumors, first to identify the specific basin of drainage (14), and subsequently to determine additionally the specific nodes within that basin most likely to harbor metastases (15, 16). Although lymphatic mapping has been applied to many tumor types, this manuscript addresses their most common uses: sentinel node localization in melanoma and breast cancer.

When injected randomly into tissue, the colloidal particles of appropriate size (in the range of approximately 2–200 nm) gain entrance to lymphatics through clefts in the walls of lymphatics, or by endocytosis through the walls. Some particles may be phagocytosed by peripheral macrophages. Intralymphatic particles may thus be either intracellular, phagocytosed by macrophages, or remain suspended in lymphatic fluid (17). In either case they are transported to the nearest draining lymph node, i.e., the sentinel node for the tissue into which they were injected. In general their rate of transport varies inversely with the size of the colloid particles, with faster transit observed for colloids with smaller particles (16, 18, 19).

Once inside a lymph node, they may be phagocytosed by macrophages or dendritic cells, which would facilitate their intranodal retention and surgical localization. In a typical injection used for sentinel node mapping however, roughly 20–100 µg, in the case of sulfur colloid, will be injected. If approximately 1% reaches the nearest draining node however, roughly 0.2 µg or 10^{10} particles would be presented to the node for potential phagocytosis. This would probably overwhelm the phagocytic cells in a single lymph node. As a result, the observed retention of colloidal tracers within sentinel lymph nodes probably also represents retention and trapping by mechanisms other than phagocytosis, including nonspecific mechanical trapping in the reticular meshwork of the node. With time

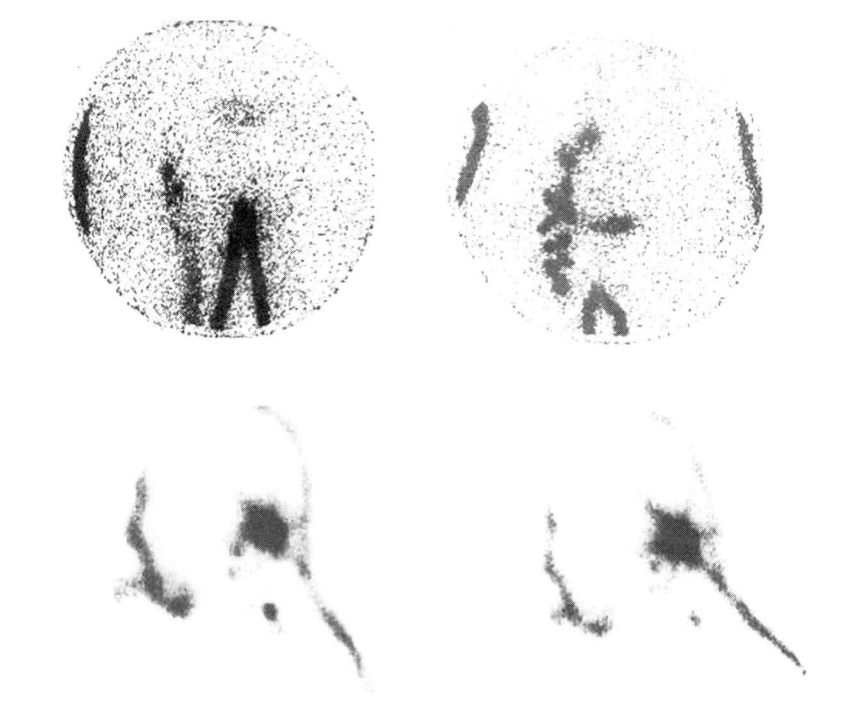

Figure 1. Variable nodal tracer uptake as a function of time in two patients. The upper two images demonstrate radiocolloid in inguinal nodes, at 5 min in the *upper left* and at 3 h in the *upper right*, after an intradermal injection in the right leg with filtered Tc99m sulfur colloid. The lower two images illustrate cervical nodes at 5 min (*lower left*) and 3 h (*lower right*) after an intradermal injection of the same radiopharmaceutical in the left ear of a different patient. The two upper images demonstrate progressive accumulation of tracer in the right inguinal nodes in time, whereas the lower images demonstrate a different, and relatively constant, retention, and uptake in left cervical and supraclavicular nodes. The nodal uptake of tracer varies in time, but often in an unpredictable manner in different patients. Used with permission from Springer – Cancer Metast Rev 2006; 25:185

however, such nonspecific trapping will allow release of particles for subsequent migration to other nodes (16). Krynyckyi et al. (20) demonstrated that colloidal preparations with higher specific activity demonstrated higher retention of radioactivity within sentinel nodes than those with lower specific activity, consistent with the concept of a limited capacity for phagocytic uptake within a single node.

It is logical to conclude that with longer time periods after injection of colloids that greater numbers of lymph nodes will be visualized using colloids. In fact there is evidence that this occurs, but there is also evidence that images acquired as long as 24 h after injection may demonstrate patterns of nodal uptake that are very similar to those observed soon after injection (21, 22). Hence there appears to be both a wash-through phenomenon as well as a mechanism for prolonged retention within nodes that receive a high flux of colloidal materials (Fig. 1).

RATIONALE OF LYMPHOSCINTIGRAPHY AND PROBE LOCALIZATION

The arguments for sentinel node procedures include accurate localization, removal, and evaluation of the node(s) most likely to harbor metastases, improved staging and prognostication, shorter and simpler surgery, reduced surgical morbidity, and the potential for adjuvant therapy and improved survival. Lymphoscintigraphy, which pictorially identifies these nodes, is extremely helpful in this effort since the drainage of tumors is often unpredictable on a clinical basis, and since unusual or unexpected patterns are common (15). For example, the variable drainage patterns of melanomas near Sappey's line, or on the head and neck, are now well recognized. Breast cancers in any part of the breast, not just in medial quadrants, can drain to internal mammary nodes (23).

Lymphoscintigraphy also portrays the temporal sequence of nodal uptake, depicting the first node to intercept lymph drainage from a tumor, i.e., the true sentinel node, which is the lymph node most likely to harbor metastatic cells. In addition to visualizing the lymphatic channels, basins, and nodes, preoperative lymphoscintigraphy can be used to apply skin marks for additional operative guidance. These considerations all support the use of preoperative lymphoscintigraphy.

GOALS OF LYMPHOSCINTIGRAPHY

(a) To identify the specific channels, nodal basin(s), and nodes of drainage
(b) To determine the temporal sequence of nodal uptake
(c) To mark the sentinel nodes and their afferent channels on the skin
(d) To generate clear, easily interpreted images for use in operating room
(e) To review findings with the surgeon preoperatively

If the above goals are met, the following clinical benefits are accrued:

(a) Shorter and simpler surgery
(b) Increased accuracy of surgery
(c) Reduced operative morbidity

RADIOPHARMACEUTICALS FOR LYMPHATIC MAPPING

The radiopharmaceuticals most commonly used for lymphoscintigraphy are colloidal and are radiolabeled with Tc99m. Colloidal tracer remains within lymphatic vessels rather than diffusing out of lymphatic vessels into the blood. Endolymphatic particles undergo subsequent mechanical and phagocytic trapping by macrophages in sinusoids of lymph nodes. Agents now commonly employed include Tc99m albumin nanocolloid and Tc99m rhenium sulfide in Europe, Tc99m antimony trisulfide colloid in Australia, and Tc99m sulfur colloid in unfiltered form or filtered through a submicron filter in the United States. No radiopharmaceuticals are currently approved by the U.S. FDA for lymphoscintigraphy.

Particle size influences colloid properties. Optimal size is in tens of nanometers, with the above agents ranging 5–250 nm. Small particles or nonparticulate agents, such Tc99m-labeled albumin (noncolloidal), migrate faster and provide better delineation of lymphatic channels (16, 18, 24), but also tend to leak into the blood pool. Small particles or nonparticulate tracers are also more likely to travel beyond the first or sentinel node, resulting in multiple hot nodes (18). This is more likely when larger numbers of particles are injected, which overwhelm the trapping capacity of macrophages in the first (sentinel) node.

Other noncolloidal lymphoscintigraphic agents specifically target lymph nodes, including radiolabeled antitumor antibodies, agents that bind to receptors in lymph nodes (7), and agents that mimic heme breakdown products, e.g., Tc99m phthalocyanine tetrasulfonate (PCTS) (25). Noncolloidal dyes (e.g., isosulfan blue or methylene blue) migrate much faster than colloids (24). Although usually used in nonradioactive form, radiolabeled noncolloidal dyes are also now being investigated (26, 27). Like PCTS, these labeled dyes offer the possibility of rapid visual, lymphoscintigraphic, and probe identification of sentinel nodes.

Despite general differences observed among tracers and techniques, considerable variation is observed in tracer kinetics between patients, particularly with breast cancer. No single imaging time is optimal for all patients. The radiopharmaceutical employed is a much less significant factor in overall accuracy than the skill, attention to detail, and understanding of the persons performing lymphatic mapping.

CONSIDERATIONS IN TECHNIQUE OF LYMPHATIC LOCALIZATION FOR CUTANEOUS MELANOMA

Techniques for lymphatic mapping are fairly well standardized for melanoma but not for breast cancer (28). Both radioisotopic and dye-based tracer methods are used. In general, most blue nodes are hot, but not all hot nodes are blue (29). In practice, nodal localization is optimized by using both visible dyes and radioactive tracers. The tracers are used both for lymphoscintigraphy and for probe localization. The overall reproducibility of cutaneous lymphoscintigraphy in melanoma has been found to be approximately 85% (30–32). Results can be affected, however, by previous surgical resections or radiation that alters migration patterns or by any process that affects epifascial tissues.

In experienced hands, cutaneous lymphoscintigraphy will identify a sentinel node in almost all patients, but nodal basin recurrence rates after sentinel node localization and surgery are higher for melanoma than for breast cancer (33). Melanoma is a particularly dangerous malignancy however, with no well-defined medical adjuvant therapies. Despite the relative ease of identification of the sentinel node in melanoma, recurrences are common, and not always fully predicted by the results and findings from lymphatic mapping (Fig. 2). In the Multicenter

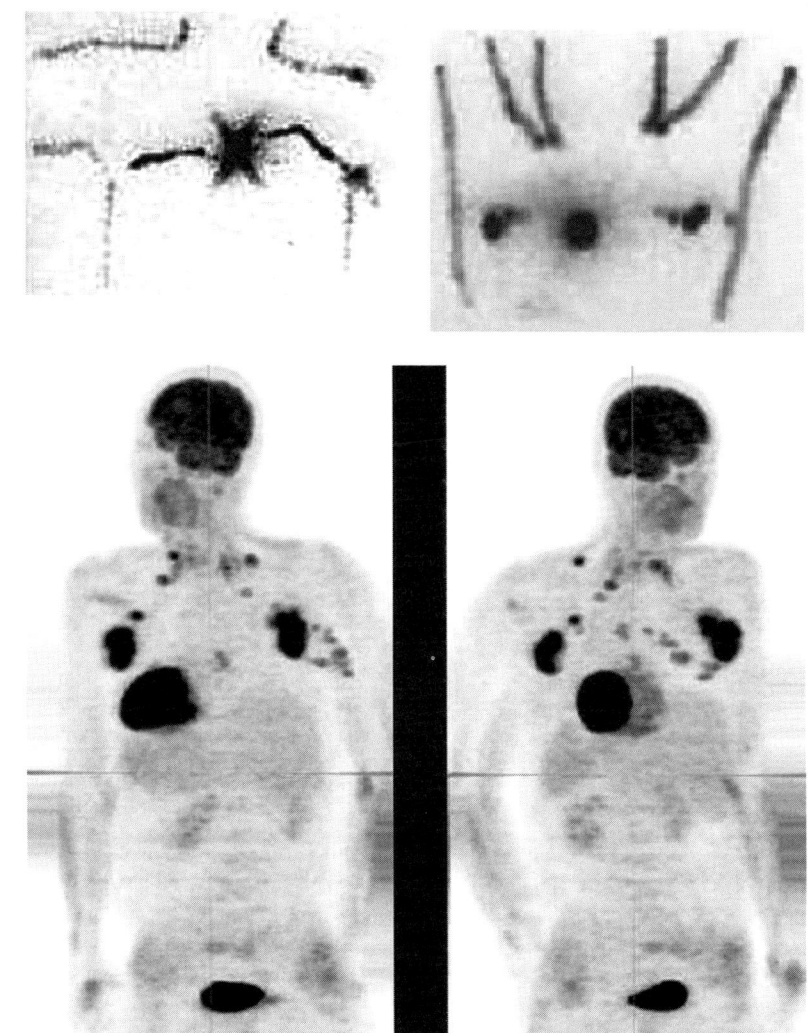

Figure 2. Upper panels show early (*upper left*) and delayed (*upper right*) images from lymphoscintigram of melanoma in midback that demonstrates bilateral axillary migration. The patient refused any axillary sampling but underwent removal of the melanoma on his back. Two years later he returned and underwent FDG PET imaging (oblique views in lower two panels) that demonstrated not only bilateral axillary metastases but also in transit metastases that probably had already seeded prior to removal of the primary after the initial lymphoscintigraphy. Supraclavicular nodal metastases are also demonstrated that were not predicted by the lymphoscintigram

Lymphadenectomy Mapping Trial I for example, the rates of recurrence and melanoma-specific mortality were 16.8 and 9.7%, respectively, at 5 years in patients without evidence of metastases in the sentinel node (34). It is essential to pay meticulous attention to detail when performing lymphatic mapping.

Other technical considerations that may influence nodal localization in melanoma include the times of imaging after injection, location and depth of the injection, positioning of the patient including arm elevation, characteristics of the radiopharmaceutical employed, including the size of the colloid particles in the injectate, and the use of adjunctive measures that modulate the flow of lymph, such as local heat and massage.

Imaging with a scintillation camera should begin immediately after intradermal (not subcutaneous) injection, in order to identify lymph channels, and to identify the first (sentinel) node(s). Subcutaneous injections result in slower and lesser migrations of tracer (24). Immediately after the injection, the site of skin puncture should be covered with a cotton ball and tape, or similar materials, to prevent seepage of tracer at that site, with resultant artifactual contamination of the skin. The use of a small-bore needle ((27) gauge or smaller) helps minimize this problem, and is also less uncomfortable for the patient. Positioning of the patient for lymphoscintigraphy should correspond, in at least some views, to the position of the patient during surgery, since lymph nodes can translate with body movement and positioning. Elevation of the arm, for example, will alter the position of axillary nodes relative to overlying skin marks. The location of the sentinel node should be determined precisely, and skin marks applied directly over the node and its afferent channel. This can be greatly facilitated by using a radiosensitive probe, after and/or during imaging in nuclear medicine. Inspection for dual channels and additional nodes that are in close proximity to the obvious ones should be carefully performed and reported. Copies of the clearest and best images should be available to the surgeon for intraoperative reference. Body outlines should be included on images to facilitate interpretation (e.g., in surgery). Body outlines should be routine in lymphoscintigraphy.

OTHER ISSUES IN THE DETECTION OF SENTINEL NODE FOR MELANOMA

Problems often encountered by less experienced users include (1) imaging too late after injection, when multiple nodes may be hot, (2) suboptimal positioning of patient (e.g., omitting oblique views of axilla with arm extended or elevated), (3) failure to perform lymphoscintigraphy at all, (4) poor communication between nuclear medicine physician and surgeon (e.g., poorly formatted images that cannot be interpreted by surgeon or others who were not involved in the generation of those images), (5) inaccurate or no skin marks over the sentinel node, and (6) failure to review the findings with the surgeon preoperatively. These problems can all result in erroneous identification of the sentinel node.

In experienced hands, cutaneous lymphoscintigraphy can successfully identify a sentinel node in almost all patients. However, the identification of lymph channels is also important in melanoma. When a separate lymph channel leading to a node is observed, that node should be regarded as a sentinel node, regardless of whether or not it is the most intense node at some later time. Additionally, knowledge of the locations of lymph channels can facilitate surgery; it directs the surgeon in the search for a blue lymphatic channel, which is often identified intraoperatively before the sentinel node itself. The channel can then be traced intraoperatively to the sentinel node. Imaging should begin immediately after injection so that lymph channels can be identified. Inspection for additional (two or more) channels and additional nodes that are in close proximity to the obvious ones should be carefully performed and reported, since additional channels may drain to additional sentinel nodes.

CONSIDERATIONS OF TECHNIQUE FOR LYMPHATIC LOCALIZATION IN BREAST CANCER

The identification of sentinel nodes in breast cancer is often more challenging than in melanoma, and techniques for lymphatic mapping are less standardized for breast cancer. Both dye-based and radioisotopic tracer methods are used, with optimal results usually obtained with the use of both techniques in combination. As with melanoma, nodes are usually, but not always both blue and hot. In general, nodes are more often hot and not blue, than blue alone (29, 35, 36). This is usually attributed to the retention of the particles by macrophages in lymph nodes, whereas blue dye is not trapped as efficiently in the node and will flow through it. Although there are usually more hot nodes than blue nodes found in the axilla, this depends on time lag after injection of either of the two tracers. Early after injection (e.g., 5–30 min), slow moving particles may not yet have arrived to the lymph basin, but the faster moving dye will have arrived, whereas later, the particles are retained, but the dye has washed out.

Techniques for breast injection differ among institutions. The best technique for injection is one of the more controversial topics in the realm of sentinel node studies. Different types of injections include parenchymal peritumoral, intratumoral, subdermal, subareolar, and periareolar injections. The relative advantages and disadvantages of the different methods are now reasonably well understood. Longer times for localization are required after parenchymal injections of radiocolloids than after dermal, subdermal, or periareolar injections, although parenchymal injections are more likely to identify nonaxillary sites of drainage, e.g., internal mammary nodes. Intratumoral or parenchymal peritumoral injections are conceptually logical. So why not always use them? The principal disadvantage of intratumoral and peritumoral injections is a lower success rates for visualization of axillary sentinel nodes. Additionally, they require longer transit times to nodes, and are somewhat more difficult to perform.

To address the problems with these parenchymal injection methods, injections into the skin or subcutaneous tissue overlying the tumor or in the periareolar region have been utilized. These methods yield higher rates of visualization of axillary nodes and are procedurally simpler. Additionally, injecting the day before surgery (21, 22) has been employed, almost assuring the identification of hot nodes by the time of surgery the next day. If only axillary nodes are to be evaluated, then the simpler nonparenchymal methods usually suffice. Cutaneous injection techniques (which use < 2 ml) can be accomplished using smaller volumes of injectate than are required by intraparenchymal peritumoral breast injections, because lymphatics are more abundant in skin than in breast tissue. An exception to the use of or need for large injectate volumes for parenchymal injections is made, however, when intratumoral injections are used for both tumor localization and identification of the sentinel node (37). In that case the radioactivity at the tumoral injection site, usually for a nonpalpable tumor, is used as a guide to delineate the tissue for excision.

The use of subareolar injections is based in part on the concept of universal lymph drainage through that region. This seems reasonable in view of the fact that the breast develops at puberty by outgrowth from subareolar tissue. This development would presumably direct lymphogenesis in the breast. Still, the concept of a single bottleneck sentinel node that drains the entire breast and overlying skin is not universally accepted (38). Kapteijn et al. (39) demonstrated, however, that drainage from breast tumors does not always proceed first to, or derive from, the areolar lymphatics. Nevertheless, periareolar injections also usually map to the same axillary nodes as other methods of injection. Indeed, same axillary nodes will usually be identified, regardless of the injection technique.

Many surgeons feel that localized parenchymal peritumoral or intratumoral injections will provide better mapping of lymphatic flow from breast tumors to internal mammary nodes (Fig. 3). Internal mammary drainage can occur from tumors located in any part of the breast, although exclusive drainage only to internal mammary nodes is uncommon (40). Deeper injections, larger tumors, and smaller breasts are more likely to demonstrate drainage to internal mammary nodes. Other methods of injection yield lower rates of identification of sentinel nodes

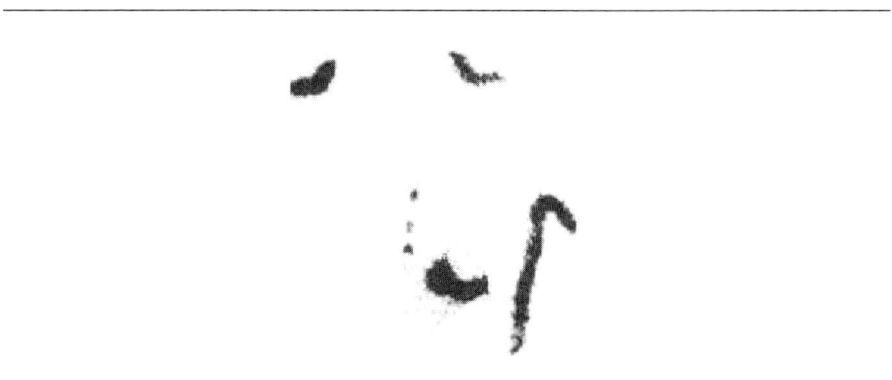

Figure 3. Early anterior view after parenchymal peritumoral injection in left breast demonstrates predominant migration to left internal mammary nodes. Although an axillary node identified at surgery, axillary sampling alone in such an individual could result in incorrect determination of nodal status

outside the axilla, particularly internal mammary nodes (39, 41–43). Subdermal or subareolar injections often fail to identify drainage to internal mammary nodes. Most surgeons and oncologists are less concerned with potential involvement of these nodes than with axillary involvement however, and many surgeons consider excising internal mammary nodes to be more difficult and dangerous than sampling axillary nodes. Internal mammary nodes are found to be exclusively positive in only a small percentage of cases, but if positive, can change staging and treatment.

Lymphoscintigraphy with a scintillation camera should begin within a few minutes after injection. Lymph channels are visualized less often with breast lymphoscintigraphy than with intradermal lymphoscintigraphy for melanoma. Identification of an afferent lymph channel is useful, however, for determining which hot nodes are sentinel nodes. Just as with melanoma, a hot node with an independent afferent channel is a sentinel node, whether located in the axilla, internal mammary chain, or elsewhere. When more than one node is recognized as hot late after injection, it is not possible to distinguish which nodes are sentinel nodes and which are second tier nodes, with significantly different likelihoods of harboring metastasis. This latter question arises when delayed imaging alone, or no imaging, is utilized. Without lymphoscintigraphy, this can be a challenging question. Sequential imaging begun early after injection maps the anatomic and temporal sequence of nodal uptake and appearance. The important first node is not always the hottest node later, and the hottest node often is not the node that contains tumor cells when only a single node is positive (35). Node size, time delay, tumor involvement of a node, and other factors affect the uptake of radiocolloid in a node.

Patient positioning during lymphoscintigraphy, at least for some of the images, should be similar or identical to that used in surgery, with the patient's arm elevated or extended in a manner similar to that to be used later during surgery, for visualization of axillary nodes. Images should include body outlines to facilitate interpretation (e.g., in surgery). The location of the sentinel node should be defined precisely as possible, and skin marks applied directly over the node as viewed from the perspective of the surgeon. Again, probe confirmation in nuclear medicine optimizes this effort. With several methods of injection, imaging, and localization now in wide use, it is probably advisable that centers become facile with more than one technique, but that the users (surgeons and nuclear medicine physicians) fully understand the relative benefits and disadvantages of each of the methods they employ.

In breast cancer, lymphoscintigraphy will localize sentinel nodes not found through use of radiosensitive probes alone in a small but significant number of cases. This derives not from any superior sensitivity of the gamma camera but from the use of imaging that visualizes the entire thorax, axilla, and lower neck. If treatment planning includes consideration of the status of internal mammary or other nonaxillary (e.g., Rotter's) nodes, lymphoscintigraphy with peritumoral injection is advisable. If only hot axillary nodes are to be considered, then the procedurally simpler nonperitumoral injections, such as in subcutaneous, dermal, or periareolar regions, with only probe localization, will usually suffice.

OTHER ISSUES: BREAST CANCER

Nonvisualization of sentinel nodes is encountered more commonly with breast cancer than with melanoma. Almost all sentinel node publications report a non-negligible failure of nodal identification in a notably variable percentage of cases of breast cancer. Failure of nodal visualization is more likely in elderly individuals (44, 45), with high body mass index (23), with fatty breasts (46), and with clinically positive palpable nodes demonstrating nodal replacement or displacement by tumor. Recognition of these tendencies for nonvisualization can be useful in planning or scheduling lymphoscintigraphy and surgery. Neoadjuvant chemotherapy can result in fibrosis within nodes containing tumor cells. The effect of such fibrosis on sentinel node localization is debated (47). The nonvisualization rates diminish with increasing experience of the team however, and most experienced centers can consistently obtain visualization of the sentinel node in over 95% of cases.

A variety of measures have been employed to mitigate the occurrence of nonvisualization. Exercise, local heat, and massage have been found to accelerate lymphatic flow rates (17, 48). The use of higher concentrations of particles (49) and tracers of higher specific activity (with fewer numbers of colloid particles per unit of radioactive tracer) (20) have also been reported to increase nodal visualization in sentinel node studies in breast cancer. The use of fewer particles with tracers of higher specific activity could presumably avoid overwhelming the limited phagocytic capacity of the finite population of macrophages in the sentinel node, resulting in more exclusive, or at least preferential, uptake in the first node encountered by particles flowing from the injection site. Also, smaller particles (e.g., Tc99m antimony colloid or filtered sulfur colloid) migrate faster than larger particles (18, 24), although they may result in more flow-through or spillover into secondary nodes. Other techniques that have been employed to optimize results with breast lymphoscintigraphy include delayed imaging (for example 6–18 h after injection (21, 22)) and use of radiosensitive probes. Although some physicians claim to have determined a single time after injection that is optimal for all women, the transit times from injection sites to sentinel nodes vary widely from patient to patient, and, logistic considerations notwithstanding, no single delay will be optimal for all women (23). Because of this variation in time of visualization, some centers have elected to perform sentinel node surgery for breast cancer the day after injection. Clinical results with the next day methods are reported as similar to those with same day surgery (21, 22).

Although lymphoscintigraphy offers many potential benefits in localizing sentinel nodes, it is not as universally employed in breast cancer as in melanoma. Lymphoscintigraphy enhances localization of sentinel nodes, but may delay surgery. Furthermore, the resultant delay can result in uptake of radioisotope in additional second tier nodes that could obfuscate intraoperative localization with a probe. Lymphoscintigraphy also adds cost. In general, lymphoscintigraphy for breast cancer is employed more widely in Europe than in the United States.

As with melanoma, difficulties often experienced by new users include (1) poor communication between nuclear medicine physician and surgeon (including images that are not interpretable by surgeon), (2) improper positioning of patient (e.g., omitting oblique views of axilla with arm elevated or allowing breast injection site to overlap the axilla), (3) failure to perform lymphoscintigraphy, (4) imaging too soon or too late after injection, (5) inaccurate or no skin marks over the sentinel node, and (6) failure to review the findings with the surgeon preoperatively. Any of these pitfalls can result in misidentification of the node most likely to harbor metastases during surgery. Many of these issues can be ameliorated by direct discussion and review of lymphoscintigraphic findings by both the surgeon and nuclear medicine physician before each surgery. Such teamwork identifies unique issues for individual patients and facilitates surgical planning. Additional comparative reviews of the operative and lymphoscintigraphic findings after surgery will also strengthen the results for that center.

Despite the relatively wide variations and greater difficulty of techniques used for sentinel node localization in breast cancer compared to melanoma, the rates of recurrence after negative sentinel node sampling are significantly lower with breast cancer than with melanoma (33, 34). This emphasizes fundamental differences in the two disease processes as well as the availability and impact of effective adjuvant therapy for breast cancer but not for melanoma.

RADIATION SAFETY

Due to the local retention of the interstitially injected doses (50), radiation doses to breast from lymphoscintigraphy are sufficient to warrant doses of Tc99m below 18 MBq (~0.5 mCi) (16, 21, 51–53). Radiation doses received by breast tissue (40–150 rem or 0.4–1.5 Sieverts) during radioactive mapping procedures are within the range of doses reported to induce an increased incidence of breast cancer (54, 55). Still, the potential or theoretical predicted increase would be well below the known recurrence rate of breast cancer after local resection (56), and the radiation dose from the radiopharmaceutical is inconsequential compared to postoperative breast radiotherapy that is routinely employed in the treatment of breast cancer.

These procedures entail the use of radioactive materials in arenas (e.g., Surgery and Pathology) where personnel have little training or experience in their use. Although measured radiation exposures to personnel in Surgery and Pathology have been quite low, a modicum of additional training, and new institutional procedures for the handling radioactive tissue specimens are appropriate (50, 52, 57–59).

Fetal exposures should not necessarily proscribe the procedure if it is otherwise clinically indicated, because the exposure to the fetus would be minimal. Nevertheless, prudence should be exercised in these patients. The higher doses of Tc99m colloid used by some surgeons (21, 22) should be avoided in pregnant patients. Full hydration and catheterization and/or frequent emptying of the bladder would be prudent for 24 h after the breast injection of the Tc99m tracer in a pregnant woman.

Sentinel node procedures require a collaborative effort between personnel in Surgery, Nuclear Medicine, Pathology, and Radiation Safety.

REFERENCES

1. Kardinal CG, Yabro JW: A conceptual history of cancer. Semin. Oncol. 1979; 6:396-408
2. Snow H: Melanotic cancerous disease. Lancet 1892; 2:872
3. Cabanas RM: An approach for the treatment of penile carcinoma. Cancer 1977; 39:456-466
4. Morton DL, Wen DR, Wong J, et al: Technical details of intraoperative lymphatic mapping for early stage melanoma. Arch Surg 1992; 127:392-399
5. Leung MY, Liu C, Koon JC, Fung KP: Polysaccharide biologic response modifiers. Immunol Lett 2006; 105(2):101-14
6. Frangioni JV: In vivo near-infrared fluorescence imaging. Curr Opin Chem Biol 2003; 7(5):626-34
7. Vera DR, Wallace AM, Hoh C, Mattrey RF: A synthetic macromolecule for sentinel node detection: (99m)Tc-DTPA-Mannosyl-Dextran. J Nucl Med 2001; 42:951-959
8. Torabi M, Aquino SL, Harasinghani MG: Current concepts in lymph node imaging. J Nucl Med 2004; 45(9):1509-18
9. Sherman AI, Ter-Pogossian M: Lymph-node concentration of radioactive colloidal gold following interstitial injection. Cancer 1953; 6:1238-40
10. Sage HH, Kizilay D, Miyazaki M, Shapiro G, Sinha B: Lymph node scintigrams. Am J Roentgenol, Rad Therapy, and Nuclear Medicine 1960; 84:666-72
11. Ege GN: Internal mammary lymphoscintigraphy. Radiology 1976; 118:101-7
12. Ariel IM, Resnick MI, Oropeza R: The intralymphatic administration of radioactive isotopes for treating malignant melanoma. Surgery, Gynecol, & Obstet 1967; 124:1-15
13. Seitzman DM, Wright R, Halaby FA, Freeman JH: Radioactive lymphangiography as a therapeutic adjunct. Am J Roentgen Rad Ther & Nucl Med. 1963; LXXXIX; 140-9
14. Bennett LR, Lago G. Cutaneous lymphoscintigraphy in malignant melanoma. Semin Nucl Med 1983; 13:61-69
15. Uren RF, Howman-Giles RB, Shaw HM, Thompson JF, McCarthy WH. Lymphoscintigraphy in high risk melanoma of the trunk: predicting drainage node groups, defining lymphatic channels, and locating the sentinel node. J Nucl Med 1993; 34:1435-1440
16. Glass EC, Essner R, Morton DL: Comparison of three lymphoscintigraphic agents in patients with cutaneous melanoma. J Nucl Med 1998; 39:1185-1190
17. Ikomi F, Hanna GK, Schmid-Schonbein GW: Mechanism of colloidal particle uptake into the lymphatic system: Basic study with percutaneous lymphography. Radiology 1995; 196:107-115
18. Tafra L, Chua AN, Ng PC, Aycock D, Swanson M, Lannin D: Filtered versus unfiltered sulfur colloid in lymphatic mapping: A significant variable in a pig model. Ann Surg Oncol 1999; 6(1):83-87
19. Bergqvist L, Strand S-E, Persson BRR: Particle sizing and biokinetics of interstitial lymphoscintigraphic agents. Semin Nucl Med 1983; XII:9-19
20. Krynyckyi BR, Zhang ZY, Kim CK, Lipszyc H, Mosci K, Machac J: Effect of high specific-activity sulfur colloid preparations on sentinel node count rates. Clin Nucl Med. 2002 Feb; 27(2):92-5
21. Babiera GV, Delpassand ES, Breslin TM, et al: Lymphatic drainage patterns on early versus delayed breast lymphoscintigraphy performed after injection of filtered Tc99m sulfur colloid in breast cancer patients undergoing sentinel lymph node biopsy. Clin Nucl Med 2005; 30:11-15
22. Gray RJ, Pockaj BA, Roarke MC: Injection of Tc99m-labeled sulfur colloid the day before operation for breast cancer sentinel node mapping is as successful as injection the day of operation. Am J Surg 2004; 188:685-689
23. Haigh PI, Hansen NM, Giuliano AE, Edwards GK, Ye W, Glass EC: Factors affecting sentinel node localization during preoperative breast lymphoscintigraphy. J Nucl Med 2000; 41:1682-1688
24. Kersey TW, Van Eyk J, Lannin DR, Chua AN, Tafra L: Comparison of intradermal and subcutaneous injections in lymphatic mapping. J Surg Res 2001 Apr; 96(2):255-259
25. El-Tamer M, Saouaf R, Wang T, Fawwaz R: A new agent, blue and radioactive, for sentinel node detection. Ann Surg Oncol 2003; 10(3):323-329
26. Sutton R, Tsopelas C, Kollias J, Coventry B, Chatterton BE: Sentinel node biopsy and lymphoscintigraphy with a technetium 99m labeled blue dye in a rabbit model. Surgery 2002; 131(1):44-9
27. Tsopelas C, Bevington K, Kollias J, Shibli S, Farshid J, Coventry B, Chatterton BE: 99mTc-Evans blue dye for mapping contiguous lymph node sequences and discriminating the sentinel lymph node in an ovine model. Ann Surg Oncol. 2006; 13(5):692-700.36
28. Nieweg OE, Tanis PJ, Rutgers EJ: Summary of the Second International Sentinel Node Conference. Eur J Nucl Med 2001 May; 28(5):646-649
29. Bostick P, Essner R, Glass EC, et al: Comparison of blue dye and probe-assisted intraoperative lymphatic mapping in melanoma to identify sentinel nodes in 100 lymphatic basins. Arch Surg 1999; 134:43-49

30. Rettenbacher L, Koller J, Kassman H, Holzmannhofer J, Rettenbacher T, Galvan G: Reproducibility of lymphoscintigraphy in cutaneous melanoma: Can we accurately detect the sentinel lymph node by expanding the tracer injection distance from the tumor site? J Nucl Med 2001; 42:424-429

31. Kapteijn BAE, Nieweg OE, Valdes Olmos RA, et al: Reproducibility of lymphoscintigraphy for lymphatic mapping in cutaneous melanoma. J Nucl Med 1996; 37:972-976

32. Mudun A, Murray DR, Herda SC, et al: Early stage melanoma: lymphoscintigraphy, reproducibility of sentinel node detection, and effectiveness of the intraoperative gamma probe. Radiology 1996; 199: 171-175

33. Nieweg OE, Rijk MC, Valdes Olmos RA, Hoefnagel CA: Sentinel node biopsy and selective lymph node clearance – impact on regional control and survival in breast cancer and melanoma. Eur J Nucl Med Mol Imaging 2005; 32:631-634

34. Morton DL, Thompson JF, Cochran AJ, Mozillo N, Elashoff R, Essner R, Nieweg O, Roses DF, Hoekstra HJ, Karakousis CP, Rientgen DS, Coventry BJ, Glass EC, Wang HJ: Sentinel node biopsy or observation in melanoma. New Engl J Med 2006; 355(13) 1307 Glass EC, Essner R, Giuliano AE: Sentinel node localization in breast cancer. Semin Nucl. Med 1999; XXIX:57-68

35. Duncan M, Cech A, Wechter D, Moonka R: Criteria for establishing the adequacy of a sentinel lymphadenectomy. Am J Surg 2004; 187:639-642

36. Woznick A, Franco M, Bendick P, Benitez PR: Sentinel lymph node dissection for breast cancer: how many nodes are enough and which technique is optimal? Am J Surg 2006; 191:330-333

37. Feggi L, Basaglia E, Corcione S, Querzoli P, Soliani G, Ascanelli S, Prandini N, Bergossi L, Carcoforo P: An original approach in the diagnosis of breast cancer: Use of the same radiopharmaceutical for both non-palpable lesions and sentinel node localization. Eur J Nucl Med 2001; 28(11):1589-96

38. Canavese G, Gioponi M, Catturic A, et al: Pattern of lymphatic drainage to the sentinel lymph node in breast cancer patients. J Surg Oncol. 2000; 74(1):69-74

39. Kapteijn BA, Nieweg OE, Petersen JL, Rutgers EJ, Hart AA van Dongen JA, Kroon BB: Identification and biopsy of the sentinel lymph node in breast cancer. Eur J Surg Oncol. 1998; 24(5):427-30

40. Byrd DR, Dunnwald LK, Mankoff DA, Anderson BO, Moe RE, Yeung RS, Schubert EK, Eary JF: Internal mammary lymph node drainage patterns in patients with breast cancer documented by lymphoscintigraphy. Ann Surg Oncol 2001; 8:234-240

41. Roumen RMH, Geuskens LM, Valkenburg JGH: In search of the true sentinel node by different injection techniques in breast cancer patients. Eur J Surg Oncol 1999; 25:347-351

42. Shen P, Glass EC, Hansen N, Giuliano AE: Dermal versus intraparenchymal lymphoscintigraphy of the breast. Ann Surg Oncol. 2001 Apr; 8(3):241-8

43. Estourgie SH, Nieweg OE, Valdes Olmos RA, Rutgers EJT, Kroon BR: Intratumoral versus intraparenchymal injection for lymphoscintigraphy in breast cancer. Clin Nucl Med 2003; 28(5):371-4

44. Tanis PJ, van Sandick JW, Nieweg OE, Valdes Olmos RA, Rutgers EJ, Hoefnagel CA, Kroon BB.: The hidden sentinel node in breast cancer. Eur J Nucl Med Mol Imaging. 2002 Mar; 29(3):305-11

45. Tafra L, Lannin DR, Swanson MS, Van Eyk JJ, Verbanac KM, Chua AN, Ng PC, Edwards MS, Halliday BE, Henry CA, Sommers LM, Carman CM, Molin MR, Yurko JE, Perry RR, Williams R: Multicenter trial of sentinel node biopsy for breast cancer using both technetium sulfur colloid and isosulfan blue dye. Ann Surg. 2001 Jan; 233(1):51-9

46. Lamonica D, Edge SB, Hurd T, Proulx G, Stomper PC: Mammographic and clinical predictors of drainage patterns in breast lymphoscintigrams obtained during sentinel node procedures. Clin Nucl Med 2003; 28(7):558-564

47. Kinoshita T, Takasugi M, Iwamoto E, Akashi-Tanaka S, Fukutomi T, Terui S: Sentinel lymph node biopsy for breast cancer patients with clinically negative axillary lymph nodes after neoadjuvant chemotherapy. Am J Surg 2006; 191:225-229

48. Avery M, Nathanson SD, Hetzel FW. Lymph flow from murine foot pad tumors before and after sublethal hyperthermia. Radiation Research 1992; 132:50-53

49. Valdes Olmos RA, Tanis PJ, Hoefnagel CA, Nieweg OE, Muller SH, Rutgers EJ, Kooi ML, Kroon BB: Improved sentinel node visualization in breast by optimizing the colloid particle concentration and tracer dosage. Nucl Med Commun 2001; 22(5):579-86

50. Waddington WA, Keshtar MR, Taylor I, Lakhani SR, Short MD, Ell PJ: Radiation Safety of the sentinel node technique in breast cancer. Eur J Nucl Med 2000; 27(4):377-391

51. Eshima D, Fauconnier T, Eshima L, Thornback JR: Radiopharmaceuticals for lymphoscintigraphy: Including dosimetry and radiation considerations. Semin Nucl Med 2000; XXX(1):56-64

52. Glass EC, Basinski JE, Krasne DL, Giuliano AE: Radiation safety considerations for sentinel node techniques. Ann Surg Oncol 1999; 6:10-1

53. Bronskill MJ: Radiation dose estimates for interstitial radiocolloid lymphoscintigraphy. Semin Nucl Med 1983; XIII: 20-25

54. Kohn HI, Fry RJM: Radiation carcinogenesis. N Engl J Med 1984; 310:504-511
55. Wanebo CK, Johnson KG, Sato K, Thorslund TW: Breast cancer after the exposure to the atomic bombings of Hiroshima and Nagasaki. N Engl J Med 1968;279: 667-671
56. Huston TL, Simmons RM: Locally recurrent breast cancer after breast conservation. Am J Surgery 2005; 189:229-35
57. Stratman SL, McCarty TM, Kuhn JA: Radiation safety with breast sentinel node biopsy. Am J Surg 1999; 178:454-7
58. Miner TJ, Shriver CD, Flicek PR, Miner FC, Jaques DP, Maniscalco-Theberge ME, Krag DN: Guidelines for the safe use of radioactive materials during the localization and resection of the sentinel lymph node. Ann Surg Oncol. Ann Surg Oncol 1999 Jan-Feb; 6(1):75-82
59. Fitzgibbons PL, LiVolsi VA: Recommendations for handling Radioactive specimens obtained by sentinel lymphadenectomy. Am J Surg Pathol 2000; 24(11):1549-51

8. TARGETED INTRODUCTION OF SUBSTANCES INTO THE LYMPH NODES FOR ENDOLYMPHATIC THERAPY

PETER HIRNLE

Central Academic Hospital, Department of Radiation Oncology, Bielefeld, Germany

INTRODUCTION

Lymph node metastases are an important prognostic factor in cancer, irrespective of where the tumour is located. Until today, treatment by surgery or irradiation may be associated with massive side effects so that efficient and safe alternatives are still required. Radical surgery to treat or prevent progressing disease usually involves the removal of the regional lymph nodes, but also of their surrounding tissue and of lymph vessels. The destruction of the adjacent structures is aggravated by the problem of discerning lymph nodes from their surrounding fatty tissue. This poor selectivity leads not only to side effects, such as secondary lymphedema, but also bears the danger to overlook lymph nodes, which increases the risk of nodal recurrence. The dimension of the problem could be demonstrated by post-operative lymphangiograms, depicting the remaining lymph nodes after radical surgery (28).

The problems involved in radiation therapy for lymph nodes are that it covers large areas of the pelvis and abdomen, unnecessarily irradiating sensitive organs. This means also that only a small percentage of the total dose reaches the lymph nodes. However, also intravenously applied cytostatic drugs have considerable side effects. Due to their toxicity, there are limits with regard to the maximum possible dose. This means that the necessary concentration can rarely be reached in lymph nodes.

The above limitations of currently used methods triggered the idea that the most efficient treatment of lymph node metastases would be to locally apply highly concentrated drugs (23). This would be a method to totally destroy lymph node metastases, while conserving the lymphatic pathways.

BASIC REQUIREMENTS OF ENDOLYMPHATIC THERAPY

Drug Carriers

When injecting water soluble drugs into lymph vessels, rapid diffusion into surrounding tissue prevents the drug from reaching the lymph nodes in clinically effective proportions (37). This effect can be minimised by using a lipoid carrier for otherwise water soluble drugs. However, transporting drugs to lymph nodes is not the only prerequisite for the clinical use of endolymphatic therapy. The carrier needs to ensure also that the drug is retained in the lymph node to expose the tumour cells to the drug as long as possible. In the best case, this drug depot acts also as a chemical barrier, preventing the tumour cells from spreading through the lymph system. Both effects should not be painful for patients.

In order to prevent unwanted side effects, the lipoid carrier needs to fulfil certain criteria. First and foremost, the carrier should not be toxic for the vessel walls and the healthy tissue of the lymph node, be non-pyrogenic and sterile. Moreover, the carrier needs to be small enough to pass the lymph system freely, and the viscosity of the preparation should be low. By this, neither the injection cannula is clotted, nor is the transport within the small lymph vessels disturbed. This reduces the risk of embolism in the lymph nodes, preventing also following complications from pulmonary embolism after discharge from the lymph system.

Until today, only pure iodised oil is in clinical use as a contrast medium for diagnostic lymphographies (21). This oil exhibits excellent properties with regard to depositing drugs in lymph nodes. Macromolecules, such as albumin, were not yet tested as drug carriers, although they do not diffuse through lymph vessel walls. However, when injected into lymph vessels, albumin was found to pass lymph nodes rapidly and virtually unchanged. Experiments demonstrated that a high percentage of the applied albumin can be found shortly after the injection in the ductus thoracicus (26). Its deposition properties are therefore low. Another reason to reject macromolecules as drug carriers is the fact that drugs get different properties when bound to them. They might even lose their cytostatic potential and are therefore not useful to transport well tested and effective drugs to lymph nodes. Due to the lack of carriers with the above specified properties, suspensions, emulsions, solutions and liposomes were tested for their potential as lipid-based endolymphatic drug carriers.

Prerequisites and Limitations of Endolymphatic Drug Application

To reach the necessary drug concentration within lymph nodes, it is necessary to flood the complete lymph system with the volume injected (Fig. 1). However, when aiming at this, it is unavoidable that a part of the injected substance reaches

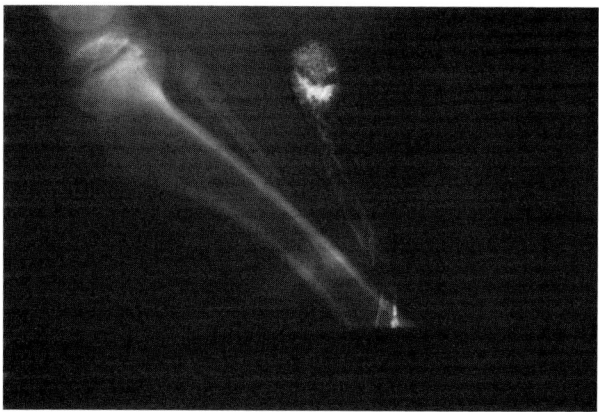

Figure 1. Filling of the dog popliteal lymph node with iodinated oil during pedal lymphography. The oil will proceed to the next nodes after complete filling of the first node

the blood via the ductus thoracicus. When applying cytostatic drugs via the lymph system, care has to be taken that the amount of the substance reaching the blood does not exceed the amount used for intravenous cytostatic therapy otherwise. As a consequence, this spillover needs to be quantifiable to make endolymphatic therapy safe. This is even more important, as the spillover varies according to the storage capacity of the lymph nodes, the kind of carrier used, the injection rate and the total amount injected. Moreover, the spillover can be increased by fluid intake and physical activity.

For the therapeutic use of endolymphatic drug application, two important factors need to be considered. First of all, as soon as the lymph flow stops, there is no way of transporting drugs through the lymph vessels. However, although completely destroyed lymph nodes cannot be reached any more by endolymphatic therapies, the endolymphatic application of cytostatic drugs has still benefits. Destroyed lymph nodes are bypassed by collateral vessels, which drain the lymph into para-aortal nodes. If endolymphatically applied cytostatic drugs circumvent bulky pelvic lymph nodes through this mechanism, at least the risk of lymphogenous tumour spread is diminished. This effect can be used as long as lymph stasis is not complete through the destruction of lymph nodes, and the insufficiency or destruction of collateral vessels. If complete lymph stasis occurs, the endolymphatic application of cytostatic drugs is contraindicated, as the storage of such drugs in dilated afferent vessels is toxic for the thin vessel walls.

The second restriction to endolymphatic therapy arises from the anatomy of the lymphatic system. Abdominal organs are partly drained into regional lymph nodes, which are sited outside the chains draining the legs. Consequently, these lymph nodes are inaccessible to pedal lymphography. However, the lymph passing though these nodes reaches the next level of lymph nodes, which are again accessible though the endolymphatic application of drugs. This is most beneficial, as this is the main route of lymphogenic tumour spread. However, additional therapies, such as surgery or irradiation of the first peripheral level of locoregional lymph nodes, form an integral part to prevent tumour spread though the lymphatic system.

Selection of Drugs for the Use in Humans

It has been previously described that there are dosage restrictions of cytostatic drugs due to their toxicity. When applying such drugs endolymphatically, the maximum dose must equal the maximum dose for intravenous use, as the unwanted escape of the drug into the blood system cannot be excluded. This might either happen by the spillover into the ductus thoracicus, or due to the total blockage of the lymph system.

As a basic requirement for endolymphatic application, cytostatic drugs need to be soluble. Pure lipid soluble substances with cytostatic properties are not routinely available, and were therefore not investigated.

For initial experiments Bleomycin was used, as it is readily soluble in water and can therefore be easily incorporated in different preparations.

Before the use of Bleomycin, experiments with model substances were carried out for safety reasons. However, such experiments can only be justified when there is a therapeutic benefit for patients. For this, dark blue dyes were introduced into the carrier systems instead of cytostatic drugs. On the one hand, dark blue dyes are not toxic for the patients. On the other hand, these agents are useful as their pre-operative endolymphatic application stains retroperitoneal lymph nodes blue and thus improves their identification and subsequent complete removal. For these initial experiments, two different substances with extremely different properties were used. Patent Blue V (Byk Gulden, Germany) is a water soluble dye, which is routinely used to stain lymph vessels before cannulation. Guajazulen is a natural plant dye, which is lipid soluble. Its safety has been proven by the mutagenicity and carcinogenicity test (10).

THE EXPERIMENTAL BASIS OF ENDOLYMPHATIC DRUG APPLICATION

Oil Suspensions

Samples of Bleomycin oil suspension (Nippon-Kayaku, Japan) were used in animal experiments (11). In these samples, the suspension was kept stable by added aluminium stearate ('Oil Bleo').

In the experiments, Oil Bleo was injected into the lymphatic vessels of the hind pad of eight related mongrel dogs. Each dog of about 13 kg ($\pm$ 1.5 kg) was injected 4 ml of the suspension over 1 h. By this, 60 mg of Bleomycin were administered each. The control group received 60 mg Bleomycin dissolved in 4 ml aqueous solution.

A self-made radioimmunoassay was used to measure the Bleomycin concentration in the biological samples. Based on previous knowledge (4), the final assay was proven to detect concentrations as low as 2 ng ml^{-1}. To demonstrate the concentration of Bleomycin, regular blood samples were taken up to 6 h after the injection. By this it was found that the Bleomycin reached with an average of 12.2 µg ml^{-1} its highest concentration 15 min after the injection. The range of the concentration was between 9.2 and 15.8 µg ml^{-1}, correlating with the respective dog's weight. With rising weight, the serum concentration gradually diminished. In contrast to the aforementioned expected findings, it was also found that the repetition of an injection into the lymphatic vessels of the opposite hind pad of the dogs led to a lower peak serum concentration. This finding was confirmed in each of the cases. Also unexpectedly, it was found that this peak was already reached directly after finishing the injection, i.e. 15 min earlier than in the first injections.

Using a haematocrit of 45.5% and a blood volume of 73 ml kg^{-1} body weight as reference values (25), the total amount of Bleomycin in the dog's blood could be calculated from the peak concentration of the drug. The calculated amount of Bleomycin in the blood represents only part of the administered drug, and was labelled 'spillover'. The spillover and its importance for the clinical use of the technique were described in the section on prerequisites and limitations of endolymphatic drug application.

From the experiments, an average spillover of 13% was found for Oil Bleo, ranging from 10.5 to 14.5%. To avoid overdosing, it is of utmost importance to know the spillover value, which is dependent on several factors. For this, the spillover must be empirically assessed and calculated separately for every species and for every agent. After empirically establishing the spillover, the following formula can be used to calculate the maximum amount of the drug for endolymphatic application

$$ML = \frac{MB \times 100}{SF},$$

where ML is the maximum amount of the drug permissible for endolymphatic injection, MB the maximum amount of the drug routinely administered intravenously (bolus) and SF the spillover factor.

If 0.5 mg Bleomycin per kilogram body weight was routinely administered intravenously (MB), and the spillover factor was 14, the calculation for a dog weighing 13 kg would look as follows:

$$ML = \frac{(13 \times 0.5\,\text{mg}) \times 100}{14} = 46.4\,\text{mg}.$$

As this value was exceeded in the experiment by about one-fourth it was concluded that the safe dosage would be 3 ml Oil Bleo. An important finding was that despite this perceived overdose, no side effects were observed. However, knowledge of the spillover factor is not the only prerequisite to determine the correct dosage of a drug. The serum concentration of Bleomycin falls below 1 µg ml^{-1} after 4 h and remains like this for at least another 2 h. A basic requirement for administering drugs endolymphatically is that the dosage of the drug leaving the lymph system during the injection and within the first 4 h after that should not exceed the routine daily dosage of the same drug prescribed for intravenous administration.

In contrast to experiments under strict laboratory conditions in animals, the situation in humans is likely to be much more complicated. Physical exercise or the consumption of large amounts of fluids was found to increase the spillover factor considerably (see further experiments), which might be caused by the overloading of lymph nodes with the injected suspension. The weight of the lymph nodes does not change after the injection of the aqueous solution.

Another important finding was that the enlargement of the lymph nodes containing Oil Bleo does not mean a uniform distribution of the drug in the lymph nodes. The highest concentration was found in the first lymph node flooded by the suspension. The lowest concentration was found in the last lymph node reached. However, this observation cannot be explained by a failure to use the correct injection technique. With 4 ml h^{-1}, the injection rate was very low. Moreover, it was assured that the lymph system was completely inundated, including the ductus thoracicus. A possible explanation for this effect is a potential filter function of lymph nodes. As common in filters, the first one retains most particles, while the subsequent ones become less and less dirty.

When transferring the above observations to humans, the findings suggest that pedal lymphography is potentially a good entrance site when inguinal lymph node metastases are targeted. However, when planning to reach intra-abdominal lymph nodes, such as the pelvic lymph nodes, an inguinal injection site might be superior.

Another factor to be considered for applying the method on humans is that the spillover in humans is likely to be lower than in dogs. The human lymph system has a much larger storage capacity due to its wealth of lymph nodes. As another consequence of the aforementioned peculiarities, in humans larger differences in drug concentrations are expected between the inguinal and the para-aortal lymph nodes. However, despite the lower drug concentration in the para-aortal lymph nodes, it remains therapeutically adequate over an extended time span. This could be demonstrated by the finding of 31 μg Bleomycin per gram tissue of para-aortal lymph nodes 1 month after the injection of Oil Bleo. Also 1 month after the endolymphatic application of Oil Bleo, it was found that the lymph nodes on the injection side were still 37% heavier than those on the non-injection side.

Another important finding was that the lymph nodes, which were flooded with Oil Bleo, contained after 1 month 140% more Bleomycin than the ones flooded with aqueous Bleomycin after 6 h. When trying to identify the reason for the increased weight of the lymph nodes treated with Oil Bleo, giant oil droplets were found in the lymph node parenchyma, which diminish in number and size over several weeks (Fig. 2). Measurements of the drug concentration showed that the drug gradually escapes from the suspension, leaving the oily part of the suspension.

When comparing 38 histologically worked-up lymph nodes containing Oil Bleo to 13 lymph nodes containing iodised oil it was found that every second lymph node after the treatment with Oil Bleo contained microscopic-sized necroses. These necrotic foci disappeared after 1 month the latest, leaving moderate fibroses in place. However, these necroses were found not to interfere with lymph circulation.

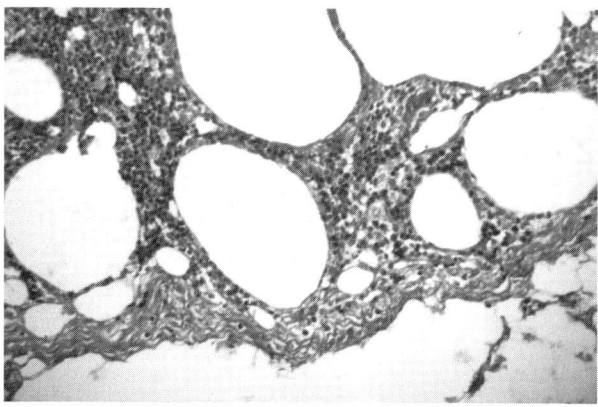

Figure 2. Popliteal lymph node of the dog 14 days after endolymphatic injection of Bleomycin oil suspension. Giant oil droplets are compressing the lymph node tissue

In contrast to that, in lymph nodes filled with Lipiodol the number of necrotic foci was three times lower. Drawing the findings from these initial experiments together, it was decided that further experiments are needed to find a more appropriate drug carrier with improved properties.

Oil Emulsions

Experiments with oil emulsions were carried out to find a way for reducing the oil content of the drug carriers. This was perceived necessary as clinical experience with lymphographies using radioactively labelled Lipiodol demonstrated that the oil reaches and finally blocks the lung capillaries via the ductus thoracicus (34). Other disadvantages of using high concentrations of oil are that the giant oil droplets, which are deposited in the lymph node parenchyma, compress the lymph node tissue to a large extent. By this, the contact of the drug with the target tissue is limited to the surface of the droplets.

To achieve the wanted reduction in oil, the drug was emulsified with different oils after initially dissolving it in water. Using this technique it was possible to use iodised oil and to preserve the diagnostic potential of such an emulsion preparation. Lipiodol Ultra-Fluid is iodinated oleum papaveris, and contains 480 mg iodine per millilitre. However, animal experiments gave evidence that the iodine content can be reduced to 350 mg ml^{-1} without compromising the diagnostic quality of X-ray images. Considering these preliminary experiments, the content of Lipiodol in the emulsion was decided to be 74%. Unfortunately, difficulties occurred in the preparation of emulsions with such a high content of iodine. Twelve emulsifiers and twelve additives were tested in 95 different combinations, before it was possible to produce two stable emulsions (15). Both stable emulsions contained Pluronic L61 + L64 as emulsifiers. For the first emulsion, Eutanol and oleum ricini were used as additives, while for the second emulsion Miglyol was used. The percentage of the additives summed up to 21.4 in each case. Also for both emulsions, a stock solution of 30 mg ml^{-1} Bleomycin was used, leading to a final content of this stock solution of 1.2% in both stable emulsions.

When testing the two above specified emulsions on an initial series of six rabbits, it was found that although the opacification of the lymph system was good in X-ray images, further investigations will not lead to clinically applicable results. Most negatively, the emulsions were stored in the popliteal lymph nodes, leading in the most prominent cases to a fourfold increase in lymph node weight. Necroses occurred in all lymph nodes treated with emulsions containing Miglyol, and in most cases treated with emulsions containing oleum ricini. Moreover, the lymph vessels appeared dilated, which might be due to the high viscosity of the emulsions. After 2 weeks, the concentration of Bleomycin in the retroperitoneal lymph nodes was only about 6% of the concentrations found in the popliteal lymph nodes.

Another four rabbits were treated with similar emulsions, containing a blue dye (Patent Blue V) instead of Bleomycin. Again the above-described negative effects occurred, thus suggesting that Bleomycin was not the agent causing the necroses. Although the use of non-iodised oil would probably solve some of the problems related to the stability and the toxicity of the emulsions, this would mean to loose the double function of the emulsions. The therapeutic properties would remain, while the diagnostic potential is likely to be lost.

Preparations Containing Guajazulen

Guajazulen-in-Lipiodol Solution

When examining 13 lymph nodes from dogs, which were treated with Lipiodol, it was found that 15% of them had necroses adjacent to the oil droplets (13). As it was not clear whether the necroses were caused by the drug dissolved in oil, or by the oil alone, further experiments were conducted.

For the experiment, the aforementioned solution containing 30% Guajazulen-in-Lipiodol was used (10). Two dogs received an injection of 4 ml into the hind leg vessels. Seven days after the injection, the lymph nodes were removed surgically. They were stained dark blue (Fig. 3).

Most negatively, it was found that all examined lymph nodes had disseminated necroses. In a later case, damage of the lymph node capsule was found. However, the total enlargement of the lymph nodes was not greater than it would be from normal lymphography.

In another experiment, the same solution was injected into the lymph vessels of rabbits. For this, 0.3 ml kg^{-1} were administered. However, results were found to be similar, with the lymph nodes having a dark blue colour after 7 days. Histological workup showed giant oil droplets and necroses after 1 and 7 days, respectively. After 17 days, the oil droplets had vanished almost completely, but fibrosis of the lymph node parenchyma occurred. Despite this, the function of the lymph nodes was not disturbed by this. After 1 day, a concentration of 5.3 µg g^{-1} was found in the lungs,

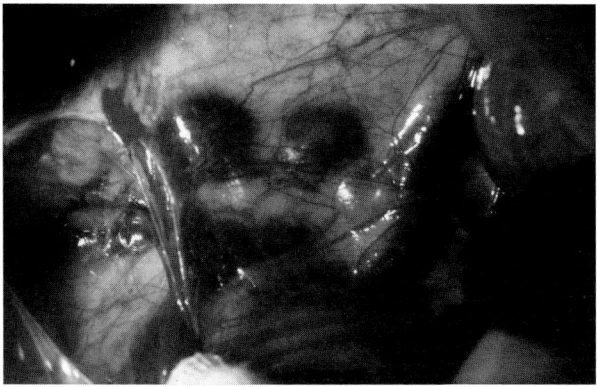

Figure 3. Dark blue staining of retroperitoneal lymph nodes 7 days after the endolymphatic injection of Guajazulen-in-Lipiodol solution

which is five times higher than in the liver and kidneys. After 7 days, the concentration declined to 1.0 μg g^{-1}, which means double the concentration found in liver and kidneys. The above results indicate that the well-known oil obstruction of the lung after lymphography also occurs with the blue solution examined in the above experiments.

Guajazulen–Tween Emulsions

For the experiments with Guajazulen–Tween emulsions, two different emulsions were prepared. The first of them consisted of 20% Guajazulen, 40% Tween 20 and 40% aqua dest. The second was composed of 10% Guajazulen and 90% Tween 80. As both emulsions caused extensive necroses when injected endolymphatically into rabbits, they were judged as being inappropriate for endolymphatic use.

Guajazulen–Lecithin Emulsion

The Guajazulen–lecithin emulsion was prepared from the following components: 10% Guajazulen, 10% lecithin, 10% ethylalcohol and 70% aqua dest. One day after the injection of this emulsion, a considerable enlargement of the lymph nodes was found. Moreover, the lymph nodes demonstrated a dark blue colour. After 3 days, macroscopic necroses were observed. At that time, the lymph vessels were found to be still dilated, of blue colour and partially destroyed due to the necroses. After these disappointing findings, the experiments with emulsions were discontinued. However, lecithin was again used in the subsequent experiments.

Experiments with Liposomes

The above-described experiments demonstrate well that classical drug carrier systems are not appropriate for endolymphatic therapy in humans. Inquiries into better carrier systems brought up the idea that liposomes might be suitable for transporting drugs to lymph nodes. This idea gained further support when considering that liposomes are constructed out of substances, which are physiologically present in lymph. For the subsequent experiments, liposomes were used consisting of 80% lecithin and 20% cholesterol.

Forty percent of the lecithin contained in lymph was found to stem directly from nutrition (32). The other 60% are either taken up from bile, or are newly synthesised. Cholesterol in lymph was found to stem from the same sources in similar proportions (6). In lymph, both substances appear in the form of chylomicrons, which are spherical structures consisting mainly of phospholipids and cholesterol. With 75%, lecithin is the most prevalent phospholipid in the chylomicrons (36). Depending on the species and the nutritional status, the size of the chylomicrons varies. In dogs, the diameter of the chylomicrons is between 180 and 200 nm (27). In rabbits, a diameter between 104 and 152 nm was found to be normal (29).

From the above-described properties of liposomes, it was concluded that liposomes are very similar with regard to size and components to the surface of chylomicrons. As a consequence, it is likely that they can be used as transportation vehicles in lymph, similar to the chylomicrons. In addition to that, liposomes can be retained in lymph node parenchyma over weeks. Due to these properties, the clinical applicability of liposomes for endolymphatic therapy appeared sufficiently likely as to justify further experiments. These are described in the following.

Experiments on Rabbits with Liposomes Containing Bleomycin

For the following experiments, liposomes were produced out of egg yolk lecithin extracted by a detergent dialysis technique based on standard methods (24). For the extraction process, the dialysis equipment Lipoprep (Dianorm, Germany) was used. The liposomes were then loaded with Bleomycin and finally centrifuged for 90 min with $195,000 \times g$. Radioimmunoassay proved that the Bleomycin content of the liposomes was 4.9 ng ml^{-1}. Extensive measures were taken to control for the quality of the liposomes. By electron microscopy, the liposomes were found to be unilamellar and homogenous, with a diameter of 170 nm. Laser light scattering (Coulter Nanosizer) proved a low polydispersity (0–1) in the liposome preparation. Moreover, a microbiological assay gave evidence that the liposomes were sterile. A test for the in vitro stability showed a vesicle disintegration of 17.7% after 25 days.

The final liposomes were then injected into the lymph system of 'Giant German' rabbits, each weighing about 7 kg (16). The injection rate was 0.07 ml min^{-1}, and a total of 0.3 ml liposomes per kilogram body weight were administered. The results achieved with these liposomes in rabbits paralleled the findings of the previous experiments. Three days after the injection, the Bleomycin concentration was 42.14 μg g^{-1} in the popliteal lymph nodes. This means that the concentration was again three times higher in the popliteal lymph nodes than in the retroperitoneal ones. The drug was retained in the lymph nodes, dropping to a concentration of 0.18 μg ml^{-1} after 1 month in the popliteal lymph nodes. This was still twice the concentration than that reached in the retroperitoneal lymph nodes.

After leaving the lymph system via the ductus thoracicus, the liposomes were mainly stored in the spleen. This might be due to the high density of reticulo-endothelial formations in this organ. After 3 days, the concentration of Bleomycin in the spleen was with 0.48 µg five times higher than the concentration of Bleomycin in the lungs. This finding demonstrates a clear advantage of using liposomes for endolymphatic drug application, compared to using pure oil. The latter was found to be mainly deposited in the lungs, where it causes major respiratory problems.

Another important finding was that 3 days after the injection, the weight of the lymph nodes treated with liposomes was still 70% higher than that of their untreated counterparts. After 4 weeks, this effect was not present any more, and the weight of the treated and the untreated lymph nodes was similar. The histological workup of the lymph nodes 3 days after the injection showed that the liposomes were stored in the lymph nodes as small droplets, which causes only a moderate compression of the lymph node tissue. Moreover, no toxic effects were found. Twenty-eight days after the injection, the droplets were found to be completely absorbed. However, minor signs of fibrosis gave evidence of the previous presence of large amounts of the drug.

Experiments on Rats with Liposomes Containing Blue Dye

Using a detergent dialysis technique, liposomes were produced, which consisted of 80% phosphatidylcholine and 20% cholesterol. Liposomat, an especially designed dialysis equipment (Dianorm, Germany), ensured the standardisation of the production process, and therefore of the liposomes. During the production process, the liposome vesicles were loaded with a mixture of Patent Blue and mixed micelle solution. Finally, a concentration of 1.6 mg ml^{-1} was reached in the vesicles, which could be detected at 630 nm.

To determine their general staining properties, these liposomes were intramuscularly injected into rats. Dark blue staining was observed in the muscle tissue around the injection site. The blue colour was still observable 28 days after the injection, when the experiment was terminated. Other important findings were that the liposomes did not cause pain, and produced no toxic changes in the muscle. The rats from the control group, which received injections of Patent Blue aqueous solution, did not show persistent staining of the muscle. Both, the high local deposition rate as proven by the persistent staining, as well as the good tissue tolerance suggested further experiments with this preparation.

Experiments on Rabbits with Liposomes Containing Blue Dye

The liposomes prepared with the same technique as those for the experiments on rats were stuffed with Patent Blue up to an internal concentration of 0.8 mg ml^{-1}. Due to the excellent staining properties of the liposomes containing 1.6 mg Patent Blue per millilitre, cutting down the concentration by 50% seemed to be justified (14). For this experiment, 0.3 ml kg^{-1} of the liposomes were endolymphatically injected into six rabbits (12). As rabbits of 7 kg body weight were chosen, 2.1 ml of the liposomes were injected each. Again, the experiment was scheduled for 28 days. After 28 days, excellent dark blue staining of the retroperitoneal lymph nodes was observed (Fig. 4).

In the stained areas, a Patent Blue concentration of 172 μg g^{-1} tissue was found, which indicates a fivefold decrease within a month. A Patent Blue concentration of more than 5 μg g^{-1} was found in the tissue around the lymph nodes. The histological workup of the lymph nodes (Fig. 5) demonstrated that no tissue damage occurred due to the injection of the above-described liposomes.

Experiments on Dogs with Liposomes Containing Blue Dye

Initially, a short-term experiment was carried out on dogs, as it was known from previous work that most of the potential complications of the endolymphatic administration of liposomes occur during or shortly after the injection. However,

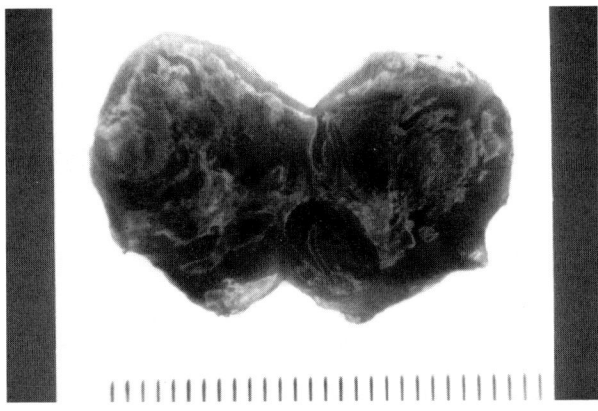

Figure 4. Dissected popliteal rabbit lymph node 28 days after endolymphatic injection of blue liposomes. The node is homogenously stained dark blue, is not enlarged and has no evidence of necrosis or inflammation

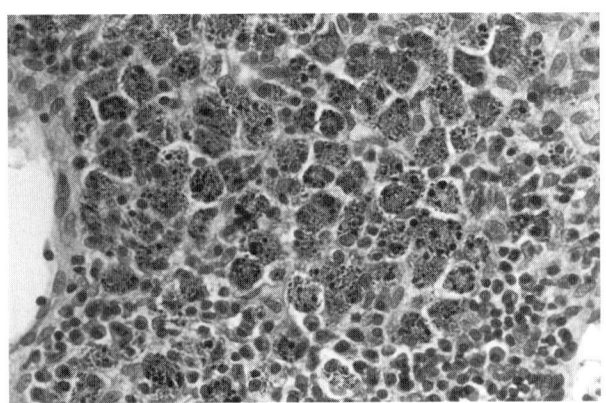

Figure 5. Histological specimen of popliteal rabbit lymph node 28 days after endolymphatic injection of blue liposomes. Accumulation of blue dye in fine granular pattern

at the time of commencing the experiment, it was hypothesised that liposomes were the best carriers for the endolymphatic administration of drugs.

As large amounts of concentrated liposomes were needed for this experiment, a new preparation technique was used. The mixed micelle solution containing 9.8 g egg yolk lecithin, 1.62 g cholesterol and 12.6 g sodium cholate was dialysed against a continuous buffer flow, using a capillary flow dialyser. Unfortunately, the thus produced liposomes appeared diluted and required a reduction of volume. By dialysing the liposomes for 3 h against 500 ml of 5% polyethyleneglycol solution (MW 40,000/Serva), the lipid concentration increased. After this second dialysis, 85 ml of concentrated liposome suspension remained. The remaining suspension was loaded with blue dye (Isosulfan blue/Sigma), using the previously described technique (17). Finally, the suspension was dialysed until a dye concentration below 0.01 mg ml^{-1} was reached.

The resulting liposomes had a final volume of 54 ml and a diameter of 75 nm ($\pm$4 nm). The suspension had a dye concentration of 2.6 mg ml^{-1}, which was proven by a measurement of the HPLC-system. Gamma-ray perturbed angular correlation technique (18) was able to demonstrate for the first time that the above liposomes remained stable over 57 h when incubated with fresh dog lymph at 37°C. This finding partially explains the good deposition properties of liposomes in lymph nodes.

A chromatographical examination demonstrated the different localisation of blue dye in the liposome suspension. The inner volume of the liposome vesicles was found to contain about 60% of the dye, with the remaining dye being stored in the outer aqueous coating of the vesicles. During dialysis, the content of the inner volume remained bound to the vesicles, while the remaining free dye in the outer compartment was reduced to below 0.01 mg ml^{-1}. The spontaneous destruction rate of liposomes in vitro was similar to previous results. After 3 months, 50% of the dye had escaped as a free drug from the inner volume of the vesicle to its outer compartment.

For the subsequent in vivo experiment, eight dogs were divided into two equal groups. The dogs within the first group were subcutaneously injected 0.5 ml of the liposome solution into the hind pad. In this group, the ductus thoracicus was surgically identified and cannulated in the left neck region before the administration of the liposomes.

In all cases it was found that some of the liposomes were drained from the subcutaneous injection site by lymphatic vessels. This was concluded from the dark blue staining of these vessels. Moreover, it was found that during a period of 10–60 min, a small percentage of liposomes were transferred to the ductus thoracicus without any sign of destruction (0.53–1.12%). However, the percentage of free dye was slightly elevated.

Following this procedure, the blue-stained lymph vessels of the hind pad were cannulated, and 4 ml of the liposomes were injected. For this, the injection was performed over 1 h. It was most interesting to find that the results of this experiment paralleled the findings from former experiments with oil suspensions. During the injection, the concentration of dye rapidly increased in the ductus thoracicus. The maximum concentration was again reached by the time of finishing the injection, reaching a concentration of 15.4% of dye in lymph on average. After the 1-h maximum, the concentration decreased rapidly for 30 min, when a plateau of below 50 $\mu g \ ml^{-1}$ was attained. At this time, 26% of the total amount of dye injected was found in the lymph. After the initial 30 min, the decrease in concentration went slower.

However, the high storage capacity of 74% of the injected substance is unstable. After reaching the basic spillover of 50 $\mu g \ ml^{-1}$, 500 ml of saline were administered over 30 min. During the infusion the lymph volume increased rapidly, as did the drug spillover. A total of 14.8% of the administered dye was found in the lymph fraction containing the peak concentration. The extra spillover caused by the saline infusion led to the increase of dye drained into the ductus thoracicus, with 64.6% of the total dye found there. This finding demonstrates well that the activation of lymph flow during drug administration should be avoided. Otherwise, harmful drug peaks in the blood occur, and the envisaged effect of the drug in the lymph nodes is lost.

In contrast to the storage capacity, the liposomes that passed through the lymph system remained stable. The initial intra-vesicle fraction of dye, which was 60%, diminished to amounts between 50.1 and 43.9%. This means that an average of 78% of the liposomes remained intact during their passage thought the ductus thoracicus into the blood. The results of the in vitro experiments using the PAC-technique could therefore be confirmed for the in vivo situation.

Also in this experiment, the lymph nodes were stained dark blue and could thus be well discriminated against the surrounding fat tissue. The naked eye cannot detect any difference in dye concentration. The observed weight difference between the treated and the untreated lymph nodes was only significant for the popliteal nodes, with the treated nodes being on average 42% heavier than their untreated counterparts (ranging from 27 to 57%). This finding compares well to previous results. The histological workup of the treated lymph nodes gave evidence of deposited dye and a dilated sinus. No other structural changes were observed.

At the outset of this experiment it was found that a small amount of liposomes reached the ductus thoracicus after subcutaneous bolus injection. This could be a hint towards the potential of liposomes for the indirect administration of drugs, without the need for a time consuming and technically challenging cannulation of lymph vessels. To explore this potential effect, the second group of dogs received a slow subcutaneous injection of liposomes into two feet. During 30 min, 2 ml of liposomes were injected into each foot. The control group of another two dogs received an aqueous dye under exactly the same conditions. However, in both the study and the control group, the uptake was poor. As a consequence, the experiments with dogs indicated that the endolymphatic application of drugs by cannulating the lymph vessels remains the only acceptable pathway for delivering highly concentrated drugs to lymph nodes.

Experiments on Pigs with Liposomes Containing Blue Dye

The direct lymphography by cannulating lymph vessels has, however, its drawbacks. It must be handled by trained experts, and would need too much time for routinely staging lymph nodes prior to surgery. It would also not be helpful for the identification of sentinel lymph node in breast cancer, because the identification and cannulation of lymphatic vessels leaving breast tumours will remain the procedure of academic interest only.

The indirect lymphography by interstitial deposition of the dye remains the only method to stain blue the sentinel lymph nodes in practical use. This technique is more successful in the breast than in other organs, because the mammary glands have a highly developed lymphatic drainage network.

To study this subject, the experiment on seven female pigs was conducted (5). In each case, a 0.5 ml depot containing 12.5 mg Patent Blue was injected into each of the four upper and lower mammary glands. On the right side, the dye was incorporated in liposomes, on the left side it was in aqueous solution.

The liposomes consisted of lecithin and cholesterol in a molar ratio of 3:1. They were produced by extrusion using membranes with thickness between 0.2 and 5 μm. Their average diameter was 172 nm.

After time intervals between 3 and 24 h, the lymph nodes of the groin, pelvis and neck were photographed in situ and then removed. The excised lymph nodes were photographed again and weighed. Each lymph node was minced to a homogenous cell suspension. This suspension was centrifuged at $1,000 \times g$ for 30 min. The concentrations of Patent Blue were measured at 635 nm by spectrophotometry.

Three hours after injection, the lymph nodes of both sides were stained. The amount of dye on the right side was 4.55 times higher compared with the left side.

Six hours after injection, staining of the lymph nodes on the left side was no more detectable with the naked eye, even when the remnants of dye were present. The amount of dye on the right side was 12.85 times higher compared to the left side. After 12 h, the difference remained nearly unchanged (10.03 times higher concentration on the right). After 24 h, the difference dropped to 4.60 times higher on the liposome side.

In all times and all regions, the staining of the lymph nodes with liposomal dye was much better. There were alterations which might have reduced the value of histological examination.

CLINICAL OUTLOOK

Liposomes are recommended as carriers of drugs dedicated to treat locally the lymphatic system and for the preoperative staining of lymph nodes. They allow sustained deposition of drugs and dyes in lymph nodes and do not reduce the accuracy of histological examinations. Their small size excludes a mechanical blockage of lung capillaries in cases with spillover from the lymphatic system.

From the information gained during the above-described animal experiments, the following conclusions are drawn for future work on humans:

1. Inject the substance as close as possible to the target lymph nodes. This will elevate the drug concentration in the area.
2. Do not inject more than the maximum dose acceptable for intravenous application. This is only acceptable after the maximum spillover is proven in humans.
3. Inject as little volume as possible. The inundation of normally sized retroperitoneal lymph nodes should be possible with 4 ml volume on each side.
4. Inject about 4 ml h^{-1}.
5. The patient should stay with as little movement as possible for about 1 day after the injection. This will lead to a longer retention of the injected substance in the lymph nodes. Do not administer bolus infusions and keep fluid intake as low as possible for the same reason.
6. If higher dosages or higher volumes are necessary, cannulate the ductus thoracicus to minimise the likelihood of adverse effects. High amounts of cytostatic agents can be administered with such an 'isolated perfusion' of the lymph system.
7. No problems from obstructed lung vessels should be observable when using liposomal cytostatic agents.
8. Liposomes for staining the lymph nodes preoperatively can be mixed with liposomes carrying drugs. Use this possibility to stain lymph nodes for more radical, but also more selective surgery.
9. Do not perform surgery earlier than 3 h after the endolymphatic application of dye. Otherwise, the dye might be still in the lymph vessels or stain the surrounding structures blue, rather than only the lymph nodes.
10. It is assumed that there is still a measurable amount of endolymphatically administered drugs after 1 month. This should prevent the lymphogenous spread of tumour cells from these lymph nodes.
11. The interstitial injection of liposomal dye is more suitable to detect sentinel lymph nodes in breast surgery than after the injection of aqueous dye.

The last point, sentinel lymphonodectomy, became already wide clinical routine, especially in melanoma (7) and breast malignancies (9). It has been shown that the histopathological examination of the sentinel node is representative enough to avoid the excision of neighbouring lymph nodes (2, 3, 31). The results in vulvar (1) or colorectal carcinoma (19) are, however, less promising because of a high false-negative rate.

Localisation of the sentinel node is possible by staining with different dyes (20, 22) by radioactive tracers (30, 35) or a combination of both (8, 33).

In opposite, the direct application of cytostatic drugs to the lymphatic system is not clinically used due to concurrent intravenous infusion, which can be performed much cheaper and without technical experience, even when the drug levels in lymph nodes are extremely low compared with liposomal preparations.

The endolymphatic treatment of malignancies which spread via the lymphatic vessels seems still the most direct option to successfully control cancer dissemination.

REFERENCES

1. Ansick, A.C., Sie Go, D., van der Velden, J. et al: Identification of sentinel lymph node in vulvar carcinoma patients with the aid of a patent blue V injection: A multicenter study. Cancer 86 (1999), 652-656
2. Bland, K.I.: Refining the optimal technical approach for sentinel node localization in breast cancer patients. Ann. Surg. Oncol.6 (1999), 418-419
3. Bostic, P.J., Giuliano, A.E.: Vital dyes in sentinel node localization. Sem.Nucl. Med. 30 (2000), 18-24
4. Broughton, A., Strong, J.E.: Radioimmunoassay of Bleomycin. Cancer Research 36 (1976), 1418
5. Dieter, M., Schubert, R, Hirnle, P.: Blue liposomes for identification of the sentinel lymph nodes in pigs. Lymphology 36 (2003), 39-47
6. Dietschy, J.M., Siperstein, M.D.: Cholesterol synthesis by the gastrointestinal tract: localisation and mechanisms of control. Journal of Clinical Investigation 44 (1965), 1311
7. Gallegos Hernanadez, J.F., Gutierrez, F., Barosso, S. et al: Identification of sentinel lymph node with patent blue V in patients with cutaneous melanoma. Gac. Med. Mex. 134 (1998), 419-422
8. Gennari, R., Soldt, H.S., Bartolomei, M. et al: Sentinel node localization: A new prospective in the treatment of nodal melanoma metastases. Intl. J. Oncol. 15 (1999), 25-32
9. Haigh, P.I., Giuliano, A.E.: Role of sentinel lymph node dissection in breast cancer. Annals of medicine 32 (2000), 51-56
10. Harzmann, R., Hirnle P., Geppert, M.: Retroperitoneal lymph nodal visualization using 20 % Guajazulen blue (chromolymphography). Lymphology 22 (1989),147-149
11. Hirnle, P.: Endolymphatic application of Bleomycin oil suspension in dog model. Lymphology 18 (1985), 56-63
12. Hirnle, P.: Histological findings in rabbit lymph nodes after endolymphatic injection of liposomes containing blue dye. J. Pharm. Pharmacol. 43 (1991), 217-218
13. Hirnle, P., Geppert, M.: Histologic changes in dog lymph nodes after endolymphatic application of bleomycin oil suspension. Lymphology 22 (1989), 100-102
14. Hirnle, P., Harzmann, R., Wright, J.K.: Patent blue V encapsulation in liposomes: potential applicability to endolymphatic therapy and preoperative chromolymphography. Lymphology 21 (1988), 187-189
15. Hirnle, P., Heide, P.E.: Iodinated emulsions of cytostatic agents for combined diagnostic and therapeutic lymphography. In: Casley-Smith, J.R., Piller, N.B. (eds.) Progress in Lymphology, University of Adelaide Press (1985), 279-281
16. Hirnle, P., Jaroni, H., Schmidt, K.-H.: Endolymphatic application of liposomes containing bleomycin in rabbits. In: Casley-Smith, J.R., Piller, N.B. (eds.) Progress in Lymphology, University of Adelaide Press (1986), 276-278
17. Hirnle, P., Schubert R.: Liposomes containing blue dye for preoperative lymph node staining: Distribution and stability in dogs after endolymphatic injection. Int J Pharmaceutics 72 (1991), 259-269
18. Hwang, K.J., Mauk, M.R.: Fate of lipid vesicles in vivo: A gamma-ray perturbed angular correlation study. Proceedings of the National Academy of Sciences (USA) 74 (1977), 4991
19. Joosten, J.A.A., Stroble, L.J.A., Wauters, C.A.P. et al: Intraoperative lymphatic mapping and the sentinel node concept in colorectal carcinoma. British J. Surgery: 86 (1999), 482-488
20. Kern, K.A.: Sentinel lymph node mapping in breast cancer using subareolar injection of blue dye. J. Am. Coll. Surg. 189 (1999), 539-545
21. Kinmonth, J.B.: The lymphatics. Surgery, lymphography and disease of the chyle and lymph system. Edward Arnold 1982
22. Lucci, A., Turner, R.R., Morton, D.L.: Carbon dye as an adjunct to isosulfan blue dye for sentinel lymph node dissection. Surgery 126 (1999), 48-53
23. Mathew, C.P., Intralymphatic chemotherapy. Case report of a successful result. Indian J. Cancer, 6, 112, 1969
24. Milsman, H.W., Schwenderer, R.A., Weder, H.G.: The preparation of large single bilayer liposomes by a fast and controlled dialysis. Biochemica et Biophysica Acta 512 (1978), 147
25. Nickel, R., Schummer, A., Seiferle, E.: Lehrbuch der Anatomie der Haustiere. Parey, Berlin, Hamburg (1976)
26. Patterson, R.M., Ballard, C.L., Wasserman, K., Mayerson, H.S.: Lymphatic permeability to albumin. American Journal of Physiology 194 (1958), 120
27. Pinter, G.G., Zilversmith, D.B.: A gradient centrifugation method for the determination of particle size distribution of chylomicrons and of fat droplets in artificial fat emulsion. Biochemica et Biophysica Acta 59 (1962),116

28. Piver, M.S., Wallace, S., Castro, J.R.: The accuracy of lymphangiography in carcinoma of the uterine cervix. American Journal of Roentgenology 111 (1971), 278

29. Redgrave, T.G., Dunne, K.B.: Chylomicron formation and composition in unanaesthetized rabbits. Atherosclerosis 22 (1975), 389

30. Roumen, R.M., Geuskens, L.M., Valkenburg, J.G.: In search of the true sentinel node by different injection techniques in breast cancer patients. Eur. J. Surg. Oncol. 25 (1999), 347-351

31. Rozenberg, S, Liebens, F., Ham, H.: False-negative rates in sentinel node in breast cancer. Lancet 354 (1999), 773-774

32. Scow, R.O., Stein, Y., Stein, O.: Incorporation of dietary lecithin and lysolecithin into lymph chylomicrons in the rat. Journal of Biological Chemistry 242 (1967), 4919

33. Wallace, A.M., Vera, D.R., Stadalnik, R.C.: Blue dye and Tc-99m-labeled human serum albumin: Sentinel node detection by magic bullets? J. Nucl. Med. 40 (1999), 1149-1150.

34. Weissleder, H., Pfannenstiel, P., Peters, P.E.: Distribution pattern of radioactive labelled Lipiodol-UF following intralymphatic application for therapy. Lymphology 9 (1976), 122

35. Wilhelm, A.J., Mijnhout, G.S., Franssen, E.J.F.: Radiopharmaceuticals in sentinel lymph node detection - an overview. Eur. J. Nucl. Med. 26 (1999), 36-42

36. Zilversmith, D.B.: The composition and structure of lymph chylomicrons in dog, rat and man. Journal of Clinical Investigation 44 (1965), 1610

37. Zweifach, B.W., Prather, J.W.: Micromanipulation of pressure in terminal lymphatics in the mesentery. American Journal of Physiology 228 (1975), 1326

9. MECHANISMS OF METASTASIS: SEED AND SOIL

ADRIANO PIRIS AND MARTIN C. MIHM, JR

Mass General Hospital, Harvard Medical School, Boston, Massachusetts, USA

INTRODUCTION

Stephen Paget published in 1889 in The Lancet a paper by the title of "The distribution of secondary growths in cancer of the breast" inspired by the work of Fuchs "Das Sarkom des Uvealtractus" in 1882 published in Graefe's Archiv Fur Ophthalmologie. Although Fuchs has written previously about the metastatic embolus and its relationship to the recipient tissue, it is Paget who spread the concept of the "seed and soil" that continues to be regarded as a major contribution to the area of cancer metastasis. The "seeds" refer to certain tumor cells with metastatic capability, and the "soil" is any organ or tissue providing a proper environment for growth of the seeds (1). Paget suggested that the spread of metastatic cells was organ specific and not merely anatomic.

Since Paget's seminal publication several other investigators have come to further validate the complex interaction between tumor cells and the host's organ microenvironment as one of the main determinants of metastatic spread of a given tumor. In the early 1900s, Ewing (2) questioned the validity of Paget's theory postulating that metastasis is a result of mechanical factors due to the vascular system's anatomy. In 1979, Sugarbaker (3) stated that regional metastases could be due to anatomical or mechanical issues (such as lymphatic drainage) but metastases to distant organs are site specific. Further work by Hart and Fidler (4) in the 1980s supported Paget's "seed and soil" theory by showing preferential homing of tumor cells of B16 melanoma in specific distant sites. More evidence for the theory surfaced, including in vitro studies showing organ-selective adhesion, invasion, and growth (5). Schakert and Fidler (6) showed different patterns of brain metastases in two separate murine melanomas injected into carotid arteries.

A modern view of the "seed to soil" hypothesis includes three principles (7). The first is that tumors are heterogenous and groups of cells have variable angiogenic, invasive, and metastatic characteristics (5, 8). The second principle is that metastasis is selective for cells that are capable of invasion, embolization, survival in circulation, and extravasation and proliferation in a distant organ (9, 10). Third and finally, the result of metastasis is dependent on the interaction of tumor and host mechanisms (7).

THE SEED

The cell or group of cells that will ultimately develop into a successful metastatic clone is the survivor of a heterogeneous population that resulted from oncogenic mutations. These mutations are the explanation to the survival advantage of the "seed."

Changes in the genome, including DNA mutations, chromosomal abnormalities, and epigenetic alterations, ultimately lead to a pool of survival traits that result in tumorigenesis.

It was originally thought that the major abnormalities in the DNA occurred in the late stage of tumor development. More recent studies have clearly shown that certain cells, since the early stages of the primary tumor, already have the genomic changes that are responsible for metastasis, in other words, the cells in the primary tumor determine the metastatic potential in the individual patient since the early stages of disease (11). There are many examples of genomic mutations among which we can cite the alterations in the retinoblastoma gene and its effect on the cell cycle, the overactivation of the Akt pathway, as well as the overexpression of cyclin D1 in some cases of acral melanoma (12).

Another example of acquired survival advantage is the ability of the cells to survive in a hypoxic environment, for example the ability of certain cells to stabilize hypoxia inducible factor-1 transcriptional complex. Cells that overexpress this transcription factor are successful in metastasis resulting from increase in angiogenesis and anaerobic metabolism, as well as increased capacity for invasion (13).

Other characteristics of the cells of the primary tumor relate to their surface molecules including cadherins, integrins, and immunoglobulin superfamily. Study of the melanoma cell has revealed that the clearest sign of a tumor cell acquiring invasive ability is the loss of E-cadherin. E-cadherin is expressed in both keratinocytes and melanocytes, and appears to be the major adhesion molecule between the epidermis and keratinocyte. Malignant transformation of the melanocytes is associated with loss of this factor than that liberates the cell from its fixed position in the epidermis so that it can become motile. The invasive cells in the dermis express N-cadherin which allows for interaction with fibroblasts, endothelial cells, and other melanoma cells.

Integrins have been shown to occur in the process of malignant transformation, for example α-6-β-4 is expressed by cancer cells and binds to the extracellular matrix protein laminin. α-v-β-3 and α-3-β-1 have been implicated in metastatic disease. α-v-β-3 in addition to binding to stromal collagen is also a ligand for Thy-1 expressed on activated endothelial cells. These changes favor primary tumor cells leaving their environment and extending to other sites (14).

For the tumor cells to reach a distant site, cell motility is necessary and requires the presence of appropriate surface markers that allow for adhesion to stromal proteins in which these cells migrate. In addition, the presence of alterations in the actin-based cytoskeleton is necessary for the cells to be motile (15).

Motility studies have shown the importance of focal adhesion kinases and their relationship to stromal components resulting in assembly and disassembly of the focal adhesion sites, which directly relates to the actin–myosin intracellular activity. In a mouse melanoma model one of the focal adhesion kinase proteins Nedd9, when overexpressed, leads to increased cell motility and subsequent invasive activity.

Podoplanin is a glycoprotein that is expressed in the advancing edge of growing tumors. This factor appears very important for invasion through effect on the anchoring protein ezrin (16).

OSTEOPONTIN

Recent studies have emphasized the importance of the angiogenetic factor Osteopontin (OPN) in the role of primary tumor metastasis. OPN has been found to have multiple effects on downstream signaling pathways associated with specific cell activity. It has directly led to inhibition of apoptosis through the P13K/Akt as well as the NFκB. The latter is shown to be important in B16F10 melanoma cell lines. This effect of OPN in the B16 melanoma has also been associated with production of MMP-2. Further effect on invasion is related to its effect on Urokinase plasminogen factor pathway. A very interesting effect on endothelial cell migration, inhibition of apoptosis, and promotion of vascular lumen formation is OPN driven partially regulated by NFκB. OPN, also an angiogenetic factor, mediates its effect as a ligand for α-v-β-3, the combination of which results in marked endothelial cell activation in rats through the NFκB pathway (17).

STEM CELLS

More and more evidence accumulates that there are indeed cancer stem cells in primary tumors. First described in the hematopoietic system, these cells have two critical features. First they self-renew and second they can lead to generations of normal hematopoietic cells. Bonnet and Dick (18) described these cells as well as the corresponding leukemic stem cells. Similar cells have now been found in other organs. This important discovery has opened avenues of investigation into further understanding tumorigenesis, the role of such cells in metastasis, and therapeutic strategies.

Self-renewal in stem cells and malignant cells have been shown to be related to the Wnt/β-catenin, Hedgehog, and Notch signaling pathways (19), targeting these pathways in a manner that affects only cancer stem cells would be a desirable approach to blocking cancer stem cell renewal.

INVASION THROUGH THE BASEMENT MEMBRANE ZONE AND MIGRATION THROUGH THE STOMA

Once the tumor cell has dissociated from its attachments to other resident epithelial cells by loss for example of E-cadherin among other factors, the tumor cell must cross or disrupt the basement membrane to reach the stroma. The basement membrane zone is composed of a variety of substances including type IV collagen and laminin among others. The passage through the basement membrane is accomplished by proteolytic substances that are released by the cancer cells. Extracellular proteases are also recruited. The matrix metalloproteinases (MMPs) have dual effects in some cases, some allowing for digestion of the stroma and others showing direct antagonism with tumor growth (20, 21).

THE STROMA AND ITS ROLE IN CANCER METASTASIS

Similar to the role of stroma in modifying mesenchyma and altering the epithelial structure during the formation of the embryo, there is evidence accumulating that there are definite interactions between tumor cells and their stroma. One very interesting example of relationship between breast cancer and its stroma relates to the discovery that the fibroblasts produce chemokine CXCL12 in association with breast cancer. The CXCL12 not only results an increase in angiogenesis, but also in some manner results in further tumor proliferation and marked increased migration. The angiogenesis component is directly a result of the interaction of CXCL12, the ligand, with its receptor CXCR4 on the surface of progenitor endothelial cells (22).

The production of IGF1 by melanoma cells stimulates fibroblast to produce both VEGF and β fibroblast growth factor that leads to angiogenesis. Furthermore fibroblasts secrete IL8 that recruits monocytes and neutrophils stimulating production of TNFα and VEGF. Furthermore the stromal fibroblasts provide a scaffold in which the tumoral cells migrate (23).

Activated macrophages have a very interesting role in tumor progression. These cells favor migration to regions of hypoxia where they are induced to secrete numerous factors that lead to angiogenesis as well as metalloproteinases and growth factors. Thus the presence of tumor-associated macrophages leads to aggressive tumor behavior.

ANGIOGENESIS AND INVASION OF BLOOD VESSELS

In the stroma the tumor cells must now proliferate, however to accomplish this the neoplasm requires a neovasculature that will extend well beyond the preexisting blood vessels, since the "native" vasculature will eventually become insufficient for the tumor.

Also, this newly formed vessel will allow the tumor cells to enter the vasculature and extend to distant sites. The term "angiogenic switch" has been introduced by

Hanahan and Folkman (24) and describes a dynamic and necessary ability of the tumors to allow for growth of new vessels as well as invasion of the vessels as part of the metastatic process. These new vessels are derived either from the preexisting blood vessels or by recruitment of circulating endothelial progenitors that express CXCR4. Lymphangiogenesis has also been noted to occur in tumors and is related to prognosis (25).

Tumor cells that have successfully invaded the blood vessels adhere to blood platelets to protect them from destructive physical forces such as hemodynamic shear and also from sensitized killer mononuclear cells. At the same time there is thrombosis with fibrin deposition (26, 27). The presence of platelets with fibrin deposition creates a tumor–platelet complex that essentially acts as an embolus.

This important complex structure apparently has a causative role for tumor cells lodging in target organs. While this phenomenon explains a possible physical mechanism for tumor cells to lodge in a host organ and develop a metastasis, there is also accumulating evidence that the receptors on malignant cells reacting to specific ligands on the host result in metastatic growth in these "specific" sites.

Several examples support this hypothesis. Melanoma cells have been shown to express high CXCR4, CCR7, and CCR10 mRNA. The respective ligands for these receptors are highly expressed in lymph node, lung, liver, bone marrow, and skin where melanoma tends to metastasize (28). In lung metastases the integrin α-3-β-1 expressed in tumor cells binds to laminin-5 in the basement membrane of pulmonary vasculature (29). The receptor CXCR4 on breast cancer cells results in preferential accumulation of these cells in lung tissue where the chemokine CXCL12 ligand is abundantly produced in lung tissue (30).

SUCCESSFUL MIGRATION FROM BLOOD VESSELS TO TARGET TISSUE

The phenomenon of extravasation includes first the attachment to the microvasculature in the target tissue or organ through adhesion receptors.

Depending on the tissue type, the metastasizing cells (seeds) may first proliferate in the intravascular space forming a mass that mechanically disrupts the vasculature (31). The role of the protein ezrin in osteosarcoma metastasis has been studied by Kahnna et al. (32). It appears that this cytoskeletal anchoring protein is important in establishing adherence between osteosarcoma cells and the vasculature. Blockage of ezrin leads to an increase in cancer cell death before extravasation.

The role of vascular permeability factors is also a crucial one. VEGF is an example of a molecule that enhances extravasation by the separation of endothelial cells by affecting the cell junctions through the Src family of kinases (33).

What is very interesting about this particular feature of colonization is that VEGF is produced by some lines of metastatic cells. This observation is another example of the complex nature of the metastatic process and also of a property giving a survival advantage to cells that are capable of producing successful metastases.

COLONIZATION

As already indicated Paget in 1889 referred to malignant cells as seeds that only would grow in certain soils. There are examples of different tumors that colonize more specifically given organs, for example, prostate cancer metastasizes to bone and only rarely to lung and liver, on the other hand breast cancer frequently colonizes bone, as well as lung, liver, and ovaries. Another remarkable example of organ-specific metastasis is the fact that malignant melanoma originating in the uvea consistently metastasizes to the liver.

A very important example of soil specificity was shown by the work where peritoneal fluid containing ovarian cancer cells was diverted to the inferior vena cava as a palliative measure in patients with wide spread metastasis in the peritoneal cavity. The absence of any significant metastases in organs continuously exposed to these tumor cells greatly emphasizes the importance of the "soil" in the metastatic process (34, 35).

To understand these phenomena it is clear that one must consider that there is a specific attractant or a special niche in the target organ or "soil." By the same token the metastasizing tumor must have the proper characteristics that allow it to reside in the niche and successfully grow.

THE SOIL

The concept of "premetastatic niche" refers to the series of changes that occur in the future site of metastasis or "soil" in preparation for the reception of the tumoral cells. These reactions start with release of chemokines and other mediators by the tumor. Among the many alterations that lead to the formation of a premetastatic niche, there have been described three main phenomena (36).

One of them is the secretion by the primary tumor of vascular endothelial growth factor A (VGEF-A) which in turns activates bone marrow-derived hematopoietic progenitor cells (HPCs), endothelial progenitor cells (EPCs), as well as mature endothelial cells. Simultaneously the premetastatic sites show an increase in fibronectin in the subcapsular region of the target organ. Additionally, there is production of metalloproteases in the recipient stroma.

These events are synchronized in the following manner. The circulating HPCs produce VLA-4 (α-4-β-1) integrin that allows their adhesion to the future sites of metastasis. This adhesion occurs thanks to the presence of recently formed fibronectin in the subcapsular region of the target organ. Simultaneously this process is facilitated by the production of metalloproteases, specifically MMP9 that render the recipient stroma more permeable to additional HPCs and to the incoming tumoral cells.

The selective migration of HPCs and EPCs to the premetastatic niche along with the increased production of fibronectin and metalloproteases contributes to a chain reaction that activates other mediators such as chemokines and integrins that ultimately promote the lodging and proliferation of tumor cells in the new microenvironment.

Even after the arrival of the HPCs in the new "soil" they maintain their undifferentiated state and continue to express markers of progenitor cells. These progenitor cells show two types of VGEF receptors. The cells that express receptor 1 (VGEFR1) promote extravasation and retention of VEGFR2 + EPCs, and in conjunction they promote metastasis and angiogenesis. The complete mechanism of recruitment of these cells vital to preparation of the special niche for the tumor cells is not fully described and further investigation is underway.

COLONIZATION: MICRO- VS. MACROMETASTASIS

The fact that tumor cells arrive and establish residence at a given organ does not mean that they will necessarily proliferate in the new location. For the successful establishment of a metastasis several crucial events must take place, among which we can cite angiogenesis and cell cycle activity. Some cells, however, cannot at a given site enter the cell cycle and remain dormant. Interestingly enough, cells that are dormant when extracted and grown in vitro can produce tumors. It is obvious then that there are intrinsic differences in genomic make up of tumor cells that have to be evaluated to understand the factors intrinsic to the cell (seed) but also the microenvironmental pressure of the soil.

A very appropriate example of the difference between micro- and macrometastasis can be found in the sentinel lymph node studies in human malignant melanoma. In the last years several studies emerged trying to predict the significance of the volume of metastatic disease found in the sentinel lymph node. It appears that there is a direct relationship between the size of the metastatic focus in the sentinel lymph node and the presence of additional metastasis in the remaining (nonsentinel) lymph nodes. In a recent study by Van Akkoi et al. the presence of deposits 0.1 mm or less in size was not associated with positive metastases in the nonsentinel lymph nodes.

The sentinel lymph node can also be used as an example of how the "soil" undergoes functional and morphological changes in the presence of a tumoral clone. Cochran et al. (37) have demonstrated that in fact there is a profound immune downregulation in the positive sentinel lymph nodes when compared to the negative ones. They showed that sentinel lymph nodes harboring metastasis have a marked diminution in their paracortical area as well as a decreased number of dendritic cells, when compared to negative lymph nodes. Furthermore the dendritic cells present in the affected lymph nodes lack the numerous dendrites needed for antigen presentation. In a more recent article (38), the same author presents the positive sentinel lymph node as a selected target made susceptible to metastasis through the production of chemical mediators by the tumor cells, adding one more example to the recently discussed phenomenon of "premetastatic niche."

The dormancy of tumor cells as evidenced by the presence of minimal residual disease is highly significant because these quiescent cells are not able to be affected by different types of eradication therapy. It would also be very important to know what factors will lead these cells after many years to give late stage metastases, sometimes as long as 20 years or more, such as in melanoma and breast cancer.

CONCLUSION

All of these studies relate to basically the genomic expression of the tumor cell of origin and how that tumor cell reacts with the environmental milieu.

It is very clear that the metastatic phenomenon is highly complex. The presence of a tumor cell changes the environment of the body by its production of soluble factors that spread to other tissues and alter completely certain specific sites to which the cell may metastasize. Finally the complex interaction that follows between the cell and its environment leads to great challenges in understanding the phenomenon but also to develop pharmacogenomic approaches to control the metastatic phenomenon. What is so important from recent investigations is that not only must the research efforts be directed at understanding the critical aspects of the tumor cell, but also the aspects in the preferred site of metastases that could be altered therapeutically so that the tumor cell would not be able to successfully attach to that site and proliferate.

REFERENCES

1. Paget S. The distribution of secondary growths in cancer of the breast. Lancet 1:571-3, 1889
2. Ewing J. Neoplastic Diseases. 6th edition. WB Saunders, Philadelphia. 1928
3. Sugarbaker EV. Cancer metastasis: a product of tumor host interactions. Curr Probl Cancer 3:1-59, 1979
4. Hart IR, Fidler IJ. Role of organ selectivity in the determination of metastatic patterns of B16 melanoma. Cancer Res 40:2281-87, 1980
5. Fidler IJ. Modulation of the organ environment for the treatment of cancer metastasis (editorial). J Natl Cancer Inst 84:1588-92, 1995
6. Schakert G, Fidler IJ. Site-specific metastasis of mouse melanomas and a fibrosarcoma in the brain or the meninges of syngeneic animals. Cancer Res 48:3478-3484, 1988b
7. Fidler IJ. Critical determinants of metastasis. Semin Cancer Biol 12:89-96, 2002
8. Fidler IJ. Critical factors in the biology of human cancer metastasis: Twenty-Eighth GHA Clowes Memorial Lecture. Cancer Res 50:6130-6138, 1990
9. Talmadge JE, Fidler IJ. Cancer metastasis is selective or random depending on the parent tumor population. Nature 297:593-4, 1982
10. Liotta LA, Steeg PS, Stetler-Stevenson WG. Cancer metastasis and angiogenesis: an imbalance of positive and negative regulation. Cell 64:327-336, 1991
11. Bernards R, Weinberg RA. A progression puzzle. Nature. 2002 Aug 22;418(6900):823
12. Miller AJ, Mihm MC Jr. Melanoma. N Engl J Med. 2006 Jul 6;355(1):51-65
13. Axelson H, Fredlund E, Ovenberger M, Landberg G, Pahlman S. Hypoxia-induced dedifferentiation of tumor cells–a mechanism behind heterogeneity and aggressiveness of solid tumors. Semin Cell Dev Biol. 2005 Aug-Oct;16(4-5):554-63. Epub 2005 Apr 26. Review
14. Wang H, Fu W, Im JH, Zhou Z, Santoro SA, Iyer V, DiPersio CM, Yu QC, Quaranta V, Al-Mehdi A, Muschel RJ. Tumor cell alpha3beta1 integrin and vascular laminin-5 mediate pulmonary arrest and metastasis. J Cell Biol. 2004 Mar 15;164(6):935-41
15. Byers HR, Etoh T, Vink J, Franklin N, Gattoni-Celli S, Mihm MC Jr. Actin organization and cell migration of melanoma cells relate to differential expression of integrins and actin-associated proteins. J Dermatol. 1992 Nov;19(11):847-52
16. Wicki A, Lehembre F, Wick N, Hantusch B, Kerjaschki D, and Christofori G. (2006). Tumor invasion in the absence of epithelial-mesenchymal transition: podoplanin-mediated remodeling of the actin cytoskeleton. Cancer Cell 9, 261-272
17. Wai PY, Guo L, Gao C, Mi Z, Guo H, Kuo PC. Osteopontin inhibits macrophage nitric oxide synthesis to enhance tumor proliferation. Surgery. 2006 Aug;140(2):132-40
18. Bonnet D, Dick JE. Human acute myeloid leukemia is organized as a hierarchy that originates from a primitive hematopoietic cell. Nat Med 1997;3:730-737
19. Beachy PA, Karhadkar SS, Berman DM. Tissue repair and stem cell renewal in carcinogenesis. Nature. 2004 Nov 18;432(7015):324-31. Review

20. Gupta GP, Massague J. Cancer metastasis: building a framework. Cell. 2006 Nov 17;127(4):679-95. Review

21. Overall CM, Kleifeld O. Tumour microenvironment - opinion: validating matrix metalloproteinases as drug targets and anti-targets for cancer therapy. Nat Rev Cancer. 2006 Mar;6(3):227-39. Review

22. Orimo A, Gupta PB, Sgroi DC, Arenzana-Seisdedos F, Delaunay T, Naeem R, Carey VJ, Richardson AL, Weinberg RA. Stromal fibroblasts present in invasive human breast carcinomas promote tumor growth and angiogenesis through elevated SDF-1/CXCL12 secretion. Cell. 2005 May 6;121(3):335-48

23. Ruiter D, Bogenrieder T, Elder D, Herlyn M. Melanoma-stroma interactions: structural and functional aspects. Lancet Oncol. 2002 Jan;3(1):35-43. Review

24. Hanahan D, Folkman J. Patterns and emerging mechanisms of the angiogenic switch during tumorigenesis. Cell 1996 Aug 9;86(3):353-64. Review

25. Dadras SS, Lange-Asschenfeldt B, Velasco P, Nguyen L, Vora A, Muzikansky A, Jahnke K, Hauschild A, Hirakawa S, Mihm MC, Detmar M. Tumor lymphangiogenesis predicts melanoma metastasis to sentinel lymph nodes. Mod Pathol. 2005 Sep;18(9):1232-42

26. Nash GF, Turner LF, Scully MF, and Kakkar AK. (2002). Platelets and cancer. Lancet Oncol. 3, 425-430

27. Ruiter DJ, van Krieken JH, van Muijen GN, de Waal RM. Tumour metastasis: is tissue an issue? Lancet Oncol. 2001 Feb;2(2):109-12. Review

28. Morales J, Homey B, Vicari AP, Hudak S, Oldham E, Hedrick J, Orozco R, Copeland NG, Jenkins NA, McEvoy LM, Zlotnik A. CTAK, a skin associated chemokine that preferentially attracts skin homing memory T cells. Proc Natl Acad Sci USA 96:14470-75, 1999

29. Wang H, Fu W, Im JH, Zhou Z, Santoro SA, Iyer V, DiPersio CM, Yu QC, Quaranta V, Al-Mehdi A, Muschel RJ. Tumor cell alpha3beta1 integrin and vascular laminin-5 mediate pulmonary arrest and metastasis. J Cell Biol. 2004 Mar 15;164(6):935-41

30. Muller A, Homey B, Soto H, Ge N, Catron D, Buchanan ME, McClanahan T, Murphy E, Yuan W, Wagner SN, Barrera JL, Mohar A, Verastegui E, Zlotnik A. Involvement of chemokine receptors in breast cancer metastasis. Nature. 2001 Mar 1;410(6824):50-6

31. Al-Mehdi, AD, Tozawa K, Fisher AD, Shientag L, Lee A, and Muschel RJ. (2000). Intravascular origin of metastasis from the proliferation of endothelium-attached tumor cells: a new model for metastasis. Nat. Med. 6, 100-102

32. Kahnna C, Wan X, Bose S, Cassaday R, Olomu O, Mendoza A, Yeung C, Gorlick R, Hewitt SM, and Helman LJ. (2004). The membrane-cytoskeleton linker ezrin is necessary for osteosarcoma metastasis. Nat. Med. 10, 182-186

33. Criscuoli ML, Nguyen M, and Eliceiri BP. (2005). Tumor metastasis but not tumor growth is dependent on Src-mediated vascular permeability. Blood 105, 1508-1514

34. Tarin D, Price JE, Kettlewell MGW, Souter RG, Vass ACR, Crossley B. Clinicopathological observations on metastasis in man studied in patients treated with peritoneovenous shunts, Br Med J 288:749-751, 1984a

35. Tarin D, Price JE, Kettlewell MGW, Souter RG, Vass ACR, Crossley B. Mechanisms of human tumor metastasis studied in patients with peritoneovenous shunts. Cancer Res 44:3584-3592, 1984b

36. Kaplan RN, Rafii S, Lyden D. Preparing the "soil": the premetastatic niche. Cancer Res. 2006 Dec 1;66(23):11089-93. Review

37. Cochran AJ, Huang RR, Lee J, Itakura E, Leong SP, Essner R. Tumour-induced immune modulation of sentinel lymph nodes. Nat Rev Immunol. 2006 Sep;6(9):659-70. Review

38. Cochran AJ, Morton DL, Stern S, Lana AM, Essner R, Wen DR. Sentinel lymph nodes show profound downregulation of antigen-presenting cells of the paracortex: implications for tumor biology and treatment. Mod Pathol. 2001 Jun;14(6):604-8

10. PRECLINICAL MODELS OF REGIONAL LYMPH NODE TUMOR METASTASIS

S. DAVID NATHANSON

Henry Ford Health System, Detroit, Michigan, USA

INTRODUCTION

Metastasis to regional lymph nodes (RLNs) is clinically important. The adverse effects of RLN metastasis on patient survival from malignant tumors was first recognized in the eighteenth and nineteenth centuries by European physicians. Surgical management of these metastatic cancers was accomplished in the late nineteenth and early twentieth centuries (1) but the overall patient survival following these technically successful operations remained fairly poor. The latest advance in the direction of simplicity and decreased morbidity is the sentinel lymph node (SLN) biopsy, an operation that revolutionized the management of melanoma and breast cancer (2–4), and has potential use in other malignancies. The anatomic and mechanical aspects of the sentinel node concept focused attention on mechanisms of RLN metastasis (5).

The quest to find causes for RLN metastasis, initially rather primitive in its scope became more sophisticated by the end of the twentieth century, aided by rapid advances in molecular biology. Critical to the emerging understanding of the mechanisms of RLN metastasis was the development of spontaneous RLN metastasis models in animals.

Most of our knowledge of human biochemistry, physiology, endocrinology, and pharmacology has been derived from initial studies in subhuman animal models (6). Much vital information about hematogenous metastasis was gleaned from animal models. The complex interactive events of tumor metastasis were largely speculated prior to Fidler's landmark studies in mice (7). Preclinical models of experimental metastasis involved injection of tumor cells directly into the blood stream, through peripheral veins, arteries, and the heart or the spleen (8). Metastases usually formed in the first organ encountered by the tumor cells in the circulation. In the most common murine models, tail vein injection resulted in metastases in the lungs. Tumor cells injected into the cardiac left ventricle commonly metastasized to bone. Tumor injected into the spleen commonly caused liver metastases (9).

Biochemical and molecular studies of metastases led to a much greater understanding of the mechanisms of hematogenous metastasis (10). In just over 30 years, we evolved from crude pathological observations of systemic metastases to an advanced understanding of the molecular events of tumor progression, invasion, tumor cell motility, adhesion molecules, proteolytic enzyme secretion, angiogenesis, systemic embolization, arrest at distant organs, and growth at the metastatic site.

Animal models have been invaluable in the continuing study of systemic metastasis of malignant tumors (10). When scientists studied the crucial steps in metastasis at a biochemical and molecular level, they were often drawn to ask whether the unique molecules that seemed important in vitro were functional in vivo. Such experiments required whole organisms and traditionally could not ethically be accomplished in humans. Effective treatment regimens developed from animal models and have been established as part of the modern management of colorectal, lung, melanoma, breast, and other human cancers. Systemic treatments directed at specific targets, identified as critical to metastasis, will likely continue to provide improved outcomes in the future.

The effectiveness of studying the experimental metastatic process is undeniable but there are steps missing that fail to mimic the natural process of metastasis in human subjects. Tumors that originate spontaneously from epithelial organ structures must first develop the capacity to proliferate and invade the local parenchyma, a process that requires a change in the genetic, molecular, and biochemical pathways in the cells (10, 11). Interaction between the tumor and the extracellular matrix, the host immune system and the host blood and lymphatic vessels are indispensable to the growth and metastasis of the tumor. These vital processes in tumor progression and metastasis are bypassed by the artificial injection of tumor directly into the vascular compartment and could possibly also affect the arrest phase of metastasis in distant organs.

Clinical and experimental lymphatic metastases have strong similarities. To study the process of RLN metastasis clinically relevant models of tumor metastasis should mimic the pathological processes observed in patients with malignant tumors (11). Animal models of RLN metastasis proved vital in dissecting the mechanisms of this common event. Spontaneous metastasis to RLNs is often seen in primary human tumors of epithelial origin (12–14), and is also observed in spontaneous nonhuman animal tumors (8). This has prompted scientists to develop clinically relevant murine models in which RLN-metastasizing tumors can be produced with uniformity.

While knowledge of hematogenous tumor metastasis expanded, the mechanisms of lymphatic metastasis remained largely uncharted and with very little hypothesis-driven research. Spontaneous metastasis proved more difficult to study in animals than experimental metastasis because tumors injected into extravascular tissues did not always metastasize (15). The experiments took longer and were more expensive to perform. Although many primary human tumors growing in various organs could invade blood vessels directly and metastasize via the hematogenous route, most invaded lymphatic capillaries and metastasized first to the SLN (2, 3, 16). In vitro and in vivo experiments yielded valuable insights about the motility, chemotaxis, adhesion receptor expression, proteolytic enzyme secretion, "homing" patterns that mimic immune cell trafficking, gene expression, proliferation, and apoptosis of tumors that metastasize to lymph nodes compared to those that do not (5). Modern molecular biology allowed researchers to identify and specifically target molecules that are overexpressed in tumors that metastasized to lymph nodes. Gene insertions or deletions were reported in the host animal or the tumor cells and spontaneous lymph node metastasis rates observed. Other types of spontaneous metastasis experiments looked at exogenous treatment of animals with drugs, antibodies, peptides, or nucleotides that blocked those molecules which were found to be differently expressed in tumors that metastasized to lymph nodes.

This chapter highlights the development of animal models of spontaneous RLN metastasis. Initial studies focused on anatomy and pathophysiology of tumor cell entry into lymphatics and spread to the nodes. From those relatively crude beginnings came models that intersected with the biochemistry of primary tumors, looking for changes in tumor cells that might explain their propensity to invade lymphatics. Tumor and molecular biology were evolving concomitantly and the importance of the extracellular matrix in tumor growth and invasion became more apparent. A critical part of the research was the identification of lymphatic endothelial markers which enabled scientists to differentiate blood and lymphatic vessels. The investigation of possible treatment modalities, such as external (physical) stimuli and drugs and/or biologicals that increase/decrease RLN metastasis resulted in a greater understanding of the mechanisms of lymph node metastasis. The review shows how vital animal experiments have been in the quest for information. The first step in this story was the development of tumor models with reproducible spread to the RLNs.

ANATOMIC ANIMAL MODELS OF REGIONAL LYMPH NODE METASTASIS

The natural history of malignant tumors depends somewhat on the primary organ involved and from which component structure of the organ the tumor originated. Models of lymphatic metastasis were initially developed to mimic clinical cancers. Human tumors arising from epithelial components of the major organs are most likely to metastasize to RLNs while sarcomas rarely do. Carr (19) developed an anatomic–pathologic model of lymph node metastasis in rats and described histologic events at the primary tumor site and in the draining lymph nodes. He showed that tumor cells penetrate lymphatic vessels by diapedesis and segmental endothelial necrosis in areas of massive perilymphangitis. Many scientists who tried to create models of RLN metastases found that the usual transplantation sites (in the subcutaneous space, usually on the back of mice or rats) did not produce RLN metastases. Transplantation into the anatomic organ of origin (orthotopic) often would mimic the clinical lymph node metastatic pattern (Fig. 1).

In many instances models were developed in which tumor cells, often from tissue culture, sometimes from blocks of tumor tissue taken from human patients, were transplanted into an intact animal. The animals were observed over a period of weeks or months and autopsy data documented, with particular attention to tumor growth rates, the incidence of metastasis to RLNs and to distant sites. Most of the experiments described in the following sections were done using syngeneic mice or rats, some in immunocompromised murine systems, and, as molecular and genetic technology developed, in genetically modified animals. Some genetically modified animals were produced with the express intention of producing spontaneous tumors after birth, usually in adults. In some experiments tumor cells were modified by insertion of genes into those cells in culture (stable transfection) that would induce overexpression of certain proteins (receptors expressed on the cell membrane or cytokines secreted by tumor cells into the locoregional spaces). Such altered cells were transplanted into intact or genetically modified animals and their metastatic growth compared to that of mock-transfected cells. In later sections of the chapter we will examine exogenous treatment of tumor-bearing animals where the effects on RLN metastasis may have been partly or wholly based on their interaction with genetic material in the growing tumors. Intact animals or animal tissues have also been used to look at particular functions thought to be important in the development of RLN metastasis, such as lymphangiogenesis and chemokinesis.

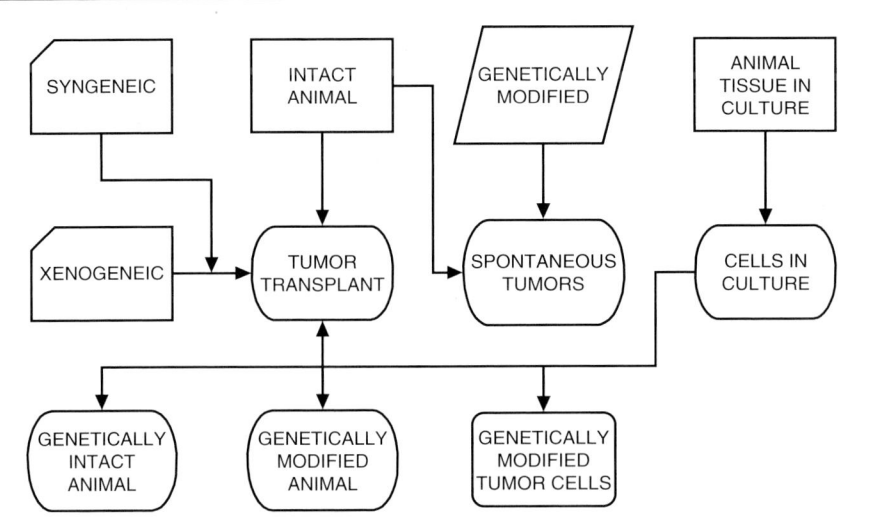

Figure 1. Summary of the evolution of animal models used to study RLN metastasis

Spontaneous tumors occur in outbred animals. Those that we know best occur in about 4% of the over 100 million pets living in the United States (8). Little is known about the molecular basis of these tumors, and there is almost no knowledge that distinguishes the mechanisms of RLN metastasis in animals from humans.

Transplant Models

Spontaneous tumors grown in highly inbred syngeneic host animals, removed surgically and placed in culture, can be transplanted into subsequent generations of naïve syngeneic hosts. Growth of tumor in these recipients inevitably skips the "normal" steps of tumor progression. Such steps could be important to the development of lymphatic metastasis. Syngeneic tumors occasionally resulted in lymph node metastases (see Table 1, with references). Certain maneuvers were found to encourage RLN metastasis. For example, B16 melanoma injected into the footpad of syngeneic C57BL/6 mice reproduced the entire cascade of RLN metastasis seen in human melanoma. Highly selected clones of the B16, such as the F10 clone, metastasized more efficiently to the RLNs (17). In other models, lymph node metastasis occurred only when the syngeneic transplant was injected orthotopically (18).

The advantage of syngeneic or xenogeneic tumor models is the rapidity with which new drugs or other treatment modalities can be evaluated in vivo. Most of the experiments described in Tables 1 and 2 were completed in 3 months or less and valuable information obtained. As is true of research in general, perhaps the most important effect of this extensive animal research was the questions that were

Table 1. Syngeneic tumors that metastasized to regional lymph nodes (RLNs)

Histology	Species	References
Prostate	Mouse	(20–26)
Prostate	Rat	(27–30)
Oral (squamous)	Hamster	(31–35)
Ear (VX2)	Rabbit	(36–41)
Colorectal	Rat	(42)
Lung (adenocarcinoma)	Mouse	(43, 44)
Lung (adenocarcinoma)	Rat	(45)
Pancreas (endocrine)	Mouse	(46)
Pancreas (exocrine)	Rat	(47)
Breast	Mouse	(48–50)
Breast	Rat	(51–53)
Skin (squamous)	Mouse	(54)
Skin (melanoma)	Mouse	(15, 17, 55)
Skin (melanoma)	Goat	(56)
Ovary	Mouse	(57)
Kidney	Mouse	(58)
Walker carcinoma	Rat	(59, 60)
Sarcoma	Rat	(45, 61)
Sarcoma	Mouse	(50)
Uterus	Rat	(62)
Liver	Mouse	(63)
Liver	Rat	(64)

Table 2. Xenogeneic (human) tumors implanted in animals that spontaneously metastasized to RLNs after transplantation

Histology	Species	References
Prostate	Mouse	(65–73)
Oral (squamous)	Mouse	(74–80)
Oral (adenoid cystic)	Mouse	(78)
Nasopharyngeal	Mouse	(81)
Colorectal	Mouse	(82–84)
Colorectal	Rat	(42)
Lung (adenocarcinoma)	Mouse	(85–88)
Pancreas (exocrine)	Mouse	(89, 90)
Breast	Mouse	(91, 92)
Lymphoma	Mouse	(93)
Testis	Mouse	(94)
Testis (nonseminoma)	Mouse	(94, 95)
Stomach	Mouse	(96, 97)
Kidney	Mouse	(98)
Cervix	Mouse	(99)

generated about the mechanisms of lymphatic metastasis. Great advances were being made in the 1980s and 1990s in understanding hematogenous metastases (10, 11) and it was assumed that these same biochemical and molecular events also occurred in tumors destined to spread to lymph nodes. But there were unique aspects of lymphatic metastasis that needed to be addressed.

It is still not clear why tumor cells preferentially enter lymphatic vessels rather than blood vessels at the site of invasion in the primary tumor. In the early days of evaluating the relationship between tumor cells and RLN metastasis, there was no good way to clearly differentiate lymphatic vessels from blood vessels. Light and electron microscopes were the only tools available to identify entry of tumor cells into vessels. Differentiation of the type of vessel (blood vessel or lymphatic) depended on the expertise of the observer, and the observations were crude. Identification of tumoral and/or peritumoral lymphatics depended on morphological criteria (5). Endothelial stains initially could not differentiate blood vessel capillaries from lymphatics.

Embryological studies identified specific lymphatic markers and this led to the identification of the molecular biology of lymphatic proliferation in and around tumors. Ligands were found that bound to lymphatic endothelium and induced proliferation, migration, sprouting, and formation of new lymphatics. The genes for these ligands and the receptors to which they bound were studied intensely. Gene and protein sequencing followed. Some tumor cells were found to spontaneously overproduce lymphangiogenic cytokines (100). Experiments that evaluated the effects of these cytokines on RLN metastasis included those that introduced genes into tumor cells. Gene expression sometimes induced a high locoregional concentration of these proteins. Transplantation of genetically engineered tumor cells that expressed high concentrations of these cytokines provided exciting information about the development of new peritumoral lymphatics, entry of syngeneic tumor cells into those lymphatics, methods that inhibit entry of cells into peritumoral lymphatics, the morphology of the lymphangion associated with the tumor, lymph flow velocity, and the rate of tumor cell entry into the SLN. Many different genes have been stably transfected into tumor cells and transplanted into rodents. Some are described in this chapter (see below).

Spontaneous Tumors in Animals

Spontaneous Tumors in Outbred Animals

Cancers occur naturally in many animals, including pets, such as cats and dogs. The large numbers of pets with cancer in the United States (in excess of 4 million) (8), many of whom are expected to visit veterinary oncologists, may provide a good source of information for RLN metastasis models from primary tumor sites. There are potential advantages to studying lymph node metastasis in dogs. These animals are genetically closer to humans than the murine systems that are commonly used (101). Tumor progression is faster than in the comparable human tumor (such as prostate, breast, lung, head and neck, melanoma) (8), and the tumors behave in ways that are similar to the human counterparts. These tumors are also likely to be similar to their human counterparts in other ways, such as the relationship to environmental factors in carcinogenesis, and the reaction of the host animal to tumor growth. However, very little lymph node metastasis research has been done in this outbred population. It is easier to study highly inbred and/or immune-compromised murine models in which metastasis progression occurs much quicker than in larger animals. Now that the dog genome has been sequenced, it is likely that molecular targets involved in this species and RLN metastasis will be pursued. This will undoubtedly enhance our understanding of the mechanisms of RLN metastasis.

Spontaneous Tumors in Transgenic Animal Models

The vast majority of spontaneously arising or transplanted tumors in murine models did not metastasize to the RLNs (8, 102). Understanding the molecular pathways that underlie spontaneous RLN metastasis allowed the generation of transgenic mouse models that are shown in Table 3.

In these models genetic manipulation not only induced carcinogenesis, but was also associated with RLN metastasis. Qian et al. (46), in an elegant pancreatic islet cell transgenic tumor progression model, showed how introduction of a gene changed the natural progression of these tumors in RipTag2 mice that normally did not metastasize to the RLNs. Creation of double transgenic mice by introduction of L-selectin produced a pancreatic islet cell tumor model with RLN metastasis.

Mandriota et al. (107) reproduced the pancreatic β cell tumors described by Qian et al. (46). In single transgenic RipTag2 mice that developed spontaneous pancreatic tumors, no RLN metastases occurred. In double transgenic mice that secreted excess VEGF-C, driven by the rat insulin promoter, the animals frequently developed lymph node metastases. These experiments produced important, perhaps irrefutable, evidence that VEGF-C is indispensable to the development of RLN metastasis, although this may not apply to all tumor systems in animals.

Table 3. Genetically engineered animal tumor models with spontaneous RLN metastasis

Gene or product	Tumor type	References
Pten	Prostate	(20)
TRAMP	Prostate	(26)
Probasin-Tag	Neuroblastoma	(103)
Cryptdin2-Tag	Prostate	(104)
T7-pkc	Squamous cell carcinoma	(54)
Mt-MET	Breast	(105)
MMTV-wnt-1	Breast	(106)
Rip-VEGF-C/RipTag	Pancreas (endocrine)	(107)
Probasin-Tag	Prostate	(108)
Kras/Ink4aKO	Pancreas	(109)
L-selectin	Pancreas (endocrine)	(46)
NCAM-deficient	Pancreas (endocrine)	(110)

The ability of scientists to incorporate genes into animals has helped advance the understanding of the mechanisms of spontaneous RLN metastasis. Potential molecular mechanisms were evaluated by insertion of genes of interest at the zygote or early embryonic stage of small animal development (see Table 3 above).

Other genetic mechanisms were also useful, such as deletion of genes in "knockout" mice. Metastasis genes have been identified in experimental metastasis models and these may also play a role in spontaneous metastasis models, although this area of research needs quite extensive work to prove this hypothesis (111, 112).

Animal Models Used to Study Biochemical Changes Associated with RLN Metastasis

The RLN metastasis literature has expanded considerably in the past three decades and biochemical alterations investigated. Table 4 shows biochemical correlates with increased invasiveness, growth, motility, and adhesion of a number of spontaneous

Table 4. Biochemical/molecular changes in cells/tumors with increased metastasis to lymph nodes

Tumor/species	Recipient	Function studied	Biochemical correlates	References
Oral/human	Mouse	Increased invasiveness	1. Increased UPA receptors 2. Increased integrin $\beta1$ 3. Increased MMP-1	(75)
Lung/human	Mouse	Increased primary tumor growth	1. Increased UPA 2. Increased MMP-2 3. Increased MMP-9	(86)
Gastric/human	Mouse	1. Increased motility 2. Increased adhesion	1. Increased integrin $\beta1\alpha2$ 2. Increased HLA 3. Increased LFA 1	(96, 97)
Uterus/rat	Rat	Increased invasion	Decreased ICAM-1	(62)
Melanoma/mouse	Mouse	Increased motility	Increased membrane laminin	(113, 160)

syngeneic and xenogeneic tumor systems that metastasized to the RLNs. The changes do not necessarily correlate specifically with the tendency for RLN metastasis, because similar up- or downregulation of proteolytic enzymes, cell membrane adhesion (and other) molecules, major histocompatability (and other) antigens have also been described in experimental metastasis systems that correlate with hematogenous metastasis. All of these changes have been studied extensively in vitro evaluating the process of invasion.

ANIMAL MODELS OF LYMPHANGIOGENESIS

Introduction: The Biology of Lymphatic Vessels

An understanding of the biology of lymphatic vessels evolved rapidly over the past 10 years because of the need to understand the mechanisms of tumor metastasis, lymphedema, immune responses to organisms and foreign antigens, obesity, and many other diseases (100).

Figure 2 summarizes the current study of lymphangiogenesis in animal model systems other than tumors. Important work in the embryonic development of the lymphatic system helped identify sequential expression of specific genes and their products that evolved over time.

In mice lymphatic endothelial cells (LECs) arise by sprouting from embryonic veins in the jugular and perimesonephric areas around embryonic day 10 (100). Prox-1 and VEGF-C are essential for migration of LECs and the formation of a primary lymphatic plexus. In VEGF-C null mice LECs initially differentiate in the cardinal veins but do not migrate to form primary lymph sacs. The receptor for VEGF-C, VEGFR-3, is also essential and its absence leads to embryonic death.

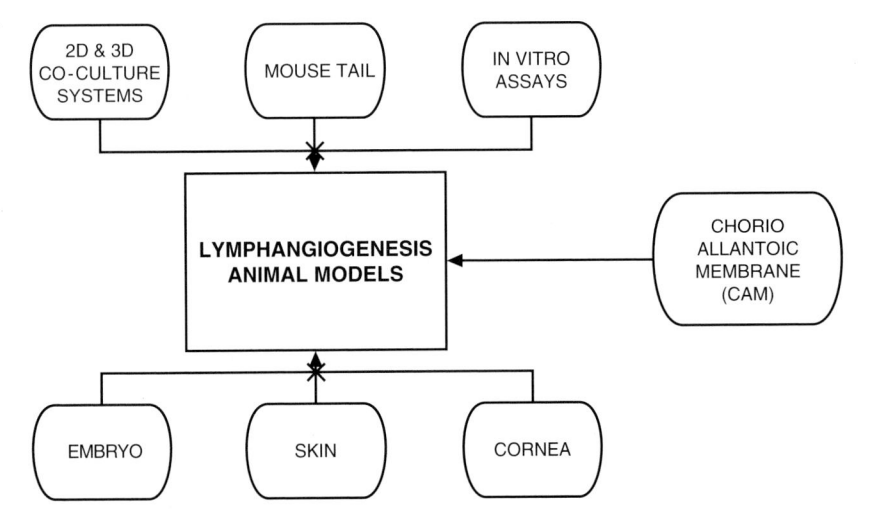

Figure 2. Animal models of lymphangiogenesis

VEGF-D, an important ligand for VEGFR-3 and 2, is not essential to the developing lymphatic system of the mouse embryo. The development of a superficial lymphatic capillary plexus and collecting lymphatic vessels is entirely related to a remodeling process in late embryogenesis and in the postnatal period. The maturation of the lymphatic vasculature requires Ang2, Ephrin B2, Foxc2, and Podoplanin. Other genes and growth factors may be involved in the development of new lymphatic vessels (102).

Jeltsch et al. (114) recognized that overexpression of VEGF-C in transgenic mice induced lymphatic vessel hyperplasia. Oh et al. (115) demonstrated the role of VEGF-C in new lymphatic vessel growth in an avian chorioallantoic membrane model. Enholm et al. (116) consolidated this important observation by administering an adenovirus vector of VEGF-C in high concentration into interstitial spaces of adult mice, producing lymphatic hyperplasia. Kubo et al. (117) blocked lymphangiogenesis in a mouse cornea model by blocking the receptor for VEGF-C and VEGFR-3. Boardman and Swartz (118) measured VEGF-C at the edge of a circumferential wound in the adult mouse tail and found new lymphatic vessels bridging the wound gap and these were associated with high tissue levels of VEGF-C. VEGF-C and VEGFR-3 are commonly coexpressed at sites where lymphatic vessels sprout endothelial cells (119). While other cytokines can stimulate new lymphatic growth in vivo, the induction of new lymphatic vessels in embryos and adult animals is highly dependent upon the concentration of VEGF-C.

Lymphangiogenesis, Tumor Growth, and Lymph Node Metastasis

The process of tumor cell entry into lymphatics was observed by light and electron microscopy (19). Sophisticated studies in animal embryos, coupled with the discovery of markers specific for LECs (120), resulted in the observation that tumors often induced new lymphatic capillary growth (lymphangiogenesis) by producing VEGF-C and other cytokines that bind to lymphatic endothelial receptors and stimulate proliferation, tube formation, and longitudinal growth (121).

RLN metastasis is a clinically vital event in the staging and management of malignancies of epithelial origin (1). We know from many clinical studies that lymphophilic dyes and radioactive colloids enter the same lymphatic capillaries that are invaded by malignant cells (16). It is easy to understand why some dyes enter those capillaries: the reasons are almost entirely size dependent. If the size of a dye particle is too big, it will stay in the injected tissue in phagocytic cells. If too small, the particles are absorbed into venous capillaries and immediately disseminate through the blood stream. It is only the intermediate-sized inanimate particles (usually between 40 and 100 nm in diameter) that are absorbed by the terminal lymphatics and swept along by a "tide of fluid" to the SLN. However, live tumor cells, larger than 100 nm in diameter, pursue the same lymphatic pathways to the identical SLN to which the inanimate dye flows (122).

Entry of tumor cells into lymphatic capillaries is much more common than the alternate route through venous capillaries in and around the tumor mass, suggesting directional mechanisms that move tumor cells in one direction rather than another. The mechanisms for the metastasis of tumor cells through lymphatic trunks are complex and involve mechanical, biochemical, and molecular interactions. Many disciplines have been involved and, as is often true in understanding biological mechanisms, connecting the preclinical animal with clinical and in vitro experiments requires a pairing of different intellectual disciplines.

One of the major disciplines necessary for the understanding of the mechanisms of RLN metastasis involves the molecular–genetic–embryologic and cell biology arenas. This has been made possible by modern DNA–RNA techniques that allow experts to identify the molecular structures of important cytokines, chemokines, receptors, enzymes, and proteins. Once lymphatic (LECs) and blood vessel endothelial cells (BECs) were accurately distinguishable by specific markers, it became possible to dissect the microscopic and submicroscopic sites of tumor cell entry into peritumoral (and, perhaps, intratumoral) lymphatics and to design experiments that might enable us to interfere with this process.

Syngeneic and xenogeneic tumor cells were genetically modified to produce growth factors. There is a distinctive and convincing association between growth factor-induced lymphangiogenesis and concomitant RLN metastasis. Pro- and antilymphangiogenic molecules can emanate from cancer cells, endothelial cells, stromal cells, blood, and extracellular matrix. VEGFs-C and D have been consistently associated with induction of lymphangiogenesis. Other growth factors were also found capable of stimulating new lymphatic growth (102). The more recent studies of lymphangiogenesis and increased RLN metastasis are summarized in Table 5. These studies showed consistency amongst the different tumor types studied. The experiments are

Table 5. Growth factors that induced lymphangiogenesis and promoted lymph node metastasis

Growth factor	Tumor type	Animal model	References
VEGF-C	Breast	MDA-MB-435 XENOGRAFT	(125)
	Breast	MCF-7 XENOGRAFT	(126)
	Breast	NM-081 XENOGRAFT	(127)
	Breast	C166 MOUSE SYNGENEIC	(128)
	Fibrosarcoma	T241 XENOGRAFT	(124)
	Gastric	AZ521 XENOGRAFT	(129)
	Lung	TKB5 XENOGRAFT	(130)
	Lung	LNM35 XENOGRAFT	(123)
	Melanoma	A375 XENOGRAFT	(131)
	Melanoma	B16F10 SYNGENEIC MOUSE	(124)
	Pancreas	RipTag MOUSE TRANSGENIC	(107)
	Prostate	PC-3 XENOGRAFT	(131)
	Rectal	DLD1 XENOGRAFT	(132)
VEGF-D	Lung	TKB5 XENOGRAFT	(130)
	Pancreas	MiaPaCa-2 XENOGRAFT	(133)
	Pancreas	Capan-1 XENOGRAFT	(133)
	Kidney	293EBNA XENOGRAFT	(134)
VEGF-A	Fibrosarcoma	T241 XENOGRAFT	(135)
	Skin	MOUSE TRANSGENIC	(136)
PDGF-BB	Fibrosarcoma	T241 XENOGRAFT	(137)

from different laboratories, in spontaneous transgenic as well as syngeneic and xenogeneic systems. Lymphangiogenesis appears necessary for most models of RLN metastasis.

He et al. (123) blocked the VEGFR-3 receptor with soluble VEGFR-3-Ig. This inhibited macrometastasis at various times during xenogeneic human lung cancer (LNM35) growth in the ears of nude mice. They showed dramatic lymphangiogenic changes, such as lymphatic sprouting and dilatation, induced by the VEGF-C-producing tumors, facilitated tumor cell entry, and spread to the RLNs. The soluble VEGFR-3-Ig inhibited macrometastasis but not micrometastasis. Initiation of lymphangiogenesis correlated with tumor lymphangiogenesis. Inhibition was not due to direct effect of the inhibitor on tumor cell growth.

Hoshida et al. (124) dissected the contribution of lymphatic vessel biology to lymphatic RLN metastasis. The gene for VEGF-C was stably transfected into B16F10 melanoma and T241 fibrosarcoma cell lines. The cytokine was overproduced by tumors in culture. The cells were also transfected with green fluorescent protein and injected into syngeneic C57Bl/6 (B16F10 melanoma model) or nude (T241 fibrosarcoma model) mice. Intravital imaging, with combined angiography and lymphangiography, showed tumor cell trafficking from the tumor to the SLN. Increased VEGF-C also induced lymphangiectasis, lymphangiogenesis, and the number of cells metastasizing from the primary tumor to the SLN. VEGF-C overexpressing tumors showed increased RLN metastasis in the cervical lymph node, stimulated peritumoral lymphatic hyperplasia, increased total volumetric flow rate in the lymphatics at the ear base, and increased tumor cell delivery to the SLN. Transport of tumor cells in lymphatic vessels was dependent on lymph flow. There was a 200-fold increase in SLN metastasis in VEGF-C overexpressing tumors compared to mock-transfected tumors (with little VEGF-C production). Peritumoral lymphatic hyperplasia and tumor cell delivery to the SLN were significantly suppressed by blocking the receptors for VEGF-C.

The increased surface area of functional lymphatics in the tumor margin may have increased the opportunity for more tumor cells to enter the lymphatics and spread to the SLN. Further studies may show whether new lymphatics are passive recipients of invasive tumor cells, or whether they play a more active role in this process.

Evidence that functional lymphatics occurred at the tumor margin and not within the tumor was first provided by Zeidman et al. (138). Padera et al. (139) produced the most convincing evidence that peritumoral lymphangiogenesis was critical in the development of RLN metastasis. Their study was done using two stable cells lines: T241 murine fibrosarcoma and B16F10 murine melanoma that overexpressed VEGF-C. The cells were transplanted into live mice. VEGF-C expression increased the lymphatic surface area in the tumor margin and also increased lymphatic metastasis in this tumor model but there were no functional intratumoral lymphatics as assessed by four independent functional assays and immunohistochemical staining. These findings suggested that the functional lymphatics in the tumor margin alone were sufficient for lymphatic metastasis. Functional lymphatics at the tumor margin increased lymphatic surface absorptive area, providing more opportunity for cancer cell intravasation. Increased peritumoral lymphatics were accompanied by increased lymphatic metastasis in VEGF-C overexpressing tumors. Tumors that lacked intratumoral lymphatics still metastasized. It is probable that the mechanical forces generated by the growing tumors collapsed intratumoral lymphatics, rendering them nonfunctional. However, the role of intratumoral lymphatics in RLN metastasis is still debated (141).

MECHANICAL ASPECTS OF TUMOR METASTASIS

Interstitial Fluid Pressure (IFP) in Tumors

A mechanical understanding of fluid dynamics in tumors has allowed us to gather further insights into the mechanisms of lymph node metastasis in animals (142). More recently, Swartz et al. (143) brought more experimental validation to this intriguing discipline. Exploration and study of IFP in tumors and surrounding tissues continued to demonstrate the importance of the interface between the primary tumor mass, the extracellular matrix, fluid efflux from tumors, lymph flow from tumors into collecting lymph vessels, and directional flow toward the RLNs. At least three biological mechanisms seem essential to this process (1) induction of new blood vessels (angiogenesis) by cytokines produced by the host and the tumor, (2) a significant increase in interstitial fluid volume (IFV) because of increased fluid leakage through the walls of morphologically abnormal tumor blood vessels, and (3) the secretion of lymphangiogenic cytokines, including VEGFs-C and D with correspondingly more peritumoral lymphatic vessels to accommodate the increased flow from the tumor into the peritumoral interstitium.

Figure 3 summarizes how interstitial hypertension may develop in tumors and how that may translate into increased lymph flow from the primary tumor to the SLN. The pressure dynamics of solid stress (144), produced by tumor cell proliferation in a confined space, adds to the hydrostatic pressure of altered fluid dynamics within tumors and is not shown in the diagram.

Tumor microvessels are leaky (145, 146). Vascular endothelial growth factor-A (VEGF-A), originally called *vascular permeability factor* (VPF), was named after one of its most important properties. Vascular endothelial growth factors (VEGFs) have potent effects on capillary permeability (147). Hyperpermeability to plasma proteins is largely attributable to VEGF-A, one of the most potent vascular permeability agents known. It is about 50,000 times more potent than histamine at inducing blood vessel leakiness (145). Fibrin, one of the proteins that leaks into the interstitial tissues, retarded clearance of edema fluid (148). Overall permeability of tumor vessels is augmented by a large number of fenestrae, disruption of perivascular basement membranes, widened interendothelial junctions, and a greater number of pinocytotic vesicles (149). Coupled with the apparent lack of functional lymphatics in tumors (139), many tumors developed interstitial hypertension.

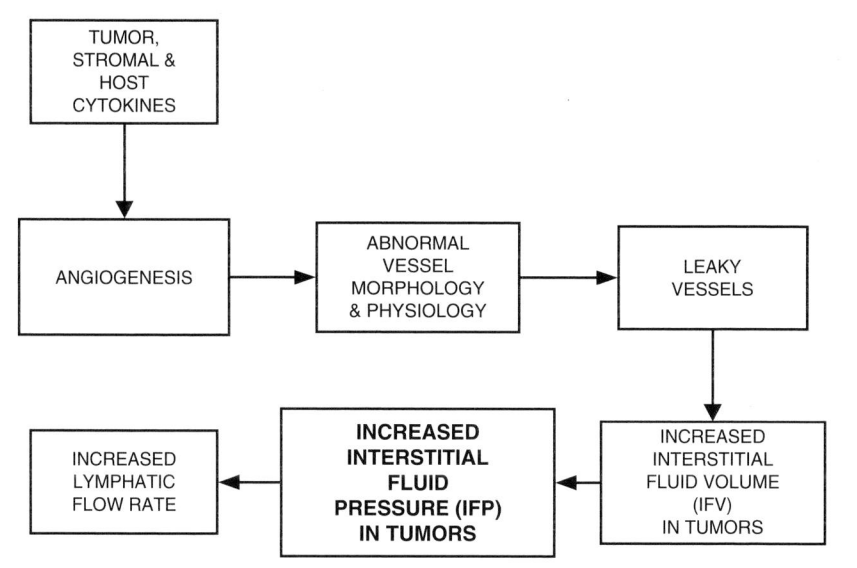

Figure 3. The process of interstitial hypertension and lymphatic flow in animal models

The IFP of normal host tissues surrounding a growing tumor was consistently low, in the range of 0 to −1 mmHg. Hydrostatic pressure in malignant tumors of epithelial origin, such as the human breast, can be as high as 30 mmHg (150, 151). The marked increase in fluid diffusion from the intravascular compartment to the interstitial space of the tumor resulted in marked increases in intratumoral interstitial fluid volume and pressure (148). Lymphatics are absorbing vessels and the rate of absorption is influenced by the capillary filtration of fluid into the interstitium. The pressure differential between the tumor and the surrounding host tissues resulted in diffusion of fluid, often seen as peritumoral edema in radiological studies or in the operating room by surgeons and pathologists, resulted in a "tide of fluid" from the tumor to the surrounding host tissues. The pressure was highest in the center of the tumor and lowest at the tumor–normal tissue interface (152); creating a gradient that encouraged fluid diffusion. The resulting increased IFV caused interstitial swelling. Malignant cells at the surface of tumors with demonstrated loss of cohesiveness to other cells (154) were carried along this "tide of fluid" toward peritumoral lymphatics (124). Tumor cells gained access to the lymphatic lumen through intercellular gaps. Initial lymphatics are particularly well adapted by ultrastructure to permit or promote the entry and exit of cells, such as tumor cells, by virtue of their lack of basement membrane. The process is aided by the specialized tethering of the LECs to the extracellular matrix, which caused the intercellular spaces to open when the host IFP was increased by the "tide of fluid" from the tumor (140, 153). Anchoring filaments prevented the lymphatic capillaries from collapsing and increase lymphatic vessel diameters and also pulled open the intercellular junctions, producing interendothelial clefts. This provided easy access to the lymphatic lumen of fluid, particles, and cells. Retrograde flow was prevented when the pressures inside and outside the lymphatic capillaries equalized, resulting in closure of the interendothelial clefts (140).

Lymphatics normally carry interstitial fluid toward the heart through the peripheral lymphatic system and they are likely to accommodate the "tide of fluid" from tumors (152), just as they do when there is an abnormal volume of fluid in tissues with other diseases. IFP in experimental tumor systems was increased proportional to tumor size (150) and size correlated with the incidence of metastasis (17). External influences on intratumor IFP, such as small doses of hyperthermia or radiation (155), also resulted in increased SLN metastasis. Therapeutic doses of these modalities decreased lymph node metastasis. The increase or decrease in the "tide of fluid" may have enabled tumor cells to enter lymphatics in or around the tumor either more or less easily, respectively. An exciting recent observation in human patients with colorectal cancer was the observation that drugs that "normalized" tumor blood vessels also decreased intratumoral IFP (156).

Transport of Lymph Through the Lymphatic System

Lymph is formed by osmotic and hydrostatic pressure dynamics that were clearly described by Starling at the end of the nineteenth century (153). A combination of IFP and the pressures produced by the existing extracellular matrix and the growing tumor created a pump-like effect that moved fluid into lymphatic capillaries (157). Movement toward the heart through lymphatic trunks was affected by skeletal motion, muscular activity, massage, respiration, minor pressure oscillations caused by neighboring arterial and arteriolar pressure pulsations, blood pressure, exercise, and some drugs (140, 153). In the human skin lymph flow velocity averages about $10 \ \mu m \ s^{-1}$, and in mice lymphatic flow from the footpad to the popliteal lymph node is in the same range (158). Lymph flow fluctuates and oscillates over a broad range of velocities.

Rates of Lymphatic Flow from Tumors

Intratumoral IFP is commonly much higher than that in the surrounding host tissues. In the C57Bl/6 mouse F10 spontaneous metastasis model (17), lymph flow rates (LFRs) from mouse footpad tumors were significantly higher than from comparable normal footpads (159). LFR rose significantly with increasing tumor size. LFR and primary melanoma tumor size also correlated directly with the incidence of RLN metastases to the popliteal and femoral lymph nodes. Lymph vessel diameters between the footpad and the popliteal lymph node also increased proportional to the size of the primary tumor, and to the incidence of RLN metastasis (160). Hoshida et al. (124), in an ear model of the B16 melanoma, confirmed these findings and also showed a relationship to the secretion of VEGF-C by tumor cells.

LFR in the B16 tumor-bearing mouse leg model was altered by the application of external physical energies, such as heat or irradiation. Local hyperthermia not only increased the flow rates, but also increased RLN metastases (113). Low dose irradiation of the primary footpad tumor increased RLN metastasis and also LFR (161). However, therapeutic doses of irradiation decreased both LFR and RLN metastases.

Intravital Microscopy

Intravital microscopy and variations of this technology have been useful in dissecting anatomical, functional, molecular, and pathophysiological processes within experimental tumors in various animals (162). This technology has recently been applied to discern the various steps of lymphatic metastasis and has provided important insights into the pathophysiology of lymphatics in and around tumors (139).

He et al. (123) examined by fluorescent microlymphangiography the functional lymphatic network surrounding xenotransplanted subcutaneous tumors in the mouse ear. They also used other in vivo imaging techniques and whole mounts of excised tissues using confocal microscopy. They were able to confirm extensive lymphatic vessel sprouting toward tumor cells secreting VEGF-C, dilatation of peritumoral lymphatics, identify lymphangiogenesis occurs at a later time than angiogenesis, the time of onset of lymph node metastasis coincided with maximal tumor lymphangiogenesis and suppressed these activities by administration of a soluble inhibitor of VEGFR-3.

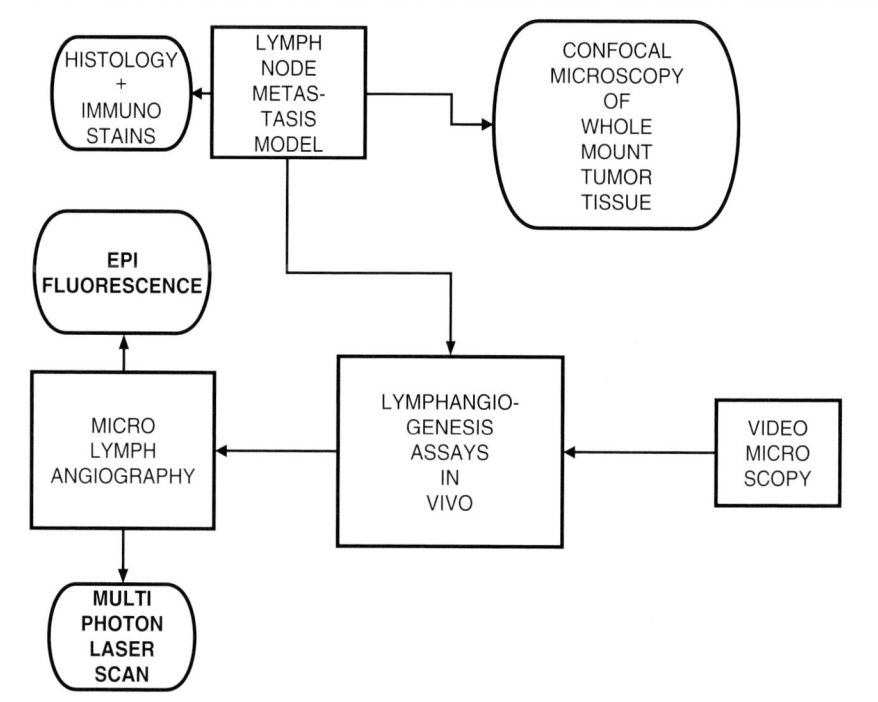

Figure 4. Methods used to study peritumoral lymphatics

Hoshida et al. (124) used epifluorescence with multiphoton laser scanning to observe peritumoral ear lymphatics. They measured lymph fluid velocity in peritumoral lymphatics by fluorescent recovery after photobleaching with spatial Fourier analysis (SFA FRAP) (163). They imaged the vasculature of both normal and tumor-bearing ears by simultaneous angiography and lymphangiography. They confirmed an increased rate of lymphatic flow induced by VEGF-C-producing tumors.

Boardman and Swartz (118), in a series of experiments in the mouse tail, suggested that increased IFP, coupled with the secretion of VEGF-C and matrix metalloproteases, might be the primary stimulus for lymphangiogenesis. The model fits the findings of tumor models in mice and suggests that lymphangiogenesis needs all three of these functional events.

Intravital videomicroscopy (IVVM) (164) is a useful technique for obtaining real-time images of the intact lymphatic vasculature that drains the region of the murine mammary fat pad. Large and small lymphatic vessels were clearly defined using oblique transillumination. RLN metastasis was observed directly. The method was also useful for observation and quantification of fluid motion within vessels and lymph nodes. Figure 4 shows methods used to study lymphatics between the primary tumor site and the SLN.

CHEMORECEPTORS AND CHEMOKINES

Tumor cells that travel in lymphatic vessels toward the RLNs may pass through the nodes and enter the blood stream through the thoracic duct–jugular vein junction in the neck, or stop and grow in the node, or pass through lymphaticovenous connections in the node into the venous blood and spread to hematogenous sites (165). Although all three of these options probably occur, it is not yet clear what entices tumor cells to stop and grow in the node. This important question has been addressed in a number of ways. The clinical implications of growth in the RLNs are vital to staging and management decisions. For example, some tumors that grow in the draining RLNs may not spread further through the hematogenous route; such a system may be a barrier to further metastatic growth by the lymph node. Clinical studies suggest that a barrier function of the draining nodes does not exist or is, at most, relatively ineffective. However, other studies show the advantage of surgical removal of tumor-bearing regional nodes in the overall survival of some melanoma patients (166).

An important question in the biology of tumor metastasis is: once the tumor cells have maneuvered their way through the lymphatic capillaries and trunks to the SLN, what makes them adhere to the structures within the node? To address this question some scientists have looked at the mechanisms whereby lymphoid and dendritic cells (DCs) "home" to certain parts of the node and stay there. Miller et al. (167) imaged the dynamic behavior of living lymphocytes deep within intact lymph nodes. They identified T and B cells after antigenic challenge. Lymphocytes injected intravenously homed straight to the lymph nodes to specific T and B cell sites. Chemoattractant cytokines (CC), such as CCL19, induced circulating T cells expressing the chemokine receptor 7 (CCR7), secreted by DCs, to enter the lymph node parenchyma following a chemokine gradient. B-lymphocytes, which express the receptor CXCR5, follow the chemoattractant BLC/CXCL13 into the B-cell-rich follicles. In contrast, Stoll et al. (168) found DCs entered the local lymph vessels that channel interstitial fluid and cells from the skin to the local lymph node. DCs, when stimulated by inflammatory cytokines, migrated from the skin following a chemoattractant gradient to RLNs.

Movement of tumor cells to RLNs resembles migration of DCs. Muller et al. (169) explored the metastasis of breast cancer in immunocompromised mice. They noted RLN metastasis when CXCR4 was expressed and inhibition of metastasis by antibodies that block this receptor.

Wiley et al. (170) found the B16/F1 syngeneic melanoma did not commonly metastasize to the RLNs. After transfection of the gene for CCR7 RLN metastasis was significantly increased. Neutralizing antibodies against either the ligand (CCL21) or the receptor abrogated the increase in RLN metastasis. The mechanism for this phenomenon of chemokinesis is demonstrable directly in vitro where chemokines stimulated chemotaxis of tumor cells with the appropriate chemoreceptors. It seems likely that tumor cells enter peritumoral lymphatics because of mechanical factors and that chemotaxis may play a directional role. RLNs have been shown to produce the ligand for the chemokine receptors.

OTHER POTENTIAL MECHANISMS: EXPERIMENTAL SYSTEMS THAT ALTER REGIONAL LYMPH NODE METASTASIS

Figure 5 summarizes an extensive literature of experiments in animal tumor models in which lymph node metastasis was increased (stimulated) or decreased (suppressed) (Table 6).

These agents are classified according to their proposed mechanism of action into endocrine, cytotoxic, antiangiogenic, anti-inflammatory, immune modulatory, or other. If we look at these potential mechanisms we might speculate that there were two major varieties of experiments that the investigators did. In essence, drugs may target the tumor cells themselves, or the biological milieu that is necessary for the maintenance of those cells, such as blood supply; these experiments would not necessarily address the mechanism of RLN metastasis. Hypothesis–driven experiments, in which a highly likely mechanism was addressed, would include those in which antiangiogenesis drugs/biologicals were used. Such experiments might interfere with lymphangiogenesis directly (for example, VEGFR-3-Ig); this has been shown by a number of investigators to decrease RLN metastasis. Drugs such as TNP-470, which target the development of new blood vessels, might have inhibited RLN metastasis by decreasing the intratumoral interstitial fluid pressure and the lymphatic flow from the tumor to the SLN. Tumor cell proliferation, known to be decreased by endocrine and cytotoxic drug administration, may have resulted in a serendipitous secondary observation of decreased RLN metastasis. Immunomodulatory

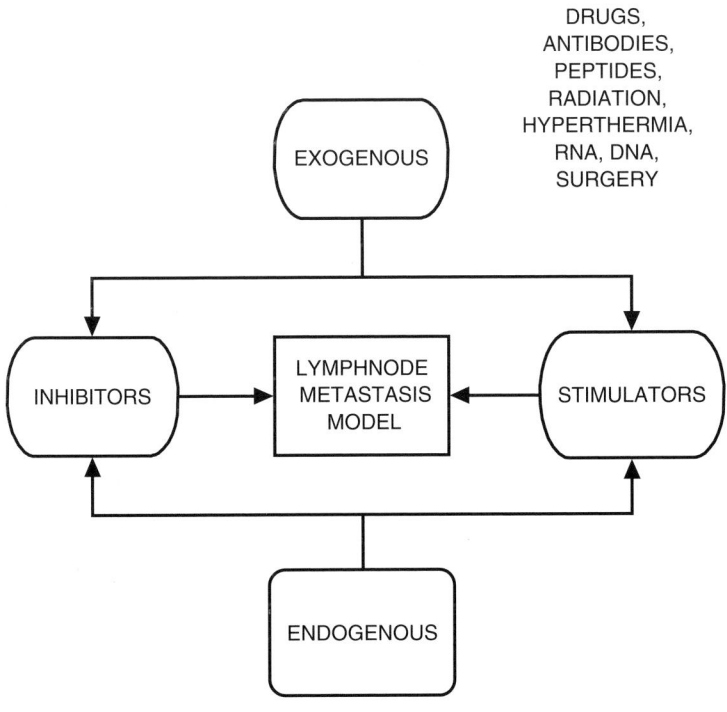

Figure 5. The figure identifies both exogenous and endogenous factors that alter the rates of lymphatic metastasis

agents, such as interleukin 2, may have similarly decreased tumor cell proliferation, and resulted in apoptosis or cell death and only secondarily decreased RLN metastasis. Anti-inflammatory agents, such as celecoxib, may similarly target tumor cells and only secondarily decrease RLN metastasis. The drugs/biologicals classified as "other" in the table may have other biological effects and the investigators also found decreased in RLN metastasis.

SUMMARY

Animal models have produced vital information regarding the mechanisms of RLN metastasis. Modern imaging and molecular techniques have made it clear that growing tumors secrete cytokines that induce invasion, angiogenesis, lymphangiogenesis, increased intratumoral IFV and IFP, increased fluid flow from the tumor to the surrounding tissues, increased lymphatic flow, an increase in the rate of entry of tumor cells into lymphatic capillaries, and an increased number of tumor cells reaching the RLN(s). This is important knowledge that will help direct translational research in human patients. We can look forward to continued improvement in the management of human tumors that metastasize to the RLNs.

Table 6. Identifies drugs or biological agents that were found to decrease RLN metastasis in mice, rat, rabbit, or hamster models of RLN metastasis

Mechanism	Drug/biological	Animal recipient	Tumor/species	References
Endocrine	Trioxefene (LY133314)	Rat	Prostate/rat	(27)
	Androgen ablation	Mouse	Prostate/mouse	(26)
	Raloxifene	Rat	Prostate/rat	(29)
	Flurbiprofen (E7869)	Mouse	Prostate/mouse	(25)
Cytotoxic	Camptothecin analogue (DX-8951f)	Mouse	Pancreas/human	(89)
	Cisplatin	Mouse	Oral squamous/ human	(79)
	Uracil/tegafur	Mouse	Colorectal/human	(83)
	Benzoporphyrin (photodynamic)	Rat	Prostate/rat	(28)
	5-Fluorocytosine	Mouse	Prostate/mouse	(24)
Antiangiogenic/ lymphangiogenic	Flt3-ligand	Mouse	Prostate/mouse	(22)
	TNP-470	Rabbit	VX2/rabbit	(37)
	Anti-α2 integrin antibody	Mouse	Gastric/human	(96)
	Combretastatin	Mouse	Lung/mouse	(45)
	VEGFR-3-Ig	Mouse	Lung/human	(171)
	ANTI-VEGF-D	Mouse	Breast/human	(172)
	ANTI-EGFR +VEGFR	Mouse	Colon/human	(176)
Anti-inflammatory	Celecoxib	Mouse	Lung/human	(173)
	E-7869	Mouse	Prostate/mouse	(25)
Immunomodulator	IL2	Mouse	Prostate/human	(174)
	OK 432 (streptococcal immunopotentiator)	Hamster	Oral/hamster	(32)
Other	Desmopressin	Mouse	Breast/mouse	(49)
	C-Met ribozyme	Mouse	Prostate/mouse	(65)
	Flaxseed	Mouse	Breast/human	(91)
	ANTI-L-selectin antibodies	Mouse	Pancreas/mouse	(46)
	Berberine	Mouse	Lung/mouse	(175)
	IkappaBalpha	Mouse	Prostate/human	(81)
	MMI 270 (MMP inhibitor)	Mouse	Lung/human	(177)
	Tyrosine kinase inhibitor	Mouse	Bladder/human	(178)

ACKNOWLEDGMENTS

Funded by the Nathanson/Rands Chair in Breast Cancer Research. Editorial assistance provided by Nandita Mani.

REFERENCES

1. Rosenberg SA (1997) Principles of cancer management: surgical oncology. In: De Vita VT Jr., Hellman S, Rosenberg SA (eds) Cancer: Principles of oncology, 5th edn. Lippicott-Raven, Philadelphia, pp295
2. Morton DL, Wen DR, Wong JH, Economou JS, Cagle LA, Storm FK, Foshag LJ, Cochran AJ (1992) Technical details of intraoperative lymphatic mapping for early stage melanoma. Arch Surg 127:392-399
3. Giuliano AE, Kirgan, DM, Guenther JM, Morton DL (1994) Lymphatic mapping and sentinel lymphadenectomy for breast cancer. Ann Surg 220:391-401

4. Krag DN, Meijer SJ, Weaver DL, Loggie BW, Harlow SP, Tanabe KK, Laughlin EH, Alex JC (1995) Minimal-access surgery for staging of malignant melanoma. Arch Surg 130:654-658
5. Nathanson SD (2003) Insights into the mechanisms of lymph node metastasis. Cancer 98:413-423
6. Leader RW, Padgett GA (1980) The genesis and validation of animal models. Am J Pathol 101 (3 suppl):S11-S16
7. Fidler IJ (1973) Selection of successive tumour lines for metastasis. Nat New Biol 242:148-149
8. Khanna C, Hunter K (2005) Modeling metastasis in vivo. Carcinogenesis 26:513-523
9. Krishnan K, Khanna C, Helman LJ (2005) The biology of metastases in pediatric sarcomas. Cancer J 11:306-313
10. Fidler IJ (1997) Molecular biology of cancer: invasion and metastasis. In: DeVita VT, Hellman S, Rosenberg SA (eds) Cancer: Principles and Practice of Oncology. Lippincott-Raven, Philadelphia, pp135-152
11. Liotta LA (1985) Mechanisms of Cancer invasion and metastasis. In: DeVita VT, Hellman S, Rosenberg SA(eds) Important Advances in Oncology. Lippincott-Raven, New York, p 28
12. McGuire WL (1987) Prognostic factors for recurrence and survival in human breast cancer. Breast Cancer Res Treat 10:5-9
13. Harrison JC, Dean PJ, el-Zeky F, Vander Zwaag R (1994) From Dukes through Jass. Pathological prognostic indicators in rectal cancer. Hum Pathol 25:498-505
14. Balch CM, Soong SJ, Gershenwald JE, Thompson JF, Reintgen DS, Cascinelli N, Urist M, McMasters KM, Ross MI, Kirkwood JM, Atkins MB, Thompson JA, Coit DG, Byrd D, Desmond R, Zhang Y, Liu PY, Lyman GH, Morabito A (2001) Prognostic factors analysis of 17,600 melanoma patients: Validation of the american joint committee on cancer melanoma staging system. J Clin Oncol 19:3622-3634
15. Mead MJ, Nathanson SD, Lee M, Peterson E (1985) Prophylactic lymphadenectomy for B16 melanoma in C57BL/6 mice. J Surg Res 38:391-327
16. Reintgen D, Cruse CW, Wells K, Berman C, Fenske N, Glass F, Schroer K, Heller R, Ross M, Lyman G (1994) The orderly progression of melanoma nodal metastases. Ann Surg 220:759-767
17. Nathanson SD, Haas GP, Mead MJ, Lee M (1986) Spontaneous regional lymph node metastases of three variants of the B16 melanoma: Relationship to primary tumor size and pulmonary metastases. J Surg Oncol 33:41-45
18. Bresalier RS, Hujanen ES, Raper SE, Roll FJ, Itzkowitz SH, Martin GR, Kim YS (1987) An animal model for colon cancer metastasis: Establishment and characterization of murine cell lines with enhanced liver-metastasizing ability. Cancer Res 47:1398-1406
19. Carr I (1983) Lymphatic metastasis. Cancer Metastasis Rev 2:307-317
20. Abate-Shen C, Banach-Petrosky WA, Sun X, Econimides KD, Desai N, Gregg JP, Borowsky AD, Cardiff RD, Shen MM (2003) Nkx3.1; Pten mutant mice develop invasive prostate adenocarcinoma and lymph node metastases. Cancer Res 63:3886-3890
21. Ciavarra RP, Holterman DA, Brown RR, Mangiotti P, Yousefieh N, Wright GL Jr, Schellmammer PF, Glass WF, Somers KD (2004) Prostate tumor microenvironment alters immune cells and prevents long-term survival in an orthotopic mouse model following flt3-ligand/CD40-ligand immunotherapy. J Immunother 27:13-26
22. Somers KD, Brown RR, Holterman, Yousefiah N, Glass WF, Wright GL Jr, Schellhammer PF, Qian J, Ciavarra RP (2003) Orthotopic treatment model of prostate cancer and metastasis in the immunocompetent mouse: Efficacy of flt3 ligand immunotherapy. Int J Cancer 107:773-780
23. Martiniello-Wilks R, Dane A, Mortensen E, Jeyakumar G, Wang XY, Russell PJ (2003) Application of the transgenic adenocarcinoma mouse prostate (TRAMP) model for pre-clinical therapeutic studies. Anticancer Res 23:2633-2642
24. Zhang Z, Yin L, Zhang Y, Zhao F (2002) In situ transduction of cytosine deaminase gene followed by systemic use of 5-fluorocytosine inhibits tumor growth and metastasis in orthotopic prostate cancer mouse models. Chin Med J 115:227-231
25. Wechter WJ, Leipold DD, Murray ED Jr, Quiggle D, McCracken JD, Barrios RS, Greenberg NM (2000) E-7869 (R-flurbiprofen) inhibits progression of prostate cancer in the TRAMP mouse. Cancer Res 60:2203-2208
26. Gingrich JR, Barrios RJ, Kattan MW, Nahm HS, Finegold MJ, Greenberg NM (1997) Androgen-independent prostate cancer progression in the TRAMP model. Cancer Res 57:4687-4691
27. Neubauer BL, McNulty AM, Chedid M, Chen K, Goode RL, Johnson MA, Jones CD, Krishnan V, Lynch R, Osborne HE, Graff JR (2003) The selective estrogen receptor modulator trioxifene (LY133314) inhibits metastasis and extends survival in PAIII rat prostatic carcinoma model. Cancer Res 63:6056-6062
28. Momma T, Hamblin MR, Wu HC, Hasan T (1998) Photodynamic therapy of orthotopic prostate cancer with benzoporphyrin derivative: Local control and distant metastasis. Cancer Res 58:5425-5431

29. Neubauer BL, Best KL, Counts DF, Goode RL, Hoover DM, Jones CD, Sarosdy MF, Shaar CJ, Tanzer LR, Merriman RL (1995) Raloxifene (LY156758) produces antimetastatic responses and extends survival in the PAIII rat prostatic adenocarcinoma model. Prostate 27:220-229
30. Rubenstein M, Saffrin R, Shaw M, Muchnik S, Guinan P (1995) Orthotopic placement of the dunning R3327 AT-3 prostate tumor in the Copenhagen X Fischer rat. Prostate 27:148-153
31. Chen S, Pan J, Liao X (2001) The experimental of pegylated liposomal doxorubicin to therapy tongue cancer and metastases lymph nodes. Zhonghua Kou Qiang Yi Xue Za Zhi 36:338-340
32. Nakajima J, Mogi M, Chino T (1996) Inhibition by streptococcal immunopotentiator OK432 of lymph-node metastasis in hamster cheek-pouch carcinoma with enhancement of tumour necrosis factor-alpha and interleukin-6 in serum. Arch Oral Biol 41:513-516
33. Ohtake K, Shingaki S, Nakajima T (1993) Histologic study on the metastatic process in the experimental model of lymph node metastasis. Oral Surg Oral Med Oral Pathol 75:472-478
34. Ohtake K, Shingaki S, Nakajima T (1990) A model for the study of lymph node metastasis from oral carcinoma by serial transplantation of metastatic tumor in hamsters. Oral Surg Oral Med Oral Pathol 69:701-707
35. Kage T, Mogi M, Katsumata Y, Chino T (1987) Regional lymph node metastasis created by partial excision of carcinomas induced in hamster cheek pouch with 9,10-dimethyl-1,2-benzanthracene. J Dent Res 66:1673-1679
36. Dunne AA, Schmidt A, Kuropkat C, Ramaswamy A, Schulz S, Werner JA (2003a) The auricular VX2 carcinoma–an animal model for the sentinel node concept. In Vivo 17:457-461
37. Seki S, Fujimura A (2003) Three-dimensional changes in lymphatic architecture around VX2 tongue cancer–dynamic changes after administration of an antiangiogenic agent. Lymphology 36:199-208
38. Dunne AA, Plehn S, Schulz S, Levermann A, Ramaswamy A, Lippert BM, Werner JA (2003b) Lymph node topography of the head and neck in New Zealand white rabbits. Lab Anim 37:37-43
39. Dunne AA, Mandic R, Ramaswamy A, Plehn S, Schulz S, Lippert BM, Moll R, Werner JA (2002) Lymphogenic metastatic spread of auricular VX2 carcinoma in New Zealand white rabbits. Anticancer Res 22:3273-3279
40. van Es RJ, Dullens HF, van der Bilt A, Koole R, Slootweg PJ (2000) Evaluation of the VX2 rabbit auricle carcinoma as a model for head and neck cancer in humans. J Craniomaxillofac Surg 28:300-307
41. Sueyoshi S (1992) Experimental study of lymph node metastasis in thoracic esophageal carcinoma–regarding lymph node metastasis and changes in lymphatic flow by ultrafine charcoal in rabbit esophageal carcinoma model. Nippon Geka Gakkai Zasshi 93:462-474
42. Dunnington DJ, Buscarino C, Gennaro D, Greig R, Poste G (1987) Characterization of an animal model of metastatic colon carcinoma. Int J Cancer 39:248-254
43. Doki Y, Murakami K, Yamaura T, Sugiyama S, Misaki T, Saiki I (1999) Mediastinal lymph node metastasis model by orthotopic intrapulmonary implantation of Lewis lung carcinoma cells in mice. Br J Cancer 79:1121-1126
44. Gao P (1993) Two high spontaneous lung and lymph node metastasis models derived from 615 mouse pulmonary adenocarcinoma (I615PAC-8811). Zhongguo Yi Xue Ke Xue Yuan Xue Bao 15:266-273
45. Hori K, Saito S, Nihei Y, Suzuki M, Sato Y (1999) Antitumor effects due to irreversible stoppage of tumor tissue blood flow: Evaluation of a novel combretastatin A-4 derivative, AC7700. Jpn J Cancer Res 90:1387-1395
46. Qian F, Hanahan D, Weissman IL (2001) L-selectin can facilitate metastasis to lymph nodes in a transgenic mouse model of carcinogenesis. Proc Nat Acad Sciences 98:3976-3981
47. Mutter D, Hajri A, Tassetti V, Solis-Caxaj C, Aprahamian M, Marescaux J (1999) Increased tumor growth and spread after laparoscopy vs laparotomy: Influence of tumor manipulation in a rat model. Surg Endosc 13:365-370
48. Van de Velde CJ, Van Putten LM, Zwaveling A (1977) A new metastasizing mammary carcinoma model in mice: Model characteristics and applications. Eur J Cancer 13:555-565
49. Giron S, Tejera AM, Ripoll GV, Gomez DE, Alonso DF (2002) Desmopressin inhibits lung and lymph node metastasis in a mouse mammary carcinoma model of surgical manipulation. J Surg Oncol 81:38-44
50. Finlay-Jones JJ, Bartholomaeus WN, Fimmel PJ, Keast D, Stanley NF (1980) Biologic and immunologic studies on a murine model of regional lymph node metastasis. J Natl Cancer Inst 64:1363-1372
51. Taback B, Hashimoto K, Kuo CT, Chan A, Giuliano AE, Hoon DS (2002) Molecular lymphatic mapping of the sentinel lymph node. Am J Pathol 161:1153-1161
52. Schirner M, Kraus C, Lichtner RB, Schneider MR, Hildebrand M (1998) Tumor metastasis inhibition with the prostacyclin analogue cicaprost depends on discontinuous plasma peak levels. Prostaglandins Leukot Essent Fatty Acids 58:311-317

53. Neri A, Welch D, Kawaguchi T, Nicolson GL (1982) Development and biologic properties of malignant cell sublines and clones of a spontaneously metastasizing rat mammary adenocarcinoma. J Natl Cancer Inst 68:507-517
54. Jansen AP, Verwiebe EG, Dreckschmidt NE, Wheeler DL, Oberley TD, Verma AK (2001) Protein kinase C-epsilon transgenic mice: A unique model for metastatic squamous cell carcinoma. Cancer Res 61:808-812
55. Trites J, Yoo J, Taylor M, Schmidt E, Morris V, MacDonald I, Chambers A, Groom A (2000) Lymph node metastasis in malignant melanoma: An in vivo animal model. J Otolaryngol 29:233-238
56. Parsons PG, Takahashi H, Candy J, Meyers B, Vickers J, Kelly WR, Smith I, Spradbrow P (1990) Histopathology of melanocytic lesions in goats and establishment of a melanoma cell line: A potential model for human melanoma. Pigment Cell Res 3:297-305
57. Ichii S, Imai Y, Irimura T (2000) Initial steps in lymph node metastasis formation in an experimental system: Possible involvement of recognition by macrophage C-type lectins. Cancer Immunol Immunother 49:1-9
58. Vandendris M, Dumont P, Semal P, Heimann R, Atassi G (1985) Investigation of a new murine model of regional lymph node metastasis: Characteristics of the model and applications. Clin Exp Metastasis 3:7-19
59. Carr J, Carr I, Dreher B, Betts K (1980) Lymphatic metastasis: Invasion of lymphatic vessels and efflux of tumour cells in the afferent popliteal lymph as seen in the Walker rat carcinoma. J Pathol 132:287-305
60. Carr I, McGinty F (1974) Lymphatic metastasis and its inhibition: An experimental model. J Pathol 113:85-95
61. Cobb RA, Steer HW (1987) Tumor cell trapping in rat mesenteric lymph nodes. Br J Exp Pathol 68:461-474
62. Hashii K, Tohya K, Kimura M, Tateyama I, Mori T, Kadota E, Hashimoto S, Tomura T (1997) Novel animal model of lymph node metastasis by intrauterine inoculation of the actively metastatic subline PL3 separated from rat Walker 256 tumor cells. Invasion Metastasis 17:149-157
63. Li HF, Ling MY, Xie Y, Xie H (1998) Establishment of a lymph node metastatic model of mouse hepatocellular carcinoma Hca-F cells in C3H/Hej mice. Oncol Res 10:569-573
64. Takazawa H, Shimuzu S (1976) An experimental model for lymphatic metastasis in rats. Gann 67:403-406
65. Kim SJ, Johnson M, Koterba K, Herynk MH, Uehara H, Gallick GE (2003) Reduced c-Met expression by an adenovirus expressing a c-Met ribozyme inhibits tumorigenic growth and lymph node metastases of PC3-LN4 prostate tumor cells in an orthotopic nude mouse model. Clin Cancer Res 9:5161-5170
66. Jenkins DE, Yu SF, Hornig YS, Purchio T, Contag PR (2003) In vivo monitoring of tumor relapse and metastasis using bioluminescent PC-3M-luc-C6 cells in murine models of human prostate cancer. Clin Exp Metastasis 20:745-756
67. Qian CN, Takahashi M, Kahnoski RJ, Teh BT (2003) Effect of sildenafil citrate on an orthotopic prostate cancer growth and metastasis model. J Urol 170:994-997
68. Bastide C, Bagnis C, Mannoni P, Hassoun J, Bladou F (2002) A Nod Scid mouse model to study human prostate cancer. Prostate Cancer Prostate Dis 5:311-315
69. Chang XH, Fu YW, Na WL, Wang J, Sun H, Cai L (1999) Improved metastatic animal model of human prostate carcinoma using surgical orthotopic implantation. Anticancer Res 19:4199-4202
70. Triest JA, Grignon DJ, Cher ML, Kocheril SV, Montecillo EJ, Talati B, Tekyi-Mensah S, Pontes JE, Hillman GG (1998) Systemic interleukin 2 therapy for human prostate tumors in a nude mouse model. Clin Cancer Res 4:2009-2014
71. Rembrink K, Romijn JC, van der Kwast TH, Rubben H, Schroder FH (1997) Orthotopic implantation of human prostate cancer cell lines: A clinically relevant model for metastatic prostate cancer. Prostate 31:168-174
72. Sato N, Gleave ME, Bruchovsky N, Rennie PS, Beraldi E, Sullivan LD (1997) A metastatic and androgen-sensitive human prostate cancer model using intraprostatic inoculation of LNCaP cells in SCID mice. Cancer Res 57:1584-1589
73. Stephenson RA, Dinney CP, Gohji K, Ordonez NG, Killion JJ, Fidler IJ (1992) Metastatic model of human prostate cancer using orthotopic implantation in nude mice. J Natl Cancer Inst 84:951-957
74. Qiu C, Wu H, He H, Qiu W (2003) A cervical lymph node metastatic model of human tongue carcinoma: Serial and orthotopic transplantation of histologically intact patient specimens in nude mice. J Oral Maxillofac Surg 61:696-700
75. Zhang X, Liu Y, Gilcrease MZ, Yuan XH, Clayman GL, Adler-Storthz K, Chen Z (2002) A lymph node metastatic mouse model reveals alterations of metastasis-related gene expression in metastatic human oral carcinoma sublines selected from a poorly metastatic parental cell line. Cancer 95:1663-1672

76. Shintani S, Mihara M, Nakahara Y, Aida T, Tachikawa T, Hamakawa H (2002) Lymph node metastasis of oral cancer visualized in live tissue by green fluorescent protein expression. Oral Oncol 38:664-669

77. Myers JN, Holsinger FC, Jasser SA, Bekele BN, Fidler IJ (2002) An orthotopic nude mouse model of oral tongue squamous cell carcinoma. Clin Cancer Res 8:293-298

78. Umeda M, Yokoo S, Komori T, Nishimatsu N, Shibuya Y, Fujioka M (2001) Experimental model of invasion and metastasis by orthotopic transplantation of oral squamous and adenoid cystic carcinomas into the tongue of nude mice. Br J Oral Maxillofac Surg 39:376-380

79. Kawashiri S, Kojima K, Kumagai S, Nakagawa K, Yamamoto E (2001) Effects of chemotherapy on invasion and metastasis of oral cavity cancer in mice. Head Neck 23:764-771

80. Kawashiri S, Kumagai S, Kojima K, Harada H, Yamamoto E (1995) Development of a new invasion and metastasis model of human oral squamous cell carcinomas. Eur J Cancer B Oral Oncol 31B:216-221

81. Huang J, Tang W, Yao Y (1998) A model of nasopharyngeal carcinoma with spontaneous highly lymphatic metastasis in nude mice and its biological characteristics. Zhonghua Yi Xue Za Zhi. 78:725-728

82. Gu J, Zhao J, Li Z, Yang Z, Zhang J, Gao Z, Wang Y, Xu G (2003) Clinical application of radioimmunoguided surgery in colorectal cancer using 125I-labeled carcinoembryonic antigen-specific monoclonal antibody submucosally. Dis Colon Rectum 46:1659-1666

83. Tsutsumi S, Kuwano H, Morinaga N, Shimura T, Asao T (2001) Animal model of para-aortic lymph node metastasis. Cancer Lett 169:77-85

84. Rashidi B, Gamagami R, Sasson A, Sun FX, Geller J, Moossa AR, Hoffman RM (2000) An orthotopic mouse model of remetastasis of human colon cancer liver metastasis. Clin Cancer Res 6:2556-2561

85. Diperna CA, Bart RD, Sievers EM, Ma Y, Starnes VA, Bremner RM (2003) Cyclooxygenase-2 inhibition decreases primary and metastatic tumor burden in a murine model of orthotopic lung adenocarcinoma. J Thorac Cardiovasc Surg 126:1129-1133

86. Mase K, Iijima T, Nakamura N, Takeuchi T, Onizuka M, Mitsui T, Noguchi M (2002) Intrabronchial orthotopic propagation of human lung adenocarcinoma–characterizations of tumorigenicity, invasion and metastasis. Lung Cancer 36:271-276

87. Yano S, Nishioka Y, Izumi K, Tsuruo T, Tanaka T, Miyasaka M, Sone S (1996) Novel metastasis model of human lung cancer in SCID mice depleted of NK cells. Int J Cancer 67:211-217

88. Wang X, Fu X, Hoffman RM (1992) A patient-like metastasizing model of human lung adenocarcinoma constructed via thoracotomy in nude mice. Anticancer Res 12:1399-1401

89. Sun FX, Tohgo A, Bouvet M, Yagi S, Nassirpour R, Moossa AR, Hoffman RM (2003) Efficacy of campothecin analog DX-8951f (Exatecan Mesylate) on human pancreatic cancer in an orthotopic metastatic model. Cancer Res 63:80-85

90. Alves F, Contag S, Missbach M, Kaspareit J, Nebendahl K, Borchers U, Heidrich B, Streich R, Hiddemann W (2001) An orthotopic model of ductal adenocarcinoma of the pancreas in severe combined immunodeficient mice representing all steps of the metastatic cascade. Pancreas 23:227-235

91. Chen J, Stavro PM, Thompson LU (2002) Dietary flaxseed inhibits human breast cancer growth and metastasis and downregulates expression of insulin-like growth factor and epidermal growth factor receptor. Nutr Cancer 43:187-192

92. Li X, Wang J, An Z, Yang M, Baranov E, Jiang P, Sun F, Moossa AR, Hoffman RM (2002) Optically imageable metastatic model of human breast cancer. Clin Exp Metastasis 19:347-350

93. Liu Q, Zhao W, Tuo C, Wang Z, Wu B, Zhang N (2002) Establishment and characteristics of orthotopically transplanted model of human primary malignant spleen lymphoma in nude mice. Zhonghua Zhong Liu Za Zhi 24:234-238

94. Koshida K, Konaka H, Kato H, Miyagi T, Egawa M, Uchibayashi T, Namiki M (2000) Correlation between expression of metastasis-related genes and lymph node metastasis in testicular cancer. Hinyokika Kiyo 46:775-781

95. Douglas ML, Boucaut KJ, Antalis TM, Higgins C, Pera MF, Stuttgen MA, Nicol DL (2001) An orthotopic xenograft model of human nonseminomatous germ cell tumour. Br J Cancer 85:608-611

96. Yamaguchi K, Ura H, Yasoshima T, Shishido T, Denno R, Hirata K (2000) Establishment and characterization human gastric carcinoma cell line that is highly metastatic to lymph nodes. J Exp Clin Cancer Res 19:113-120

97. Fujihara T, Sawada T, Hirakawa K, Chung YS, Yashiro M, Inoue T, Sowa M (1998) Establishment of lymph node metastatic model for human gastric cancer in nude mice and analysis of factors associated with metastasis. Clin Exp Metastasis 16:389-398

98. An Z, Jiang P, Wang X, Moossa AR, Hoffman RM (1999) Development of a high metastatic orthotopic model of human renal cell carcinoma in nude mice: Benefits of fragment implantation compared to cell-suspension injection. Clin Exp Metastasis 17:265-270

99. Cairns RA, Hill RP (2004) Acute hypoxia enhances spontaneous lymph node metastasis in an orthotopic murine model of human cervical carcinoma. Cancer Res 64:2054-2061

100. Alitalo K, Tammela T, Petrova TV (2005) Lymphangiogenesis in development and human disease. Nature 438:946-953
101. Kirkness EF, Bafna V, Halpern AL, Levy S, Remington K, Rusch DB, Delcher AL, Pop M, Wang W, Fraser CM, Venter JC (2003) The dog genome: Survey sequencing and comparative analysis. Science 301:1898-1903
102. Achen MG, Stacker SA (2006) Tumor lymphangiogenesis and metastatic spread – new players begin to emerge. Int J Cancer 119:1755-1760
103. Asamoto M, Hokaiwado N, Cho YM, Ikeda Y, Takahashi S, Shirai T (2001) Metastasizing neuroblastomas from taste buds in rats transgenic for the Simian virus 40 large T antigen under control of the probasin gene promoter 2. Toxicol Pathol 29:363-368
104. Garabedian EM, Humphrey PA, Gordon JI (1998) A transgenic mouse model of metastatic prostate cancer originating from neuroendocrine cells. Proc Natl Acad Sci USA 95:15382-15387
105. Jeffers M, Fiscella M, Webb CP, Anver M, Koochekpour S, Vande Woude GF (1998) The mutationally activated met receptor mediates motility and metastasis. Proc Natl Acad Sci USA 95:14417-14422
106. Li Y, Hively WP, Varmus HE (2000) Use of MMTV-Wnt-1 transgenic mice for studying the genetic basis of breast cancer. Oncogene 19:1002-1009
107. Mandriota SJ, Jussila L, Jeltsch M, Compagni A, Baetens D, Prevo R, Banerji S, Huarte J, Montesano R, Jackson DG, Orci L, Alitalo K, Christofori G, Pepper MS (2001) Vascular endothelial growth factor-C-mediated lymphangiogenesis promotes tumor metastasis. EMBO J 20:672-682
108. Masumori N, Thomas TZ, Chaurand P, Case T, Paul M, Kasper S, Caprioli RM, Tsukamoto T, Shappell SB, Matusik RJ (2001) A probasin-large T antigen transgenic mouse line develops prostate adenocarcinoma and neuroendocrine carcinoma with metastatic potential. Cancer Res 61:2239-2249
109. Aguirre AJ, Bardeesy N, Sinha M, Lopez L, Tuveson DA, Horner J, Redston MS, DePinho RA (2003) Activated Kras nad Ink4a/Arf deficiency cooperate to produce metastatic pancreatic ductal adenocarcinoma. Genes Dev 17:3112-3126
110. Crnic I, Strittmatter K, Cavallaro U, Kopfstein L, Jussila L, Alitalo K, Christofori G (2004) Loss of neural cell adhesion molecule induces tumor metastasis by up-regulating lymphangiogenesis. Cancer Res 64:8630-8638
111. Ramaswamy S, Ross KN, Lander ES, Golub TR (2003) A molecular signature of metastasis in primary solid tumors. Nat Genet 33:49-54
112. van't Veer LJ, Dai H, van de Vijver MJ, He YD, Hart AA, Mao M, Peterse HL, van der Kooy K, Marton MJ, Witteveen AT, Schreiber GJ, Kerkhoven RM, Roberts C, Linsley PS, Bernards R, Friend SH (2002) Gene expression profiling predicts clinical outcome of breast cancer. Nature 415:530-536
113. Nathanson SD, Cerra RF, Hetzel FW, Zarbo RJ, Crissman JD, Page R, Anaya P, Westrick P (1990) Changes associated with metastasis in B16-F1 melanoma cells surviving heat. Arch Surg 125:216-219
114. Jeltsch M, Kaipainen A, Joukov V, Meng X, Lakso M, Rauvala H, Swartz M, Fukumura D, Jain RK, Alitalo K (1997) Hyperplasia of lymphatic vessels in VEGF-C transgenic mice. Science 276:1423-1425
115. Oh SJ, Jeltsch MM, Birkenhager R, McCarthy JE, Weich HA, Christ B, Alitalo K, Wilting J (1997) VEGF and VEGF-C: Specific induction of angiogenesis and lymphangiogenesis in the differentiated avian chorio-allantoic membrane. Dev Biol 188:96-109
116. Enholm B, Karpanen T, Jeltsch M, Kubo H, Stenback F, Prevo R, Jackson DG, Yla-Herttuala S, Alitalo K (2001) Adenoviral expression of vascular endothelial growth factor -C induces lymphangiogenesis in the skin. Circ Res 88:623-629
117. Kubo H, Cao R, Brakenhielm E, Makinen T, Cao Y, Alitalo K (2002) Blockade of vascular endothelial growth factor receptor-3 signaling inhibits fibroblast growth factor-2-induced lymphangiogenesis in mouse cornea Proc Natl Acad Sci USA 99:8868-8873
118. Boardman KC, Swartz MA (2003) Interstitial flow as a guide for lymphangiogenesis. Circ Res 92:801-808
119. Alitalo K, Carmeliet P (2002) Molecular mechanisms of lymphangiogenesis in health and disease Cancer Cell 1:219-227
120. Tammela T, Enholm B, Alitalo K, Paavonen K (2005) The biology of vascular endothelial growth factors. Cardiovasc Res 65:550-563
121. Saharinen P, Tammela T, Karkkainen MJ, Alitalo K (2004) Lymphatic vasculature: development, molecular regulation and role in tumor metastasis and inflammation. Trends Immunol 25:387-395
122. Nathanson SD, Wachna DL, Gilman D, Karvelis K, Havstad S, Ferrara J (2001) Pathways of lymphatic drainage from the breast. Ann Surg Oncol 8:837-843
123. He Y, Rajantie I, Pajusola K, Jeltsch M, Holopainen T, Yla-Herttuala S, Harding T, Jooss K, Takahashi T, Alitalo K (2005) Vascular endothelial growth factor receptor 3-mediated activation of lymphatic endothelium is crucial for tumor cell entry and spread via lymphatic vessels. Cancer Res 65:4739-4746
124. Hoshida T, Isaka N, Hagendoorn J, diTomaso E, Chen YL, Pytowski B, Fukumura D, Padera TP, Jain RK (2006) Imaging steps of lymphatic metastasis reveals that vascular endothelial growth factor-C increases

metastasis by increasing delivery of cancer cells to lymph nodes: therapeutic implications. Cancer Res 66:8065-8075

125. Skobe M, Hawighorst T, Jackson DG, Prevo R, Janes L, Velasco P, Riccardi L, Alitalo K, Claffey K, Detmar M (2001) Induction of tumor lymphangiogenesis by VEGF-C promotes breast cancer metastasis. Nat Med 7:192-198

126. Mattila MM, Ruohola JK, Karpanen T, Jackson DG, Alitalo K, Harkonen PL (2002) VEGF-C induced lymphangiogenesis is associated with lymph node metastasis in orthotopic MCF-7 tumors. Int J Cancer 98:946-951

127. Krishnan J, Kirkin V, Steffen A, Hegen M, Weih D, Tomarev S, Wilting J, Sleeman JP (2003) Differential in vivo and in vitro expression of vascular endothelial growth factor (VEGF)-C and VEGF-D in tumors and its relationship to lymphatic metastasis in immunocompetent rats. Cancer Res 63:713-722

128. Chen Z, Varney ML, Backora MW, Cowan K, Solheim JC, Talmadge JE, Singh RK (2005) Down-regulation of vascular endothelial cell growth factor-C expression using small interfering RNA vectors in mammary tumors inhibits tumor lymphangiogenesis and spontaneous metastasis and enhances survival. Cancer Res 65:9004-9011

129. Yanai Y, Furuhata T, Kimura Y, Yamaguchi K, Yasoshima T, Mitaka T, Mochizuki Y, Hirata K (2001). Vascular endothelial growth factor C promotes human gastric carcinoma lymph node metastasis in mice. J Exp Clin Cancer Res 20:419-428

130. Ishii H, Yazawa T, Sato H, Suzuki T, Ikeda M, Hayashi Y, Takanashi Y, Kitamura H (2004) Enhancement of pleural dissemination and lymph node metastasis in intrathoracic lung cancer cells by vascular endothelial growth factors (VEGFs). Lung Cancer 45:325-337

131. Lin J, Lalani AS, Harding TC, Gonzalez M, Wu WW, Luan B, Tu GH, Koprivnikar K, VanRoey MJ, He Y, Alitalo K, Jooss K (2005) Inhibition of lymphogenous metastasis using adeno-associated virus-mediated gene transfer of a soluble VEGFR-3 decoy receptor. Cancer Res 65: 6901-6909

132. Kawakami M, Yanai Y, Hata F, Hirata Y (2005) Vascular endothelial growth factor C promotes lymph node metastasis in a rectal cancer orthotopic model. Surg Today 35:131-138

133. Von Marschall Z, Scholz A, Stacker SA, Achen MG, Jackson DG, Alves F, Schirner M, Haberey M, Thierauch KH, Wiedenmann B, Rosewicz S (2005) Vascular endothelial growth factor-D induces lymphangiogenesis and lymphatic metastasis in models of ductal pancreatic cancer. Int J Oncol 27:669-679

134. Stacker SA, Caesar C, Baldwin ME, Thornton GE, Williams RA, Prevo R, Jackson DG, Nishikawa SI, Kubo H, Achen MG (2001) VEGF-D promotes the metastatic spread of tumor cells via lymphatics. Nat Med 7:186-191

135. Bjorndahl MA, Cao R, Burton JB, Brakenhielm E, Religa P, Galter D, Wu L, Cao Y (2005) Vascular endothelial growth factor-A promotes peritumoral lymphangiogenesis and lymphatic metastasis. Cancer Res 65:9261-9268

136. Hirakawa S, Kodama S, Kunstfeld R, Kajiya K, Brown LF, Detmar M (2005) VEGF-A induces tumor and sentinel lymph node lymphangiogenesis and promotes lymphatic metastasis. J Exp Med 201:1089-1099

137. Cao R, Bjorndahl MA, Religa P, Clasper S, Garvin S, Galter D, Meister B, Ikomi F, Tritsaris K, Dissing S, Ohhashi T, Jackson DG, Cao Y (2004) PDGF-BB induces intratumoral lymphangiogenesis and promotes lymphatic metastasis. Cancer Cell 6:333-345

138. Zeidman I, Copeland BE, Warren S (1955) Experimental studies on the spread of cancer in the lymphatic system: II. Absence of a lymphatic supply in carcinoma. Cancer 8:123-127

139. Padera TP, Kadambi A, di Tomaso E, Carreira CM, Brown EB, Boucher Y, Choi NC, Mathisen D, Wain J, Mark EJ, Munn LL, Jain RK (2002) Lymphatic metastasis in the absence of functional intratumoral lymphatics. Science 296:1883-1886

140. Schmid-Schonbein GW (1990) Microlymphatics and lymph flow. Physiol Rev 70:987-1028

141. Clarijs R, Ruiter DJ, de Waal RM (2001) Lymphangiogenesis in malignant tumors: Does it occur? J Pathol 193:143-146

142. Gullino PM, Clark SH, Grantham FH (1964) Interstitial fluid of solid tumors. Cancer Res 24:780-794

143. Swartz MA, Kaipainen A, Netti PA, Brekken C, Boucher Y, Grodzinsky AJ, Jain RK (1999) Mechanics of interstitial-lymphatic fluid transport: Theoretical foundation and experimental validation. J Biomech 32:1297-1307

144. Hoon DSB, Kitago M, Kim J, Mori T, Piris A, Szyfelbein K, Mihm MC Jr., Nathanson SD, Padera TP, Chambers AF, Vantyghem SA, MacDonald IC, Shivers SC, Alsarraj M, Reintgen DS, Passlick B, Sienel W, Pantel K (2006) Molecular mechanisms of metastasis. Cancer Metastasis Rev 25:203-220

145. Senger DR, Galli SJ, Dvorak AM, Perruzzi CA, Harvey VS, Dvorak HF (1983) Tumor cells secrete a vascular permeability factor that promotes accumulation of ascites fluid. Science 219:983-985

146. Senger DR, Perruzzi CA, Feder J, Dvorak HF (1986) A highly conserved vascular permeability factor secreted by a variety of human and rodent tumor cell lines. Cancer Res 46:5629-5632

147. Dvorak HF (2002) Vascular permeability factor/vascular endothelial growth factor: a critical cytokine in tumor angiogenesis and a potential target for diagnosis and therapy. J Clin Oncol 20:4368-4380
148. Boucher Y, Jain RK (1992) Microvascular pressure is the principal driving force for interstitial hypertension in solid tumors: Implications for vascular collapse. Cancer Res 52:5110-5114
149. Peterson HI (1991) The microcirculation of tumors. In: Orr FW, Buchanan MR, Weiss L (eds) Microcirculation in cancer metastases. CRC Press, Ann Arbor, MI, pp 277-298
150. Nathanson SD, Nelson LT (1994) Interstitial fluid pressure in breast cancer, benign breast conditions and breast parenchyma. Ann Surg Oncol 1:333-338
151. Jain RK (1989) Delivery of novel therapeutic agents in tumors: Physiological barriers and strategies. J Natl Cancer Inst 81:570-576
152. Jain RK (1987) Interstitial transport in tumors. Adv Microcirc 13:266-284
153. Witte MH, Jones K, Wilting J, Dictor M, Selg M, McHale N, Gershenwald JE, Jackson DG (2006) Structure function relationships in the lymphatic system and implications for cancer biology. Cancer Metastasis Rev 25:159-184
154. Liotta LA, Kohn EC (2001) The microenvironment of the tumour-host interface. Nature 411:375-379
155. Nathanson SD, Nelson L, Anaya P, Havstad S, Hetzel FW (1991) Development of lymph node and pulmonary metastases after local irradiation and hyperthermia of footpad melanomas. Clin Exp Metastasis 9:377-392
156. Willett CG, Boucher Y, di Tomaso E, Duda DG, Munn LL, Tong RT, Chung DC, Sahani DV, Kalva SP, Kozin SV, Mino M, Cohen KS, Scadden DT, Hartford AC, Fischman AJ, Clark JW, Ryan DP, Zhu AX, Blaszkowsky LS, Chen HX, Shellito PC, Lauwers GY, Jain RK (2004) Direct evidence that the VEGF-specific antibody bevacumab has antivascular effects in human rectal cancer. Nat Med 10:145-147
157. Aukland K, Reed RK (1993) Interstitial-lymphatic mechanisms in the control of extracellular fluid volume. Physiol Rev 73:1-78
158. Nathanson SD, Nelson L, Karvelis KC (1996) Rates of flow of technetium 99m-labeled human serum albumin from peripheral injection sites to sentinel lymph nodes. Ann Surg Oncol 3:329-335
159. Avery M, Nathanson SD and Hetzel FW (1992) Lymph Flow from murine footpad tumors before and after sublethal hyperthermia. Radiat Res 132:50-53
160. Nathanson SD, Avery M, Anaya P, Sarantou T, Hetzel FW (1997) Lymphatic diameters and lymph clearance rates in a murine melanoma model. Arch Surg 132:311-315
161. Nathanson SD, Westrick P, Anaya P, Hetzel FW, Jacobsen G (1989) Relationship of spontaneous regional lymph node metastases to dose of local irradiation of primary B16 melanomas. Cancer Res 49:4412-4416
162. Jain RK, Munn LL, Fukumura D (2002) Dissecting tumour pathophysiology using intravital microscopy. Nat Rev Cancer 2:266-276
163. Brown EB, Boucher Y, Nasser S, Jain RK (2004) Measurement of macromolecular diffusion coefficients in human tumors. Microvasc Res 67:231-236
164. MacDonald IC, Groom AC, Chambers AF (2002) Cancer spread and micrometastasis development: Quantitative approaches for in vivo models. Bioessays 24:885-893
165. Leong SPL (2006) Cancer metastasis and the lymphovascular system: Basis for rational therapy. Cancer Metastasis Rev 25:157-294
166. Morton DL, Thompson JF, Cochran AJ, Mozzillo N, Elashoff R, Essner R, Nieweg OE, Roses DF, Hoekstra HJ, Karakousis CP, Reintgen DS, Coventry BJ, Glass EC, Wang HJ, MSLT Group (2006) Sentinel-Node Biopsy or Nodal Observation in Melanoma. N Engl J Med 355:1307-1317
167. Miller MJ, Wei SH, Parker I, Calahan MD (2002) Two-photon imaging of lymphocyte motility and antigen response in intact lymph nodes. Science 296:1869-1873
168. Stoll S, Delon J, Brotz TM, Germain RN (2002) Dynamic imaging of T cell-dendritic cell interactions in lymph nodes. Science 296:1873-1876
169. Muller A, Homey B, Soto H, Ge N, Catron D, Buchanan ME, McClanahan T, Murphy E, Yuan W, Wagner SN, Barrera JL, Mohar A, Verastegui E, Zlotnik A (2001) Involvement of chemokine receptors in breast cancer metastasis. Nature 410:50-56
170. Wiley HE, Gonzalez EB, Maki W, Wu M, Hwang ST (2001). Expression of CC chemokine receptor 7 and regional lymph lymph node metastasis of B16 murine melanoma. J Natl Cancer Inst 93:1638-1643
171. He Y, Kozaki K, Karpanen T, Koshikawa K, Yla-Herttuala S, Takahashi T, Alitalo K (2002) Suppression of tumor lymphangiogenesis and lymph node metastasis by blocking vascular endothelial growth factor receptor 3 signaling. J Natl Cancer Inst 94:819-825
172. Stacker SA, Caesar C, Baldwin ME, Thornton GE, Williams RA, Prevo R, Jackson DG, Nishikawa S, Kubo H, Achen MG (2001) VEGF-D promotes the metastatic spread of tumor cells via the lymphatics. Nat Med 7:186-191

173. Diperna CA, Bart RD, Sievers EM, Ma Y, Starnes VA, Bremner RM (2003) Cyclooxygenase-2 inhibition decreases primary and metastatic tumor burden in a murine model of orthotopic lung adenocarcinoma. J Thorac Cardiovasc Surg 126:1129-1133

174. Triest JA, Grignon DJ, Cher ML, Kocheril SV, Montecillo EJ, Talati B, Tekyi-Mensah S, Pontes JE, Hillman GG (1998) Systemic interleukin 2 therapy for human prostate tumors in a nude mouse model. Clin Cancer Res 4:2009-2014

175. Mitani N, Murakami K, Yamaura T, Ikeda T, Saiki I (2001) Inhibitory effects of berberine on the mediastinal lymph node metastasis produced by orthotopic implantation of Lewis lung carcinoma. Cancer Lett 165:35-42

176. Yokoi K, Thaker PH, Yazici S, Rebhun RR, Nam DH, He J, Kim SJ, Abbruzzese JL, Hamilton SR, Fidler IJ (2005) Dual inhibition of epidermal growth factor receptor and vascular endothelial growth factor receptor phosphorylation by AEE788 reduces growth and metastasis of human colon carcinoma in an orthotopic nude mouse model. Cancer Res 65:3716-3725

177. Nakamura ES, Koizumi K, Kobayashi M, Saiki I (2004) Inhibition of lymphangiogenesis-related properties of murine lymphatic endothelial cells and lymph node metastasis of lung cancer by the matrix metalloproteinase inhibitor MMI270. Cancer Sci 95:25-31

178. Drevs J, Hofmann I, Hugenschmidt H, Wittig C, Madjar H, Muller M, Wood J, Martiny-Baron G, Unger C, Marme D (2000) Effects of PTK787/ZK 222584, a specific inhibitor of vascular endothelial growth factor receptor tyrosine kinases on primary tumor, metastasis, vessel density, and blood flow in a murine renal cell carcinoma model. Cancer Res 60:4819-4824

11. A NEW BREAST CANCER MODEL FOR LYMPHATIC METASTASIS

MICHAEL M. LIZARDO[1,4], IAN C. MACDONALD[1,2], ALAN B. TUCK[2,3,4], AND ANN F. CHAMBERS[1,2,4]

[1]Department of Medical Biophysics, [2]Department of Oncology, University of Western Ontario, London, Ontario, Canada, [3]Department of Pathology, London Health Sciences Center, [4]London Regional Cancer Program, London Health Sciences Center, London, Ontario, Canada

INTRODUCTION

Lymphatic vessels provide one of the main anatomical routes by which invasive tumor cells can disseminate from the primary tumor. Certain types of cancer, breast cancer in particular, have a propensity to disseminate via the lymphatics. Yet despite the prevalence of lymphatic metastasis, experimental work elucidating the underlying biology, until recently, has been relatively limited. In the past several years, experimental metastasis research has experienced a surge in the number of studies examining the molecular determinants of lymphatic metastasis, as well as in vivo imaging of its progression in animal models. The following review aims to highlight recent preclinical experimental work that contributes to our basic understanding of lymphatic metastasis in breast cancer, and to describe a recently developed human cell model for lymphatic metastasis. Before continuing, however, a brief overview of clinical and pathological studies that detail the natural history of lymphatic metastasis in breast cancer will set the disease model, which experimental models must mimic.

NATURAL HISTORY OF LYMPHATIC METASTASIS IN BREAST CANCER

Physicians have described the spread of breast cancer to axillary lymph nodes and patient treatment as early as the eighteenth century (41). Since then, a multitude of clinical and pathological studies have been published, suggesting that the lymphatic spread of breast cancer cells and formation of axillary lymph node metastases are common events in the natural history of the disease. With respect to the prevalence of lymphatic metastasis in breast cancer, 30–50% of patients with invasive disease have lymph node metastases, and lymph node status is one of the strongest prognostic indicators for breast cancer (12). Upon review of the current literature, it is evident that there are at least three potentially clinically relevant steps in lymphatic metastasis (1) lymphangiogenesis, (2) lymphatic invasion, and (3) lymph node metastasis.

LYMPHANGIOGENESIS

Neovascularization contributes to the dissemination of tumor cells by increasing the likelihood of tumor cell intravasation into vessels (11). In the context of lymphatic metastasis, it is reasonable to presume that increased lymphatic vessel density as a result of lymphangiogenesis would increase the likelihood of tumor cell invasion into lymphatic vessels. Indeed, there are clinical studies supporting this notion. Nakamura and colleagues (26) examined archived and fresh frozen patient-tissue samples, and demonstrated that elevated expression levels of vascular endothelial growth factor C (VEGF-C) was associated with increased lymphatic vessel density, lymph node metastases, and decreased patient survival. To add to these findings, Schoppmann and colleagues (36) analyzed archival tissue from patients with invasive breast cancer and found a significant association between VEGF-C expression from tumor-associated macrophages (TAMs) and lymphatic microvessel density (LMVD), as well as LMVD and lymphovascular invasion. These findings support the idea that the local peritumoral inflammatory reaction, which contains VEGF-C expressing macrophages, may contribute to lymphangiogenesis, thereby increasing the likelihood of lymphatic invasion by tumor cells (9).

LYMPHATIC INVASION

Tumor cell intravasation into lymphatic vessels is requisite for the initiation of lymphatic metastasis (27). Lymphatic or vascular invasion, a sign of poor prognosis in breast cancer, is commonly referred to as "lymphovascular invasion," and means any involvement of an endothelial-lined space (20). Although it has been said that differentiating between vascular and lymphatic space involvement is not important in terms of prognostic value (both are felt to be associated with poor outcome), the use of this definition precludes the ability to tease out the relative significance of a lymphatic vs. a vascular route of metastasis. The development of new and improved markers of lymphatic endothelium, however, have allowed the specific evaluation of tumor cells found within lymphatic vessels, as defined by positive staining for markers such as lymphatic vessel endothelial hyaluronan receptor-1 (LYVE-1) (2), podoplanin (3), D2-40 (17), or Prox-1 (42, 43). Using dual-color immunofluorescence staining for LYVE-1 and podoplanin, Schoppmann and colleagues (35) demonstrated that lymphatic invasion was associated with an increased risk of developing lymph node metastasis, as well as lower overall patient survival. The same authors also found a correlation between high LMVD and lymphatic invasion. This supports Folkman's notion that increased vessel density increases the likelihood of tumor cell intravasation, in the context of lymphatic vessels.

LYMPH NODE METASTASIS

The prognostic value of axillary lymph node metastasis has been well known, and provides one of the strongest prognostic factors in breast cancer (7, 10, 12, 19, 30, 31). This is very well established for metastatic nodal deposits >2.0 mm (15). With lesser degrees of nodal involvement, the association with outcome is less clear. The preponderance of the literature would suggest that micrometastatic nodal involvement (that recognizable on routine H&E stained slides, as >0.2 mm, but not >2.0 mm) is also significant, but perhaps with a lesser degree of impact on prognosis (pN1mi by AJCC 6th edition staging criteria) (13, 23). The clinical significance of nodal deposits no greater than 0.2 mm, however (referred to as isolated tumor cells, pN0i+ by AJCC 6th edition staging criteria), is controversial (33, 37).

THE PROGRESSION OF LYMPHATIC METASTASIS

As with stepwise progression of hematogenous (blood-borne) metastasis, lymphatic metastasis is presumed to be a stepwise phenomenon (6). From the aforementioned clinical data, we can model that lymphatic metastasis can occur in five steps as illustrated in Fig. 1.

The steps depicted in Fig. 1 manifest as distinct histopathological entities, some of which have prognostic significance (e.g., lymphatic invasion and lymph node

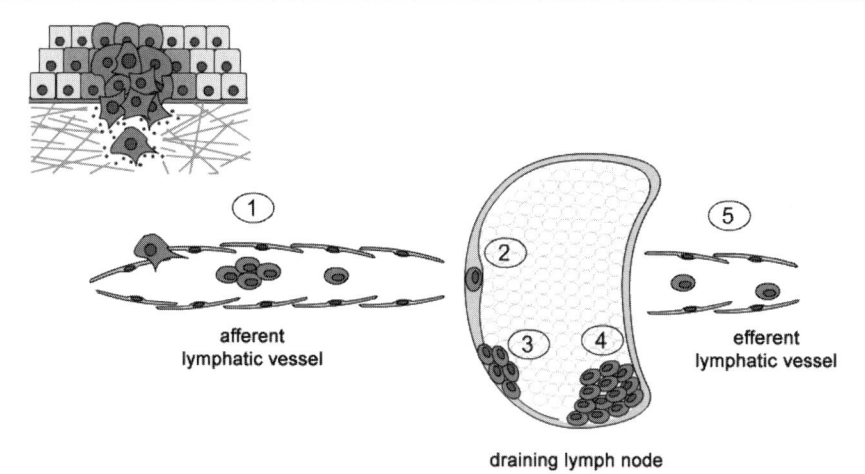

Figure 1. Events during the progression of lymphatic metastasis (*1*) tumor cell entry and transit within lymphatics (lymphatic invasion), (*2*) arrest in the draining lymph node (ITCs; "isolated tumor cells"), (*3*) formation of micrometastasis in the lymph node, (*4*) establishment of macrometastasis in the lymph node, and (*5*) further dissemination to downstream lymphatic vessels and lymph nodes

metastasis). However, whether the model represents a true continuous progression has yet to be ascertained. Questions still remain with respect to minimal nodal involvement. For example, do all ITCs develop into micrometastases, or only a small proportion? Similarly with micrometastases, what proportion of micrometastases develops into lymph node macrometastases?

Questions such as these can be addressed by using the experimental tools that were used to ascertain the timing of events and molecular determinants of *hematogenous* metastasis, and applying them to the study of the *lymphatic* metastasis. For example, Luzzi and colleagues (21), through the use of intravital videomicroscopy (IVVM), have demonstrated that tumor cells that are introduced into the systemic circulation arrest and extravasate into secondary organs with high efficiency. However, only a small proportion of these cells was able to establish growth at the secondary site. More strikingly, Naumov and colleagues (28, 29) employed IVVM to demonstrate the presence of "dormant" single nondividing cells that have extravasated into the liver parenchyma and have survived up to 11 weeks after injection. More recently, Heyn et al. (14) employed magnetic resonance imaging (MRI) to study the fate of breast cancer cells in a mouse model of brain metastasis. Their work corroborates the notion that only a small proportion of tumor cells that arrive in a secondary site have the capacity to establish metastases. Applying these imaging techniques to monitor the spread of tumor cells into the lymphatic system in vivo, in a longitudinal fashion, will provide insight into which step(s) of lymphatic metastasis tumor cells accomplish with low efficiency, thereby elucidating the rate-limiting step(s) of the process. Strategies to use IVVM methodologies to image hematogenous and lymphatic metastasis are discussed further by MacDonald et al. (22) and Jain (16).

BIOLOGICAL MODELS OF LYMPHATIC METASTASIS IN BREAST CANCER

The ideal biological model would accurately recapitulate the progression of lymphatic metastasis, whereby cells from a primary tumor metastasize to a defined lymph node(s) that drains the tumor, in a reliable and predictable manner (6). Once established, these models can be used to determine which biological and genetic factors contribute to a cancer cell's ability to preferentially spread via the lymphatics. Moreover, such models will help determine which step(s) in the progression of lymphatic metastasis offer a therapeutic window in which tumor cells are susceptible.

HISTORICAL WORK

With respect to experimental studies of lymphatic metastasis in breast, earlier work in the 1970s by Ian Carr merits discussion. At the University of Saskatchewan, Carr and colleagues studied a series of rat mammary carcinomas that reproducibly metastasized to the popliteal lymph node when injected into the foot pad. In one study using Rd/3 cells, Carr and associates demonstrated that the primary tumor in the footpad continually seeds the popliteal lymph node with tumor cells, leading to the occurrence of progressive lymphatic metastasis. However, if the footpad was removed at 24 h postinjection, progressive lymphatic metastasis did not occur (5). In another study using Walker rat carcinoma cells, cannulation of the lymphatic trunk efferent to the primary tumor revealed a progressive rise, with time, in the number of tumor cells leaving the primary tumor (4).

EXPERIMENTAL MODELS OF LYMPHANGIOGENESIS

To model tumor-associated lymphangiogenesis, Skobe and associates (38) engineered MDA-MB-435 human breast cancer cells to overexpress VEGF-C. These cells were able to significantly increase intratumoral lymphangiogenesis when implanted in nude mice. Moreover, overexpression of VEGF-C was also associated with a 60% increase in the incidence of lymph node metastasis. Similar findings have been demonstrated using MCF-7 human breast cancer cells (18, 24).

CHEMOKINES AND CHEMOKINE RECEPTORS

There is mounting evidence suggesting that tumor cells may actively migrate toward, and intravasate into, lymphatic vessels by conscripting the same mechanisms of adhesion and migration that leukocytes use for entry into the lymphatic system. In a seminal paper by Muller and associates (25), the authors provide clinical and experimental data suggesting that breast cancer cells express chemokine receptors (e.g., CXCR-4) that actively promote tumor cell migration into lymphatics and draining lymph nodes. In their experimental mouse studies, the inhibition of CXCR-4 with neutralizing anti–CXCR-4 antibodies significantly inhibited metastasis to the inguinal and axillary lymph nodes and lung.

A NEW MODEL OF LYMPHATIC METASTASIS IN BREAST CANCER

Vantyghem and colleagues (40) have established a new variant of the MDA-MB-468 human mammary adenocarcinoma cell line, called 468LN, which aggressively and preferentially spreads via lymphatic vessels, producing extensive lymph node metastases. This model will provide a powerful tool for permitting details of lymphatic metastasis to be elucidated.

The MDA-MB-468 parental cell line is tumorigenic but poorly metastatic (32, 44). In contrast, injection of 468LN cells into the second thoracic mammary fat pad of 7- to 8-week-old nude mice produces lymph node metastasis in 100% of the mice in 12 weeks ($n = 10$). Nodal involvement is apparent both above and below the diaphragm, including the axillary, cervical, periscapular, peritracheal, periaortic, inguinal mammary fat pad, perirenal, and pelvic lymph nodes.

In a preliminary analysis of molecular differences between 468LN and parental MDA-MB-468 cells, 468LN cells were found to express higher levels of the protein osteopontin (OPN), as well as increased levels of β_1, β_3, $\alpha v \beta_5$, and $\alpha_9 \beta_1$ integrins. OPN is a secreted, integrin-binding, glycophosphoprotein that has been shown to have important functional role in various aspects of malignancy, particularly tissue invasion and metastasis (8, 34, 39). More recently, Allan and associates (1) have demonstrated a functional relationship between OPN's β_3 integrin binding domain and the capacity for lymphatic spread. MDA-MB-468 breast cancer cells expressing a mutant form of OPN (lacking the RGD amino acid sequence) showed decreased lymphovascular invasion and lymph node metastases when compared with cells expressing wild-type OPN. These experiments demonstrate how additional molecules, other than lymphangiogenic factors and chemokine signaling, can contribute to the lymphatic metastatic phenotype.

The consistent ability of 468LN cells to metastasize to lymph nodes provides an excellent model to study the molecular determinants of lymphatic metastasis. When compared with the poorly metastatic parental 468 cells, differences can be observed at the molecular level. The contrast in molecular characteristics between these two cell lines will permit the elucidation of biological molecules (e.g., OPN and the $\alpha_9\beta_1$ integrin) that may influence the progression of lymphatic metastasis. Such studies will lead to a better understanding of the biology of lymphatic metastasis, and may enable the development of novel molecular-targeted therapies that reduce or inhibit the incidence of lymphatic metastasis.

UNANSWERED QUESTIONS

The recent discoveries in lymphatic biology and lymphatic metastasis are indeed proving this to be an exciting time in this field. Such studies are important in addressing questions regarding the progression of lymphatic metastasis. For example, during tumor progression, how many cells are shed into the lymphatics? What proportion of these tumor cells survives to form lymph node metastases? To what degree do lymph node metastases contribute (if at all) to systemic dissemination? What biological factors affect the progression of lymph node metastases? Such questions not only aim to determine the biological significance of ITCs and micrometastases, but to also find biological markers that have predictive value when assessing patient outcome.

At the cellular level, the interaction between breast cancer cells and the lymphatic endothelial cells and vessels may provide information about the rate-limiting step(s) of lymphatic metastasis. Is there molecular crosstalk, or adhesive interactions, between tumor cells and lymphatic endothelial cells? Does the disruption of these interactions affect the progression of lymphatic metastasis?

These unanswered questions underscore the need for more models of lymphatic metastasis. Current experimental research is beginning to uncover the molecular determinants of lymphatic metastasis. However, at the same time, it is also important to develop additional imaging strategies that permit the in vivo longitudinal imaging of the progression of lymphatic metastasis. The intersection between imaging and biological modeling of lymphatic metastasis will provide an innovative approach to discovering the in vivo dynamics of lymphatic metastasis; and more importantly, such models will permit the noninvasive and longitudinal evaluation of the efficacy of antilymphatic metastatic therapeutics.

CONCLUDING REMARKS

It is evident during the progression of lymphatic metastasis that several key events (lymphatic invasion, lymphangiogenesis, and lymph node metastasis) can clinically impact on patient outcome. The biological significance of histopathological entities such as ITCs and micrometastases in the lymph node has yet to be ascertained. Current preclinical experimental models aim to elucidate the molecular determinants that underlie lymphatic metastasis. Such studies may provide information with regards to molecular targets in which novel molecular-targeted therapies can be developed to antagonize the lymphatic spread of breast cancer cells.

ACKNOWLEDGMENTS

This research was supported in part by grant no. 016506 from the Canadian Breast Cancer Research Alliance, with special funding support from the Canadian Breast Cancer Foundation and The Cancer Research Society.

REFERENCES

1. Allan AL, George R, Vantyghem SA, Lee MW, Hodgson NC, Engel CJ, Holliday RL, Girvan DP, Scott LA, Postenka CO, Al-Katib W, Stitt LW, Uede T, Chambers AF, Tuck AB (2006) Role of the integrin-binding protein osteopontin in lymphatic metastasis of breast cancer. Am J Pathol 169:233-246
2. Banerji S, Ni J, Wang SX, Clasper S, Su J, Tammi R, Jones M, DG Jackson (1999) LYVE-1, a new homologue of the CD44 glycoprotein, is a lymph-specific receptor for hyaluronan. J Cell Biol 144:789-801
3. Breiteneder-Geleff S, Soleiman A, Kowalski H, Horvat R, Amann G, Kriehuber E, Diem K, Weninger W, Tschachler E, Alitalo K, Kerjaschki D (1999) Angiosarcomas express mixed endothelial phenotypes of blood and lymphatic capillaries: podoplanin as a specific marker for lymphatic endothelium. Am J Pathol 154:385-394
4. Carr J, Carr I, Dreher B, Betts K (1980) Lymphatic metastasis: invasion of lymphatic vessels and efflux of tumour cells in the afferent popliteal lymph as seen in the Walker rat carcinoma. J Pathol 132: 287-305
5. Carr I, McGinty F (1976) Neoplastic invasion and metastasis within the lymphoreticular system. Advances in Experimental Medicine and Biology 73(Pt B):319-329
6. Carr I, Carr J (1982) Tumor Invasion and Metastasis: Experimental models of lymphatic metastasis. In: Liotta LA, and IR Hart (eds) Developments in Oncology 7. Martinus Nijhoff Publishers, Boston, pp 189-206
7. Contesso G, Rouesse J, Petit JY, Mouriesse H (1977) Les facteurs anatomo-pathologiques du pronostic des cancers du sein. Bulletin du Cancer 64:525-236
8. Cook AC, Tuck AB, McCarthy S, Turner JG, Irby RB, Bloom GC, Yeatman TJ, Chambers AF (2005) Osteopontin induces multiple changes in gene expression that reflect the six "hallmarks of cancer" in a model of breast cancer progression. Molecular Carcinogenesis 43:225-236
9. Coussens LM, Werb Z (2002) Inflammation and cancer. Nature 420:860-867
10. Fisher ER, Sass E, Fisher B (1984) Pathological findings from the NSABP Protocol 4: discriminants for tenth year treatment failure. Cancer 53:712-723
11. Folkman J (1992) The role of angiogenesis in tumor growth and metastasis. Seminars in Oncology 6 supplement 6:15-18
12. Foster RS (1996) The biologic and clinical significance of lymphatic metastasis in breast cancer. Surgical Oncology Clinics of North America 5:79-104
13. Greene FL, Page DL, Fleming ID, Fritz AG, Balch CM, Haller DG, Morrow M (2002) AJCC Cancer Staging Manual 6th ed. New York: Springer
14. Heyn C, Ronald JA, Ramadan SS, Snir JA, Barry AM, MacKenzie LT, Mikulis DJ, Palmieri D, Bronder JL, Steeg PS, Yoneda T, MacDonald IC, Chambers AF, Rutt BK, Foster PJ (2006) In vivo MRI of cancer cell fate at the single-cell level in a mouse model of breast cancer metastasis to the brain. Magnetic Resonance in Medicine 56:1001-1010
15. Huvos AG, Hutter RV, Berg JW (1971) Significance of axillary macrometastases and micrometastases in mammary cancer. Annals of Surgery 173:44-46

16. Jain RK (2002) Angiogenesis and lymphangiogenesis in tumors: insights from intravital microscopy. Cold Spring Harb Symp Quant Biol 67:239-248
17. Kahn HJ, Bailey D, Marks A (2002) Monoclonal antibody D2-40, a new marker of lymphatic endothelium, reacts with Kaposi's sarcoma and a subset of angiosarcomas. Modern Pathology 15:434-440
18. Karpanen T, Egeblad M, Karkkainen MJ, Kubo H, Yla-Herttuala S, Jaattela M, Alitalo K (2001) Vascular endothelial growth factor C promotes tumor lymphangiogenesis and intralymphatic tumor growth. Cancer Res 61:1786-1790
19. Koscielny S, Le MG, Tubiana M (1989) The natural history of human breast cancer: The relationship between involvement of axillary lymph nodes and the initiation of distant metastases. Br J Cancer 59:775-782
20. Lauria R, Perrone F, Carlomagno C, De Laurentiis M, Morabito A, Gallo C, Varriale E, Pettinato G, Panico L, Petrella G, et al (1995) The prognostic value of lymphatic and blood vessel invasion in operable breast cancer. Cancer 76:1772-1778
21. Luzzi KJ, MacDonald IC, Schmidt EE, Kerkvliet N, Morris VL, Chambers AF, Groom AC (1998) Multistep nature of metastatic inefficiency: dormancy of solitary cells after successful extravasation and limited survival of early micrometastases. Am J Pathol 153:865-873
22. MacDonald IC, Groom AC, Chambers AF (2002) Cancer spread and micrometastasis development: quantitative approaches for in vivo models. Bioessays 24:885-893
23. Maibenco DC, Dombi GW, Kau TY, Severson RK (2006) Significance of micrometastases on the survival of women with T1 breast cancer. Cancer 107:1234-1239
24. Mattila MM, Ruohola JK, Karpanen T, Jackson DG, Alitalo K, Harkonen PL (2002) VEGF-C induced lymphangiogenesis is associated with lymph node metastasis in orthotopic MCF-7 tumors. Int J Cancer 98:946-951
25. Muller A, Homey B, Soto H, Ge N, Catron D, Buchanan ME, McClanahan T, Murphy E, Yuan W, Wagner SN, Barrera JL, Mohar A, Verastegui E, Zlotnik Z (2001) Involvement of chemokine receptors in breast cancer metastasis. Nature 410:50-56
26. Nakamura Y, Yasuoka H, Tsujimoto M, Imabun S, Nakahara M, Nakao K, Nakamura M, Mori I, Kakudo K (2005) Lymph vessel density correlates with nodal status, VEGF-C expression, and prognosis in breast cancer. Breast Cancer Research and Treatment 91:125-132
27. Nathanson SD, Anaya P, Avery M, Hetzel FW, Sarantou T, Havstad S (1997) Sentinal lymph node metastasis in experimental melanoma: relationships among primary tumor size, lymphatic vessel diameter, and 99mTc-labeled human albumin clearance. Annals of Surgical Oncology 4:161-168
28. Naumov GN, Wilson SM, MacDonald IC, Schmidt EE, Morris VL, Groom AC, Hoffman RM, Chambers AF (1999) Cellular expression of green fluorescent protein, coupled with high-resolution in vivo videomicroscopy, to monitor steps in tumor metastasis. J Cell Science 112:1833-1842
29. Naumov GN, MacDonald IC, Weinmeister PM, Kerkvliet N, Nadkarni KV, Wilson SM, Morris VL, Groom AC, Chambers AF (2002) Persistence of solitary mammary carcinoma cells in a secondary site: a possible contributor to dormancy. Cancer Res 62:2162-2168
30. Nemoto T, Vana J, Bedwani RN, Baker HW, McGregor FH, Murphy GP (1980) Management and survival of female breast cancer: results of a national survey by the American College of Surgeons. Cancer 45:2917-2924
31. Peloquin A, Poljicak M, Falardeau M, Gravel D, Moisescu R, Peloquin L (1991) Cancer of the breast: a study of 1520 consecutive patients operated on between 1960 and 1980. Canadian Journal of Surgery 34:151-156
32. Price JE, Zhang RD (1990) Studies of human breast cancer metastasis using nude mice. Cancer Metastasis Reviews 8:285–297
33. Querzoli P, Pedriali M, Rinaldi R, Lombardi AR, Biganzoli E, Boracchi P, Ferretti S, Frasson C, Zanella C, Ghisellini S, Ambrogi F, Antolini L, Piantelli M, Iacobelli S, Marubini E, Alberti S, Nenci I (2006) Axillary lymph node nanometastases are prognostic factors for disease-free survival and metastatic relapse in breast cancer patients. Clin Cancer Res 12:6696-6701
34. Rittling SR, Chambers AF (2004) Role of osteopontin in tumour progression. Br J Cancer 90:1877-1881
35. Schoppmann, SF, Bayer G, Aumayr K, Taucher S, Geleff S, Rudas M, Kubista E, Hausmaninger H, Samonigg H, Gnant M, Jakesz R, Horvat R, and Austrian Breast and Colorectal Cancer Study Group (2004) Prognostic value of lymphangiogenesis and lymphovascular invasion in invasive breast cancer. Annals of Surgery 240:306-312
36. Schoppmann SF, Fenzl A, Nagy K, Unger S, Bayer G, Geleff S, Gnant M, Horvat R, Jakesz R, Birner P (2006) VEGF-C expressing tumor-associated macrophages in lymph node positive breast cancer: impact on lymphangiogenesis and survival. Surgery 139:839-846

37. Singletary SE, Greene FL (2003) Revision of breast cancer staging: the 6th edition of the TNM Classification. Seminars in Surgical Oncology 21:53-59
38. Skobe M, Hawighorst T, Jackson DG, Prevo R, Janes L, Velasco P, Riccardi L, Alitalo K, Claffey K, Detmar M (2001) Induction of tumor lymphangiogenesis by VEGF-C promotes breast cancer metastasis. Nature Medicine 7:192-198
39. Tuck AB, Chambers AF (2001) The role of osteopontin in breast cancer: clinical and experimental studies. Journal of Mammary Gland Biology and Neoplasia 6:419-429
40. Vantyghem SA, Allan AL, Postenka CO, Al-Katib W, Keeney M, Tuck AB, Chambers AF (2005) A new model for lymphatic metastasis: development of a variant of the MDA–MB-468 human breast cancer cell line that aggressively metastasizes to lymph nodes. Clinical and Experimental Metastasis 22:351-61
41. Weiss L (2000) Metastasis of cancer: A conceptual history from antiquity to the 1990s. Cancer and Metastasis Reviews 19:219-234
42. Wigle JT, Oliver G (1999) Prox1 function is required for the development of the murine lymphatic system. Cell 98:769-78
43. Wilting J, Papoutsi M, Christ B, Nicolaides KH, von Kaisenberg CS, Borges J, Stark GB, Alitalo K, Tomarev SI, Niemeyer C, Rossler J (2002) The transcription factor Prox1 is a marker for lymphatic endothelial cells in normal and diseased human tissues. FASEB Journal 16:1271-1273
44. Zhang RD, Fidler IJ, Price JE (1991) Relative malignant potential of human breast carcinoma cell lines established from pleural effusions and a brain metastasis. Invasion Metastasis 11:204-215

12. LYMPH NODE MICROMETASTASES IN LUNG CANCER

KATHARINA E. EFFENBERGER[1], WULF SIENEL[2], AND KLAUS PANTEL[1]

[1]Institute of Tumor Biology, University Medical Center, Hamburg Eppendorf Hamburg, Germany,
[2]Department of Thoracic Surgery, Albert-Ludwigs-University Freiburg, Freiburg, Germany

INTRODUCTION

Lung cancer remains the most common cause of cancer-related death in Europe and the United States (9, 10). Nonsmall-cell lung cancer (NSCLC) affects approximately 80% of all lung cancer patients (5, 9). Surgery remains the gold standard treatment for locoregional NSCLC, and pathological lymph node (pN) status has remained the strongest clinical prognostic characteristic in early stages of operable NSCLC (21, 23). However, even in early stages, the 5-year survival rate of N0 patients remains at only 60–70% after complete resection of the primary tumor (7, 17). This suggests that tumor cell dissemination occurs early and occult micrometastases or single disseminated tumor cells (DTC), which are not discovered by conventional histopathologic methods, may be present in the lymph nodes at the time of surgery (6, 16, 18, 22, 26). Detection of these cells might potentially improve clinical lymph node staging and help to identify patients who could benefit from adjuvant or neoadjuvant therapy.

DTC are defined as single tumor cells or small cell clusters that can be detected in regional lymph nodes, peripheral blood, or organs remote from the primary tumor (e.g., bone marrow). These cells can be identified by sensitive immunohistochemical and molecular techniques (25).

DETECTION METHODS AND FREQUENCIES OF DTC IN REGIONAL LYMPH NODES

Immunohistochemistry

DTC in regional lymph nodes can be reliably detected using sensitive immunohisto-chemical techniques with monoclonal antibodies (mAb) against epithelium-specific proteins. Our group used mAb Ber-Ep 4 directed against epithelial cell adhesion molecule (EpCAM) to detect micrometastatic tumor cells (12, 14). The antibody does not react with mesenchymal tissue, including lymphoid tissue (19). In order to compare the effectiveness of the immunohistochemical analyses directly with the conventional hematoxylin–eosin (HE) method, two additional sections consecutive to those displaying Ber-Ep 4-positive cells were either stained by the routine HE method or by Ber-Ep 4. Both sections were then compared with the original positive section by an experienced pathologist without knowledge of the initial results. As a control, consecutive sections from Ber-Ep 4-negative lymph nodes were stained under the same conditions. Repeated immunostaining resulted in the redetection of Ber-Ep 4-positive cells in a neighboring section in 93.3% of the nodes and in 90.9% of the patients, respectively. In contrast, repeated HE-staining and histopathologic examination did not reveal any tumor cells.

The incidence of DTC detected by immunohistochemical staining with Ber-Ep 4 was 6.2% (35/565) in lymph nodes, which were negative by routine histopathology, and in 27 (21.6%) of 125 patients with resectable NSCLC (12). These cells occurred either as isolated, single cells, or as cell clusters of up to three cells present in the sinuses (60%) and the lymphoid tissue of the node (40%). In most patients, DTC were found in more than one of the three lymph node sections (31%), or more than one lymph node (55%). By conventional histopathology, 70 of 125 patients were staged as having pN0 disease and 55 as having pN1–2 disease according to the International Union Against Cancer (UICC) TNM classification (20). In pN1–2 patients, immunohistochemical staining detected tumor cell dissemination in 16 cases (29.1%). This was clearly higher than in pN0 patients, who had Ber-Ep 4-positive cells in their lymph nodes in 11 cases (15.7%) ($p = 0.019$). Other pathological characteristics were not associated with an increased rate of DTC.

Other immunohistochemical staining methods have been applied in order to screen histopathologically negative lymph nodes for micrometastases. Cytokeratins (CK) are intermediate filaments of the cytoskeleton of epithelial cells, and they serve for the detection of DTC originating from solid epithelial tumors (25). At least 20 different types of CK have been identified on the basis of differences in molecular weight and pH. Previously, the anti-CK monoclonal antibody AE1/AE3 has been used for immunostaining of lymph node sections (36). Five lymph nodes from each of 20 NSCLC patients were cut into three pieces and analyzed by immunohistochemical staining, flow cytometry (for both AE1/AE3 was used), and by conventional HE-staining (8). HE-staining revealed 8/100 positive lymph nodes in 4 (20%) patients, whereas immunohistochemistry resulted in 33/100 positive lymph nodes on 13 (65%) patients, and flow cytometry detected DTC in 38/100 lymph nodes in 14 (70%) patients. Ito et al. also found a correlation between flow cytometric and immunohistochemical detection of CK-positive cells within the lymph nodes, and the sensitivity of these two methods was greater than that of standard HE-staining. In a study performed by Yasumoto et al. (38), 34 of 216 (15.7%) stage I NSCLC patients had DTC in their hilar and mediastinal lymph nodes. They were detected immunocytochemically by the AE1/AE3 antibody as well.

Furthermore, AE1/AE3 antibody was used in combination with an anti-p53 protein antibody DO-1 by Gu et al. In total, 22 of 49 (44.9%) stage I (= pN0) NSCLC patients had to be upgraded (7). Patients with DTC displayed a poorer prognosis than those whose lymph nodes were free of DTC. Maruyama et al. (18) applied another monoclonal anti-CK antibody (CAM-5.2) to investigate 973 regional lymph nodes from 44 NSCLC patients. 70.5% patients had to be upstaged N1 and N2 as 91 lymph nodes showed CK-positive cells. Similar findings were reported by Chen et al. (2) in a recent retrospective study, in which 17% of the lymph nodes and 63% of the patients were considered as DTC-positive.

We conclude that serial sectioning and immunohistochemical staining improve the sensitivity of detecting DTC (24). The incidence of immunohistochemically positive lymph node specimens varies between 30 and 70% depending on the immunohistochemical staining and the primary monoclonal antibody used for DTC detection. However, immunohistochemistry is laborious, time consuming, and skilled observers are required for an objective evaluation, but a great advantage lies in the fact that IHC offers the possibility to further characterize DTC by molecular and biochemical methods (25).

Molecular Methods

Reverse transcriptase polymerase chain reaction (RT-PCR)-based tumor cell detection is in principle an observer-independent and rapid method for detecting DTC. The theory is that minute amounts of vital cancer cells can be detected in clinical samples by the amplification of specific messengerRNA (mRNA) transcripts ("markers"), selectively expressed in the cancer cells of interest but not in normal tissues. The major problem associated with RT-PCR is illegitimate transcription, which is transcription of marker genes at a minimal basic level in normal tissues without necessarily being translated into detectable amounts of protein (39). Quantitative RT-PCR (qRT-PCR) has the potential to solve this problem by setting a cut-off value using control samples to differentiate illegitimate marker gene transcription from cancer-specific expression. However, the marker transcript might be downregulated in cancer cells (e.g., CK19) and it might therefore be difficult to find an appropriate cut-off level suitable for a broad range of samples from different cancer patients with heterogeneous primary tumors.

A study performed by Salerno and coworkers (32) used a RT-PCR assay to detect occult tumor cells in lymph nodes of 28 patients with NSCLC. A total of 88 pathohistologically tumor-free nodes were examined for the expression of mRNA transcripts for mucin-1 (MUC1). MUC1 mRNA was detected in 33 (37.5%) of 88 nodes of lung cancer patients, and based on this result 16 (70%) of 23 patients had to be restaged. However, subsequent studies revealed the ubiquitous presence of MUC1 mRNA in lymph nodes and other tissues (1), diminishing its value as a tumor marker in RT-PCR studies.

A recent study applied carcinoembryonic antigen (CEA) as a marker for DTC detection (3). CEA is a 200 kDa cell-surface glycoprotein involved in cell-to-cell adhesion. Twenty-three control lymph nodes from six patients without malignancy were tested and CEA mRNA was not detected in any of the control lymph nodes analyzed. In contrast, Bostick et al. (1) found CEA mRNA in normal lymph nodes. The technology of automated quantitative real-time RT-PCR (qRT-PCR) allows rapid processing of many samples. The qRT-PCR assay for CEA mRNA was performed in such an automated real-time PCR machine, allowing quantitation of DTC in lymph nodes. The median cell number was 7,190 tumor cells per lymph node station. No statistical difference was observed between adenocarcinomas (median 7,425 tumor cells), squamous cell carcinomas (median 11,165 tumor cells), and undifferentiated tumors (median 7,190 tumor cells). Furthermore, of 232 apparently tumor-free lymph nodes from 53 stage I NSCLC patients analyzed for CEA mRNA by qRT-PCR, 59 (25.4%) were positive, revealing DTC in 30 (56.6%) patients. Similarly, Maeda and coworkers (16) observed DTC by qRT-PCR for CEA mRNA in 25% of histopathologically negative lymph nodes (52/211) and 64% of node-negative NSCLC patients (14/22).

Another study carried out by Nosotti et al. (22) evaluated the detection of DTC in histologically tumor-free lymph nodes by CEA mRNA through qRT-PCR as well as its prognostic value. In 44 NSCLC patients classified stage I, all primary tumors were positive for CEA mRNA. Of 261 analyzed lymph nodes, 35 (13.4%) showed elevated CEA mRNA levels compared with control lymph nodes and 16 (36.4%) patients were subsequently considered to have "micrometastatic" nodes.

Using qRT-PCR for creating a cut-off value to differentiate illegitimate marker gene transcription from cancer-specific expression also allowed to use cytokeratin 19 (CK19) as a marker for the detection of DTC in lymph nodes of NSCLC-patients with resectable tumors (35). CK19 is a specific cytoskeletal structure of simple epithelia, including bronchial epithelial cells. CK19 is an abundantly expressed polypeptide of epithelial cells but it can be downregulated in solid tumors. On the other hand, a low level transcription of CK19 was observed in lymph nodes of patients without malignancy (1, 35). Using qRT-PCR, out of 94 tumor-free lymph nodes, staged by the pathologist, CK19 transcripts were detected in 26 (28%) nodes, resulting in 13 (56.5%) patients that were considered as DTC-positive.

Saintigny et al. (31) tested 84 histologically negative lymph nodes of 19 patients for CK7 and CK19 mRNA by real-time RT-PCR. In the event of two (10.5%) patients (and six lymph nodes), the staging had to be changed as lymph nodes were positive for at least one marker. In another study, histopathology, immunohistochemistry, and RT-PCR were compared for 254 mediastinal lymph nodes of 49 patients suffering from NSCLC (15). Of 225 nontumoral lymph nodes based on histopathological screening, 32 (14.2%) were positive for CK19 mRNA by RT-PCR, and 16 (32.7%) patients were upstaged. Seventeen patients remained pN0 (negative by RT-PCR and HE) and 16 were classified pN2 on histopathology. IHC did not provide significant additional information.

Another study included 40 lung cancer patients (261 lymph nodes) and compared the standard HE-staining to RT-PCR for CK19 (6). In 18 patients, regional lymph node metastases were found by both HE and RT-PCR, whereas in the other 22 patients who were pathologically lymph node-negative, DTC were detected by RT-PCR in six (27%) cases.

In summary, the reported rates of DTC in lymph nodes of patients with apparently tumor-free lymph nodes range from 10 to 70%. The range of the reported rates might depend on tumor characteristics and could be influenced by specificity and sensitivity of the different applied RT-PCR methods. Compared with conventional HE-staining, RT-PCR facilitates a more sensitive assessment of the "micrometastatic status" of lymph nodes in lung cancer patients, regardless of the marker used. Moreover, the frequencies of DTC detected by qRT-PCR and those reported in immunohistochemical studies were similar. Applying molecular methods, 10.5–64.0% of the patients (i.e., 7.1–28.0% lymph nodes were DTC-positive) had to be upstaged, and 21.6–70.5% of the patients by IHC (i.e., in 6.2–33.0% of lymph nodes DTC were found), respectively. There are only a few studies directly comparing the clinical value of both technical approaches. At present, it can be concluded that both immunohistochemical and molecular detection of DTC in lymph nodes may serve as a supplement for current tumor staging in lung carcinoma. However, larger multicenter trials are needed to establish these tests in clinical practice.

PROGNOSTIC RELEVANCE OF DTC IN REGIONAL LYMPH NODES

The detection of DTC in lymph nodes by IHC is associated with a poor prognosis in patients with resectable lung cancer. Our own study on NSCLC patients revealed that after an observation time of 64 months, patients with immunohisto-chemically proven DTC in regional lymph nodes had a significantly reduced overall survival ($p = 0.0001$) (12). Correspondingly, patients with DTC experienced a higher rate of disease relapse than patients without such cells ($p = 0.0001$). Because of the elevated frequency of Ber-Ep 4-positive cells in higher pN-stages, stratification for pN-stage was done. In pN0 disease, patients with DTC had a significant overall survival disadvantage compared with those without DTC ($p = 0.010$). In pN1–2 disease, the overall survival rate was also definitely reduced in the presence of DTC and the impact of minimal tumor cell spread on overall survival was comparably strong ($p = 0.027$). A Cox regression model was applied to analyze the influence of lymphatic DTC, pT-stage, pN-stage, and age on overall survival. The multivariate analysis showed a 2.5-times increased risk of shorter survival and a 2.7-times increased risk of tumor relapse in patients with DTC vs. patients without such cells.

Pathological N-stage had a prognostic value for reduced survival in the same range (relative risk 2.3).

Maruyama et al. (18) reported that relapse-free survival was significantly shorter in patients with immunohistochemically identifiable DTC in lymph nodes than in those with DTC-negative nodes ($p = 0.004$), mainly due to distant relapse. In another Japanese study (4), paraffin-embedded specimens from 315 lymph nodes of 31 pN0 patients with completely resected (R0) NSCLC, whose primary tumors were positive for the tumor-suppressor gene product p53, were reexamined immunohistochemically using a monoclonal anti-p53 antibody. Cells positive for p53 were detected in 26 (8%) of 315 lymph nodes from 14 (45%) of the 31 patients. Once again, the finding of occult nodal tumor cells had a significant impact on survival ($p = 0.0001$).

Le Pimpec-Barthes et al. (15) used a nonquantitative CK19 RT-PCR. In their study, patients with molecularly detected DTC in lymph node had significantly reduced survival. The 2-year cancer-related death survival of the pN0 patients (100%) and the upstaged patients (64.5%) due to DTC in their lymph nodes was significantly different ($p = 0.04$). The relative risk of recurrence in the patients with DTC detected by RT-PCR compared to the pN0 patients, evaluated by the Cox model multivariate analysis, was 5.61 ($p = 0.02$). In a comparative analysis of apparently tumor-free lymph nodes between conventional HE-staining and again RT-PCR for CK19, the median observation time was 26 months (range 4–60 months) (6). Patients with DTC in the lymph nodes showed significant shorter disease-free survival duration than node-negative patients (log-rank test, $p = 0.001$). Finding of CK19 mRNA also correlated to tumor size and tumor grading. The results diagnosed by HE had no significant effect on prognoses ($p = 0.455$). A survival analysis of patients with DTC detected by an elevated CEA mRNA level through qRT-PCR revealed that patients with DTC in lymph nodes suffered from more recurrences than patients without CEA mRNA-positive lymph nodes (22).

In addition, Yasumoto et al. (38) also found a poor prognosis for those stage I NSCLC patients with immunocytochemically detected DTC in the lymph nodes by univariate ($p = 0.004$) and multivariate ($p = 0.018$) analysis. Taken together, the majority of studies investigating DTC in lymph nodes demonstrated a prognostic impact (22). This information might be used for stratification of patients in future clinical trials investigating new forms of adjuvant therapy.

TUMOR BIOLOGY OF DTC IN REGIONAL LYMPH NODES

The biology of early micrometastatic spread to lymph nodes is largely unknown. In esophageal cancer, a permanent cell line was established from a DTC-positive lymph node classified as tumor-free by routine histopathology. The cells of this cell line had characteristic features of malignant epithelial tumor cells, and they were tumorigenic and micrometastatic in vivo when transplanted in mice with severe combined immunodeficiency (33).

Genetic heterogeneity of the primary tumor is a well-known phenomenon. So far, it remains unclear which genes might be responsible for the early release of DTC into the blood or lymphatic system. In breast cancer, we found specific signatures associated with hematogenous or lymphatic spread of tumor cells (37). These signatures showed little overlap, suggesting different mechanisms leading to these two routes of dissemination. In lung cancer, similar studies are ongoing. Using array-CGH (comparative genomic hybridization) for genetic screening, our pilot study indicates the existence of certain genomic aberrations linked to micrometastatic spread to BM and some overlap with the aberrations associated to lymph node metastasis was observed (11).

Another approach is to directly characterize DTC using single cell technologies (25, 27). So far little is known about the molecular features of DTC in lymph nodes, but several groups, including ours, have used such techniques to assess DTC in bone marrow and blood. A summary of these interesting data is far beyond the scope of this review but one of the hallmarks of DTC is their dormant (i.e., non-proliferating) state (28). This "tumor cell dormancy" is characteristic for the latency period between the time from tumor cell dissemination and the development of clinically overt metastases, and the underlying mechanisms are poorly understood.

The nonproliferating state of DTC favors immunotherapeutic or other targeted therapies over S-phase-specific chemotherapeutic agents. In this context, the EpCAM antigen used for detection of DTC appears also to be an interesting therapeutic target. EpCAM is a cell adhesion molecule expressed on the cell membrane of different epithelial tumor cells, including disseminated NSCLC cells (29). Other targets for immunotherapeutic interventions belong to the class of MAGE (melanoma-associated antigen) antigens (13, 30, 34), which are the most specifically expressed tumor antigens known so far. MAGE antigens are also expressed on NSCLC cells including DTC (13). First clinical trials using vaccination strategies against MAGE antigens are ongoing.

In conclusion, the detection and characterization of DTC may lead to (a) an improved tumor staging, (b) the discovery of new therapeutic targets to eradicate minimal residual disease, and (c) novel insights into the biology of early tumor cell dissemination in cancer patients.

REFERENCES

1. Bostick PJ, Chatterjee S, Chi DD, Huynh KT, Giuliano AE, Cote R, Hoon DS (1998) Limitations of specific reverse-transcriptase polymerase chain reaction markers in the detection of metastases in the lymph nodes and blood of breast cancer patients. J Clin Oncol 16(8):2632-40
2. Chen ZL, Perez S, Holmes EC, Wang HJ, Coulson WF, Wen DR, Cochran AJ (1993) Frequency and distribution of occult micrometastases in lymph nodes of patients with non-small-cell lung carcinoma. J Natl Cancer Inst 85:493–498
3. D'Cunha J, Corfits AL, Herndon JE 2nd, Kern JA, Kohman LJ, Patterson GA, Kratzke RA, Maddaus MA (2002) Molecular staging of lung cancer: Real-time polymerase chain reaction estimation of lymph node micrometastatic tumor cell burden in stage I nonsmall cell lung cancer–preliminary results of Cancer and Leukemia Group B Trial 9761. J Thorac Cardiovasc Surg 123: 484–491; discussion 491, 2002

4. Dobashi K, Sugio K, Osaki T, Oka T, Yasumoto K (1997) Micrometastatic P53-positive cells in the lymph nodes of non-smallcell lung cancer: Prognostic significance. J Thorac Cardiovasc Surg 114: 339–346

5. el-Torky M, el-Zeky F, Hall JC (1990) Significant changes in the distribution of histologic types of lung cancer. A review of 4928 cases. Cancer 65: 2361–2367

6. Ge MJ, Wu QC, Wang M, Zhang YH, Li LB (2005) Detection of disseminated lung cancer cells in regional lymph nodes by assay of CK19 reverse transcriptase polymerase chain reaction and its clinical significance. J Cancer Res Clin Oncol 131(10):662-8

7. Gu CD, Osaki T, Oyama T, Inoue M, Kodate M, Dobashi K, Oka T, Yasumoto K (2002) Detection of micrometastatic tumor cells in pN0 lymph nodes of patients with completely resected nonsmall cell lung cancer: Impact on recurrence and Survival. Ann Surg 235:133–139

8. Ito M, Minamiya Y, Kawai H, Saito S, Saito H, Imai K, Ogawa J (2005) Intraoperative detection of lymph node micrometastasis with flow cytometry in non-small cell lung cancer. J Thorac Cardiovasc Surg 130(3):753-8

9. Janssen-Heijnen ML, Gatta G, Forman D, Capocaccia R, Coebergh JW (1998) Variation in survival of patients with lung cancer in Europe, 1985–1989. EUROCARE Working Group. Eur J Cancer 34: 2191–2196

10. Jemal A, Murray T, Ward E, Samuels A, Tiwari RC, Ghafoor A, Feuer EJ, Thun MJ (2005) Cancer statistics, 2005. CA Cancer J Clin 55:10–30, 2005

11. Kraemling M, Ruosaari S, Ylstra B, Pantel K, Wikman H (2006) Genomic profiles associated with early micrometastatic spread in lung cancer. AACR abstract, AACR #1830

12. Kubuschok B, Passlick B, Izbicki JR, Thetter O, Pantel K (1999) Disseminated tumor cells in lymph nodes as a determinant for survival in surgically resected non-small-cell lung cancer. J Clin Oncol 17: 19–24

13. Kufer P, Zippelius A, Lutterbuse R, Mecklenburg I, Enzmann T, Montag A, Weckermann D, Passlick B, Prang N, Reichardt P, Dugas M, Kollermann MW, Pantel K, Riethmuller G (2002) Heterogeneous e pression of MAGE-A genes in occult disseminated tumor cells: a novel multimarker reverse transcription-polymerase chain reaction for diagnosis of micrometastatic disease. Cancer Res 1;62(1):251-61

14. Latza U, Niedobitek G, Schwarting R, Nekarda H, Stein H (1990) Ber-EP4: New monoclonal antibody which distinguishes epithelia from mesothelial. J Clin Pathol 43:213–219

15. Le Pimpec-Barthes F, Danel C, Lacave R, Ricci S, Bry X, Lancelin F, Leber C, Milleron B, Fleury-Feith J, Riquet M, Bernaudin JF (2005) Association of CK19 mRNA detection of occult cancer cells in mediastinal lymph nodes in non-small cell lung carcinoma and high risk of early recurrence. Eur J Cancer 41:306–312

16. Maeda J, Inoue M, Okumura M, Ohta M, Minami M, Shiono H, Shintani Y, Matsuda H, Matsuura N (2006) Detection of occult tumor cells in lymph nodes from non-small cell lung cancer patients using reverse transcription-polymerase chain reaction for carcinoembryonic antigen mRNA with the evaluation of its sensitivity. Lung Cancer 52(2):235-40

17. Martini N, Bains MS, Burt ME, Zakowski MF, McCormack P, Rusch VW, Ginsberg RJ (1995) Incidence of local recurrence and second primary tumors in resected stage I lung cancer. J Thorac Cardiovasc Surg 109:120–129

18. Maruyama R, Sugio K, Mitsudomi T, Saitoh G, Ishida T, Sugimachi K (1997) Relationship between early recurrence and micrometastases in the lymph nodes of patients with stage I non-small cell lung cancer. J Thorac Cardiovasc Surg 114:535–543

19. Momburg F, Moldenhauer G, Hammerling GJ, Moller P (1987) Immun histochemical study of the expression of a Mr 34,000 human epithelium-specific surface glycoprotein in normal and malignant tissues. Cancer Res 47: 2883–2891

20. Mountain CF (1997) Revisions in the international system for staging lung cancer. Chest 111: 1710–1717

21. Mountain CF, Dresler CM (1997) Regional lymph node classification for lung cancer staging. Chest 111: 1718–1723

22. Nosotti M, Falleni M, Palleschi A, Pellegrini C, Alessi F, Bosari S, Santambrogio L (2005) Quantitative real-time polymerase chain reaction detection of lymph node lung cancer micrometastasis using carcinoembryonic antigen marker. Chest 128(3):1539-44

23. Okada M, Nishio W, Sakamoto T, Harada H, Uchino K, Tsubota N (2003) Long-term survival and prognostic factors of five-year su vivors with complete resection of non-small cell lung carcinoma. J Thorac Cardiovasc Surg 126: 558–562

24. Oosterhuis JW, Theunissen PH, Bollen EC (2001) Improved preoperative mediastinal staging in non-small-cell lung cancer by serial sectioning and immunohistochemical staining of lymph-node biopsies. Eur J Cardiothorac Surg 20:335–338

25. Pantel K, Brakenhoff R (2004) Dissecting the metastatic cascade. Nat Rev Cancer 4(6):448-56

26. Pantel K, Woelfle U (2004) Micrometastasis in breast cancer and other solid tumors. J Biol Regul Homeost Agents 18(2):120-5
27. Pantel and Panabières (2006) aceepted by Nature Clinical Practice Oncology
28. Pantel K, Schlimok G, Braun S, Kutter D, Lindemann F, Schaller G, Funke I, Izbicki JR, Riethmuller G (1993) Differential expression of proliferation-associated molecules in individual micrometastatic carcinoma cells. J Natl Cancer Inst 85:1419–1424
29. Passlick B, Sienel W, Seen-Hibler R, Wockel W, Thetter O, Pantel K (2000) The 17-1A antigen is expressed on primary, metastatic and disseminated non-small cell lung carcinoma cells. Int J Cancer 87: 548–552
30. Putz E, Witter K, Offner S, Stosiek P, Zippelius A, Johnson J, Zahn R, Riethmuller G, Pantel K (1999) Phenotypic characteristics of cell lines derived from disseminated cancer cells in bone marrow of patients with solid epithelial tumors: establishment of working models for human micrometastases. Cancer Res 59(1):241-8
31. Saintigny P, Coulon S, Kambouchner M, Ricci S, Martinot E, Danel C, Breau JL, Bernaudin JF (2005) Real-time RT-PCR detection of CK19, CK7 and MUC1 mRNA for diagnosis of lymph node micrometastases in non small cell lung carcinoma. Int J Cancer 115(5):777-82
32. Salerno CT, Frizelle S, Niehans GA, Ho SB, Jakkula M, Kratzke RA, Maddaus MA (1998) Detection of occult micrometastases in non-small cell lung carcinoma by reverse transcriptase-polymerase chain reaction. Chest 113:1526–1532
33. Scheunemann P, Izbicki JR, Pantel K (1999) Tumorigenic potential of apparently tumor-free lymph nodes. N Engl J Med 340:1687
34. Sienel W, Varwerk C, Linder A, Kaiser D, Teschner M, Delire M, Stamatis G, Passlick B (2004) Melanoma associated antigen (MAGE)-A3 expression in Stages I and II non-small cell lung cancer: results of a multi-center study. Eur J Cardiothorac Surg 25(1):131-4
35. Wang XT, Sienel W, Eggeling S, Ludwig C, Stoelben E, Mueller J, Klein CA, Passlick B (2005) Detection of disseminated tumor cells in mediastinoscopic lymph node biopsies and lymphadenectomy specimens of patients with NSCLC by quantitative RT-PCR. Eur J Cardiothorac Surg 28:26–32
36. Wiedswang G, Borgen E, Karesen R, Kvalheim G, Nesland JM, Qvist H, Schlichting E, Sauer T, Janbu J, Harbitz T, Naume B (2003) Detection of isolated tumor cells in bone marrow is an independent prognostic factor in breast cancer. J Clin Oncol 21(18):3469-78
37. Woelfle U, Cloos J, Sauter G, Riethdorf L, Janicke F, van Diest P, Brakenhoff R, Pantel K (2003) Molecular signature associated with bone marrow micrometastasis in human breast cancer. Cancer Res 63(18):5679-84
38. Yasumoto K, Osaki T, Watanabe Y, Kato H, Yoshimura T (2003) Prognostic value of cytokeratin-positive cells in the bone marrow and lymph nodes of patients with resected nonsmall cell lung cancer: a multi-center prospective study. *Ann Thorac Surg 76(1):194-201; discussion 202*
39. Zippelius A, Kufer P, Honold G, Kollermann MW, Oberneder R, Schlimok G, Riethmuller G, Pantel K (1997) Limitations of reverse-transcriptase polymerase chain reaction analyses for detection of micrometastatic epithelial cancer cells in bone marrow. J Clin Oncol 15:2701–2708

13. EFFECTS OF CHEMOKINES ON TUMOR METASTASIS

HIROYA TAKEUCHI[1], MINORU KITAGO[2], AND DAVE S. B. HOON[2]

[1]Department of Surgery, Keio University School of Medicine, Tokyo, Japan, [2]Department of Molecular Oncology, John Wayne Cancer Institute, Saint Johns Health Center, Santa Monica, California, USA

INTRODUCTION

One of the puzzling questions in the study of cancer metastasis has been: "Why do tumor cells metastasize preferably to specific organs and not to others?" The mechanism of cancer metastasis has been debated for several decades after the "seed and soil" theory, which was described by Paget (1). Paget theorized that cancer metastasis preferentially occur to organs or sites that support the growth of cancer cells. On the other hand, Ewing (2) described "anatomical mechanical theory" to account for cancer metastasis. He theorized that the patterns of blood flow from the primary tumor can predict the first metastasized organs. Recent progress in cancer metastasis biology has introduced development of a new concept, "homing theory," which incorporates the previous two theories to describe the mechanics associated with cancer metastasis. It is *hypothesized* that cancer cells are drawn to specific organ sites as a result of complex signaling between the tumor cells and the cells of the organ (3).

One of the highly important key factor recently identified in the homing theory is the chemokine receptor–ligand axis. Chemokines are small molecular weight chemotactic cytokines that are involved in a myriad of cell trafficking events. The chemokines are currently grouped into four major subfamilies (CC, CXC, CX3C, and C) based on the arrangement of the two NH_2-terminal cysteine residues (4, 5). There are more than 50 chemokine family members to date, with at least 18 chemokine receptors defined containing seven transmembrane-spanning G-protein domains (6). Chemokines, which are induced by inflammation or pathogenic stimulation, activate the migration of leukocytes, dendritic cells (DCs), and other hematopoietic cells to specific sites (7, 8). Chemokine signaling is known to activate cell motility, invasion, interaction with the extracellular matrix, and modify overall disease outcome (6, 9). Chemokine receptors can bind and activate heterotrimeric G proteins. The activated G-protein subunits stimulate multiple signal transduction pathways, such as phosphoinositide-3 kinases (PI3K), phospholipase Cβ (PLCβ), Src family kinases, and cytoskeleton-related elements. Tumor cells of different origins bear different chemokine receptors. Similarly, many embryonic and fetal cells of different origins are known to express specific chemokine receptors. In this chapter, we will focus on CCR7 and CXCR4, since they are the most predominantly studied chemokine receptors studied in human cancers.

CCL21/SLC

Of particular interest in tumor progression to lymph nodes is chemokine CCL21/SLC, also referred to as 6Ckine or exodus, which is involved in recruiting naïve T-cells, memory T-cells, natural killer cells, and DCs (7–12). CCL21/SLC is constitutively expressed in the high endothelial venules (HEV) of lymph nodes, Peyer's patches, and thymus, spleen, and mucosal tissue (11, 13). It has a high affinity for its receptor, CCR7, a member of the chemokine receptor family (14–17). CCR7 is prevalent in various subsets of T-cells of different differentiation sites and DCs. The release of CCL21/SLC by HEV cells recruits CCR7(+) cells to draining lymph nodes. Abnormal expression of CCL21/SLC affects lymphocyte circulation and recruitment to lymph nodes. Lymphocytes and DCs of the DDD/1-plt/plt (paucity of lymph node T-cells) mouse do not migrate into peripheral lymph nodes because these nodes express no detectable SLC (18). Antigen-stimulated lymph nodes, when activated, express CCL21/SLC, which can attract of CCR7(+) immune cells such as DCs, T-cells, specific subsets of activated T-cells, and naïve T-cells (11, 12, 17). This is a very significant mechanism whereby tumor-draining lymph nodes can orchestrate and accentuate tumor immunity. Without this mechanism of immune cell recruitment, lymph nodes would likely have limited capacity to control tumor progression.

Studies have demonstrated that tumor cells of different embryonic organs can express functional chemokine receptors and respond to specific chemokine ligands (19). Chemokine physiological effects on tumor cells have been shown to be similar to effects on hemopoietic-derived cells. The chemokine receptor–ligand axis is a highly complicated but efficient physiological mechanism whereby immune cells can be induced to rapidly migrate to distant organ sites where injury or infection has occurred. Tumor cells appear to have taken advantage of this same physiological mechanism to migrate to specific organ sites. This may be a mechanism that is inherently programmed in cells recapitulating events during embryonic and fetal development. The focus of our laboratory has been on studying how human tumor cells may utilize these chemokine signals to facilitate tumor cell metastasis from the primary tumor to the sentinel lymph nodes (SLNs) or distal sites in the body. The SLN is the first tumor-draining lymph node and site if metastatic disease was to establish in the regional draining node basin. We have found that metastatic tumor cells, which express functional chemokine receptors, respond to specific chemokine ligands in regional and distant organ sites. Understanding these events that promote tumor metastasis is highly important in that the tumor involvement status of the draining lymph node basin is one of the most important prognostic factors in many tumor types, such as breast, colorectal, gastric, esophageal, and melanoma.

MELANOMA

We previously reported that human melanoma cells express functional chemokine receptors CCR7 and CXCR4 (20–23). At first, we hypothesized that CCL21/SLC regulates the migration of CCR7-bearing melanoma cells from a primary lesion to the SLN. We demonstrated that melanoma cell lines and microdissected tumor tissues have heterogeneous expression of CCR7 mRNA as assessed by quantitative RT-PCR assay (20). Some melanoma cells did not express CCR7. This indicated that CCR7 receptor expression level may determine the fate of melanoma cells. There was strong functional correlation between CCR7 mRNA expression and cell migration induced by CCL21/SLC. CCL21/SLC did not induce migration of CCR7(−) cells. However, cell lines with higher CCR7 mRNA expression had a greater response to CCL21/SLC. These studies indicated the functional CCL21–CCR7 axis in human melanoma cells. Immunohistochemical (IHC) staining, a flow cytometry analysis, verified CCR7 protein expression in melanoma cells. CCR7 expression levels in primary melanomas significantly correlated with increasing Breslow thickness, which is one of the most important factors in determining prognosis of primary melanomas in patients.

CXCR4

Melanoma cell lines and metastatic melanoma in liver were shown to express various levels of CXCR4 as assessed by quantitative RT-PCR assays and IHC (21, 22). There was a significant correlation between CXCR4 mRNA expression and melanoma cell migration induced by its ligand, CXCL12. CXCR4 mRNA expression was observed in 24 of 27 (89%) melanoma liver metastases, and metastatic melanoma cells were demonstrated by IHC for immunostaining of CXCR4 (22). The ligands for CXCR4, CXCL12/SDF, are highly expressed in liver, and results suggest that CXCL12 may specifically attract melanoma CXCR4(+) cells and promote tumor progression. CXCL12/SDF are expressed by other organs, including lymph nodes as well.

EPIGENETIC REGULATION OF CHEMOKINE RECEPTORS

Variable expression of CXCR4 and CCR7 was observed in melanoma cell lines. We hypothesized that epigenetic events may regulate these receptors. One type of epigenetic event is the methylation of the promoter region of CpG islands, which can cause gene silencing (24). Another epigenetic event is the deacetylation of chromatin regions in the promoter area of the gene. To investigate this, we assessed the effect of 5-aza-2-deoxycytidine (5-Aza) and trichostatin A (a histone deacetylase inhibitor; TSA) treatment of melanoma cells in culture, and then assessed receptor expression by flow cytometric analysis and quantitative real-time RT-PCR. From these studies, we observed that the two reagents could reactivate expression and enhance function CXCR4 and CCR7 on melanoma cells (21). However, this was variable with individual cell lines. For several cell lines, enhancement of chemokine receptors was quite significant. The results strongly suggested that an epigenetic mechanism may endogenously regulate chemokine receptor expression on melanoma cells and that melanoma cells are capable of expressing very high levels of the receptors. The internal or external cell mechanisms of turning these receptors on and off are still not fully understood. However, this suggests that microenvironment factors around tumor cells may promote chemokine receptor activation.

TUMOR-DRAINING LYMPH NODES

Lymph nodes are known to produce the chemokines CCL21/SLC and CXCL12. These chemokines are elevated during inflammation and immune responses of tissue site draining lymph nodes. We assessed the expression of these chemokines in the SLN of melanoma patients with and without micrometastasis. In our results, CCL21/SLC and CXCL12 production in the SLN correlated with level of metastasis involvement. Most interestingly, chemokines were more suppressed as metastatic tumor burden increased in the SLN. There is likely to be a feedback mechanism by which CCL21/SLC production is inhibited in the lymph nodes to prevent further recruitment of T-cells and DCs/LCs. However, metastatic cells in the SLN may also directly downregulate CCL21/SLC expression via immune suppressive factors to inhibit recruitment of DCs and naïve T-cells, thus providing a mechanism for escaping destruction. Future investigations are needed to determine the mechanism of suppression of these chemokines in lymph nodes with melanoma metastasis. Chemokine suppression in lymph nodes may be a very critical event in regulating immune responses and preventing overexpression of these secondary lymphoid organs. Suppression of key regulatory immune cells such as DCs to the lymph node would significantly dampen any major attack to metastatic tumor cells. Mechanisms involved in chemokine regulation may be useful in developing more effective immunotherapeutic strategies for augmenting regional tumor immunity.

COLORECTAL CANCER

Liver metastasis is the predominant factor affecting colorectal cancer (CRC)-related high mortality. Previous studies have shown that cellular extracts from liver parenchyma have high concentrations of CXCL12, the ligand specific to CXCR4. Our *hypothesis* is that the high levels of CXCL12 in the liver could provide a specific homing target for CXCR4-bearing CRC cells, and the CXCR4 expressed by CRC is a prognostic factor for poor disease outcome. We assessed the CXCR4 expression in CRC primary and metastatic tumor specimens in the liver (22, 25). High CXCR4 expression in primary tumor specimens ($n = 57$) from AJCC stage I/II CRC patients was significantly correlated with increased risk for local recurrence and/or distant metastasis (risk ratio 1.35; 95% CI 1.09–1.68; $p = 0.0065$). High CXCR4 expression in primary tumors ($n = 35$) from AJCC stage IV patients significantly correlated with worse overall median survival (9 vs. 23 months; risk ratio 2.53; 95% CI 1.19–5.40; $p = 0.016$). CXCR4 expression was significantly higher in liver metastases ($n = 39$) compared to primary CRC tumors. Moreover, low vs. high CXCR4 expression in CRC liver metastases correlated with a significant difference in overall survival ($p = 0.036$). This suggested that the CXCL12–CXCR4 axis signaling mechanism may be clinically relevant for patients with CRC. Primary and metastatic CRC tumor cells demonstrated focal immunoactivity for CXCR4 protein in both the cytoplasm and cell membrane. Other studies using IHC have also demonstrated the prognostic significance of CXCR4 in CRC (26, 27).

CHEMOKINE RECEPTORS ON CARCINOMAS

CXCR4 has been demonstrated to be expressed by many types of carcinomas, and is associated with tumor progression and poor prognosis (4, 28). CCR7 expression has been reported for breast cancer, nonsmall-cell lung cancer, gastric cancer, and esophageal cancer (29–32). CCR7 expression in various carcinomas, in general, appears to correlate with lymph node metastasis and worse prognosis. Melanoma cells have been reported to express not only CXCR4 and CCR7, but also CCR10 and CXCR2 (19, 33). CCR10 may be related to skin metastasis of melanoma cells. CCR3 and CCR4, which are expressed in T-cell lymphomas, have been reported to correlate with tumor progression and poor prognosis of disease (34, 35).

Interestingly, sites of metastasis can be controlled by transfection of the cancer cells with different chemokine receptors in mouse B16 melanoma models (36–38). Transfection with CCR7 resulted in lymph node metastasis, transfection with CXCR4 caused lung metastasis, and transfection with CCR10 resulted in skin metastasis. Chemokine receptors on cancer cells and chemokines expressed in target organs may strongly support the "seed and soil" theory for organ-specific metastasis.

MICROENVIRONMENT

Tumor cells expressing specific chemokine receptors are likely to be more progressive in an organ microenvironment that produces specific chemokine ligands. Tumor cell adaptation to the microenvironment would promote metastasis. Tissue insult and inflammation would activate chemokine production, whereby tumor cells circulating or invading would take advantage of this favorable type of microenvironment. This chemokine receptor-axis physiological mechanism is highly effective in rapid orchestration of hematopoietic cells to specific sites. We often associate chemokine-induced migration of tumor cells to distant sites. However, migration within an organ via chemokines also is likely to occur as the microenvironment may facilitate this intraorgan dissemination. This is observable particularly in lymph nodes and in the liver. Metastasis colonization within a tissue organ is poorly understood. Chemokines as well as blood/lymphatic drainage are likely to play a significant role in this process. Once a metastatic cell reaches a distant organ site its success depends on many factors such as migration and invasion both of which are likely to be regulated by chemokine gradients status in the organ at that time.

TARGETS FOR CANCER THERAPY

Chemokines and their respective receptors are now becoming attractive molecular targets for cancer therapy. Blocking agents for chemokine receptors or the chemokines themselves may contribute significantly to suppressing tumor invasion and metastasis. For instance, anti-CXCR4 monoclonal antibody significantly inhibits the metastasis of human breast cancer cells to the lymph nodes, as well as the growth of non-Hodgkin lymphoma cells in various animal models (19, 39). A small molecule CXCR4 antagonist, AMD 3100, developed for the treatment of AIDS, has been indicated in new cancer therapy. AMD 3100 inhibited the growth of intracranial glioblastoma and medulloblastoma in a xenograft model (40). However, clinical applications of these CXCR4 inhibitors must be closely monitored because CXCL12–CXCR4 signaling plays significant roles in the development and migration of hematopoietic stem cells and immune cells. Further studies on the cancer chemokine receptor network will reveal new therapeutic approaches for the treatment of malignant tumors. Similarly, identification of new chemokine receptor–ligand axis mechanisms defined in tumor cells will likely move this field further.

CONCLUSION

There is now sufficient observation reported in multiple human tumor systems to indicate that the chemokine receptor–ligand axis is a critical component of the metastatic process. Although the chemokine receptor–ligand axis is often associated with migration, other physiological functions are turned on. Observation to date strongly suggests the chemokine receptor–ligand response of tumors appears to be related to the aggressive tumor cell phenotype. The physiological properties of metastatic solid tumor cells are very similar to hematopoietic cells during metastasis. This also suggests that regulating tumor cell metastasis may be a significant problem at various stages of progression. As we understand the chemokine receptor–ligand axis as it applies to tumor metastasis, it will open new potential approaches of targeted therapy.

REFERENCES

1. Paget S (1889) The distribution of secondary growths in cancer of the breast. Lancet 1: 571-573
2. Ewing, J (1928) Neoplastic Diseases, 6th edn. Saunders, Philadelphia
3. Stetler-Stevenson WG, Kleiner DE Jr (2001) Molecular biology of cancer: invasion and metastasis. In: DeVita VT Jr, Hellman S, Rosenberg SA (eds) Cancer: Principles and Practice of Oncology. Lippincott Williams & Wilkins, Philadelphia, pp 123-136
4. Balkwill F. Cancer and the chemokine network (2004) Nat Rev Cancer 4: 540-550
5. Zlotnik, A., and Yoshie, O (2000) Chemokines: a new classification system and their role in immunity. Immunity 12: 121-127
6. Tanaka T, Bai Z, Srinoulprasert Y, Yang BG, Hayasaka H, Miyasaka M (2005) Chemokines in tumor progression and metastasis. Cancer Sci 96: 317-322
7. Weninger W, von Andrian UH (2003) Chemokine regulation of naïve T cell traffic in health and disease. Semin Immunol 15: 257-270
8. Gunn MD (2003) Chemokine mediated control of dendritic cell migration and function. Semin Immunol 15: 271-276
9. Locati M, Deuschle U, Massardi ML, Martinez FO, Sironi M, Sozzani S, Bartfai T, Mantovani A (2002) Analysis of the gene expression profile activated the CC chemokine ligand 5/RANTES and by lipopolysaccharide in human monocytes. J Immnol 168: 3557-3562
10. Förster R, Schubel A, Breitfeld D, Kremmer E, Renner-Muller I, Wolf E, Lipp M (1999) CCR7 coordinates the primary immune response by establishing functional microenvironments in secondary lymphoid organs. Cell 99: 23-33
11. Willimann K, Legler DF, Loetscher M, Roos RS, Delgado MB, Clark-Lewis I, Baggiolini M, Moser B (1998) The chemokine SLC is expressed in T cell areas of lymph nodes and mucosal lymphoid tissues and attracts activated T cells via CCR7. Eur J Immunol 28: 2025-2034
12. Moretta A (2002) Natural killer cells and dendritic cells:rendezvous in abused tissues. Nat Rev Immunol 2: 957-965
13. Gunn MD, Tangemann K, Tam C, Cyster JG, Rosen SD, Williams LT (1998) Chemokine expressed in lymphoid high endothelial venules promotes the adhesion and chemotaxis of naive T lymphocytes. Proc Natl Acad Sci USA 95: 258-263
14. Yoshida R, Nagira M, Kitaura M, Imagawa N, Imai T, Yoshie O (1998) Secondary lymphoid-tissue chemokine is a functional ligand for the CC chemokine receptor CCR7. J Biol Chem 273: 7118-7122
15. Yoshida R, Nagira M, Imai T, Baba M, Takagi S, Tabira Y, Akagi J, Nomiyama H, Yoshie O (1998) EBI1-ligand chemokine (ELC) attracts a broad spectrum of lymphocytes: activated T cells strongly up-regulate CCR7 and efficiently migrate toward ELC. Int Immunol 10: 901-910
16. Geissmann F, Dieu-Nosjean MC, Dezutter C, Valladeau J, Kayal S, Leborgne M, Brousse N, Saeland S, Davoust J (2002) Accumulation of immature Langerhans cells in human lymph nodes draining chronically inflamed skin. J Exp Med 196: 417-430
17. Yanagihara S, Komura E, Nagafune J, Watarai H, Yamaguchi Y (1998) EBI1/CCR7 is a new member of dendritic cell chemokine receptor that is up-regulated upon maturation. J Immunol 161: 3096-3102
18. Gunn MD, Kyuwa S, Tam C, Kakiuchi T, Matsuzawa A, Williams LT, and Nakano H (1999) Mice lacking expression of secondary lymphoid organ chemokine have defects in lymphocyte homing and dendritic cell localization. J Exp Med 189: 451-460
19. Muller A, Homey B, Soto H, Ge N, Catron D, Buchanan ME, McClanahan T, Murphy E, Yuan W, Wagner SN, Barrera JL, Mohar A, Verastegui E, Zlotnik A (2001) Involvement of chemokine receptors in breast cancer metastasis. Nature 410: 50-56
20. Takeuchi H, Fujimoto A, Tanaka M, Yamano T, Hsueh E, Hoon DS (2004) CCL21 Chemokine regulates chemokine receptor CCR7 bearing malignant melanoma cells. Clin Cancer Res 10: 2351-2358
21. Mori T, Kim J, Yamano T, Takeuchi H, Huang S, Umetani N, Koyanagi K, Hoon DS (2005) Epigenetic upregulation of CCR7 and CXCR4 chemokine receptor expression in melanoma cells. Cancer Res 65: 1800-1807
22. Kim J, Mori T, Chen SL, Amersi FF, Martinez SR, Kuo C, Turner RR, Ye X, Bilchik AJ, Morton DL, Hoon DS (2006) Chemokine receptor CXCR4 expression in patients with melanoma and colorectal cancer liver metastases and the association with disease outcome. Ann Surg 244: 113-120
23. Hoon DS, Kitago M, Kim J, Mori T, Piris A, Szyfelbein K, Mihm MC Jr, Nathanson SD, Padera TP, Chambers AF, Vantyghem SA, MacDonald IC, Shivers SC, Alsarraj M, Reintgen DS, Passlick B, Sienel W, Pantel K (2006) Molecular mechanisms of metastasis. Cancer Metastasis Rev 25:203-220
24. Hoon DS, Spugnardi M, Kuo C, Huang SK, Morton DL, Taback B (2004) Profiling epigenetic inactivation of tumor suppressor genes in tumors and plasma from cutaneous melanoma patients. Oncogene 23:4014-22

25. Kim J, Takeuchi H, Lam ST, Turner RR, Wang HJ, Kuo C, Foshag L, Bilchik AJ, Hoon DS (2005) Chemokine receptor CXCR4 expression in colorectal cancer patients increases the risk for recurrence and poor survival. J Clin Oncol 23:2744-2753

26. Ottaiano A, Franco R, Aiello Talamanca A, Liguori G, Tatangelo F, Delrio P, Nasti G, Barletta E, Facchini G, Daniele B, Di Blasi A, Napolitano M, Ierano C, Calemma R, Leonardi E, Albino V, De Angelis V, Falanga M, Boccia V, Capuozzo M, Parisi V, Botti G, Castello G, Vincenzo Iaffaioli R, Scala S (2006) Overexpression of both CXC chemokine receptor 4 and vascular endothelial growth factor proteins predicts early distant relapse in stage II-III colorectal cancer patients. Clin Cancer Res 12:2795-803

27. Schimanski CC, Schwald S, Simiantonaki N, Jayasinghe C, Gonner U, Wilsberg V, Junginger T, Berger MR, Galle PR, Moehler M (2005) Effect of chemokine receptors CXCR4 and CCR7 on the metastatic behavior of human colorectal cancer. Clin Cancer Res 11:1743-50

28. Balkwill F. The significance of cancer cell expression of CXCR4 (2004) Semin Cancer Biol 14:171-179

29. Till KJ, Lin K, Zuel M, Cawley JC (2002) The chemokine receptor CCR7 and α4 integrin are important for migration of chrmonic lymphocytic leukemia cells into lymph nodes. Blood 99: 2977-2984

30. Takanami I (2003) Overexpression of CCR7 mRNA in nonsmall cell lung cancer: correlation with lymph node metastasis. Int J Cancer 105:186-189

31. Mashino K, Sadanaga N, Yamaguchi H, Tanaka F, Ohta M, Shibuta K, Inoue H, Mori M (2002) Expression of chemokine receptor CCR7 is associated with lymph node metastasis of gastric carcinoma. Cancer Res 62:2937-2941

32. Ding Y, Shimada Y, Maeda M, Kawabe A, Kaganoi J, Komoto I, Hashimoto Y, Miyake M, Hashida H, Imamura M (2003) Association of CC chemokine receptor 7 with lymph node metastasis of esophageal squamous cell carcinoma. Clin Cancer Res 9:3406-3412

33. Dhawan P, Richmond A (2002) A role of CXCL1 in tumorigenesis of melanoma. J Leukoc Biol 72: 9-18

34. Kleinhans M, Tun-Kyi A, Gilliet M, Kadin ME, Dummer R, Burg G, Nestle FO (2003) Functional expression of the eotaxin receptor CCR3 in CD30+ cutaneous T-cell lymphoma. Blood 101:1487-1493

35. Ishida T, Utsunomiya A, Iida S, Inagaki H, Takatsuka Y, Kusumoto S, Takeuchi G, Shimizu S, Ito M, Komatsu H, Wakita A, Eimoto T, Matsushima K, Ueda R (2003) Clinical significance of CCR4 expression in adult T-cell leukemia/lymphoma: its close association with skin involvement and unfavorable outcome. Clin Cancer Res 9:3625-3634

36. Wiley HE, Gonzalez EB, Maki S, Wu MT, Hwang ST (2001) Expression of CC chemokine receptor-7 and regional lymph node metastasis of B16 murine melanoma. J Natl Cancer Inst 93:1638-1643

37. Murakami T, Maki W, Cardones AR, Fang H, Tun Kyi A, Nestle FO, Hwang ST (2002) Expression of CXC chemokine receptor-4 enhances the pulmonary metastatic potential of murine B16 melanoma cells. Cancer Res 62:7328-7334

38. Murakami T, Cardones AR, Finkelstein SE, Restifo NP, Klaunberg BA, Nestle FO, Castillo SS, Dennis PA, Hwang ST (2003) Immune evasion by murine melanoma mediated through CC chemokine receptor-10. J Exp Med 198:1337-1347

39. Bertolini F, Dell'Agnola C, Mancuso P, Rabascio C, Burlini A, Monestiroli S, Gobbi A, Pruneri G, Martinelli G (2002) CXCR4 neutralization, a novel therapeutic approach for non-Hodgkin's lymphoma. Cancer Res 62:3106-12

40. Rubin JB, Kung AL, Klein RS, Chan JA, Sun Y, Schmidt K, Kieran MW, Luster AD, Segal RA (2003) A small-molecule antagonist of CXCR4 inhibits intracranial growth of primary brain tumors. Proc Natl Acad Sci U S A 100:13513-13538

14. REGIONAL LYMPH NODE METASTASES, A SINGULAR MANIFESTATION OF THE PROCESS OF CLINICAL METASTASES IN CANCER: CONTEMPORARY ANIMAL RESEARCH AND CLINICAL REPORTS SUGGEST UNIFYING CONCEPTS

BLAKE CADY

Brown Medical School, Providence, Rhode Island, USA and Comprehensive Breast Center, Rhode Island Hospital, Providence, Rhode Island, USA

Metastases:
1. "The shifting of a disease or its local manifestation from one part of the body to another . . ."
2. "The spread of a disease process from one part of the body to another, as in the appearance of neoplasms in parts of the body remote from the site of the primary tumor; results from dissemination of tumor cells by the lymphatics or blood vessels . . ."

Stedman's Medical Dictionary
Williams & Wilkins, Philadelphia 2000

INTRODUCTION

Extensive animal research into the process of metastatic development of cancers over recent years provides insight into clinical findings in patients. Clinical research and reports provide strong support for the translation of these research conclusions from the laboratory and animals to human cancers (1–6), particularly in understanding the role of lymph node metastases but also more distant metastases in almost all human epithelial cancers (2, 3). The following chapter describes an interpretation of the generic issues in metastatic development by using specific clinical examples and reports, and summarizing laboratory and animal research, whether cancer cells that result in eventual clinical metastases begin their initial journey via the lymphatic or hematogenous route.

Regional lymph node metastases have always been of concern to surgeons, since they are usually removed as part of the primary cancer resection, and the presence or absence of lymph node metastases frequently foretell in statistical probability the future risk or current presence of distant vital organ metastases. Thus, surgeons have focused their clinical energies on removing and analyzing lymph nodes, and their

Reprinted with kind permission of Springer Science and Business Media, Ann Surg, March 2007; Volume 14, issue 6, pp. 1790–1800 research interest in understanding the relationship of lymph node metastases to distant organ metastases and survival. In contemporary surgical reports of cancers from a variety of organs, surgeons frequently continue to assume that lymphatics have the primary role as the principal pathway for the cancer to spread to other distant sites, a biological view espoused 100 years ago by Halsted in breast cancer (8), Moynihan in colorectal cancer (9), and Snow in melanoma (10). However, critical appraisal of the massive amount of clinical and laboratory research indicates that metastatic cells probably spread simultaneously via lymphatics and/or hematogenously. Lymph node metastases that are manifestations of the lymphatic route are by themselves nonlethal, as regional lymph nodes do not contribute an essential life-sustaining function. Uncommon exceptions occur in the lymphatics (not lymph nodes) where lethal lymphangitic pulmonary carcinoma may cause death; such extensive lymphatic vessel spread also may occur locally in inflammatory breast cancer, "encurassé" chest wall recurrent breast cancer, primary linitis plastica gastric cancer, or extensive lymphatic vessel involvement in melanoma. By secondary narrowing of an adjacent hollow lumen, lymph node metastases themselves occasionally contribute to death such as with biliary, esophageal, bronchial, or ureteral obstruction. This assumption of nonlethal behavior confirms and elaborates laboratory conclusions regarding the lymphatic metastatic process and provides the rationale for adapting a far more restrictive role for the surgical approach to lymph node resection (11). Recent research also elaborates the metastatic cascade to more distant vital organs (2–6) as well as lymph nodes (1) and suggests similar metastatic mechanisms and phenomenon seen in regional lymph nodes (usually excised), and in vital organs (not initially removed) and thus suggests a commonality to metastatic development.

Ultimately, of course lymph flows into the vascular system through the thoracic duct or lymphovascular shunts in more peripheral regions, thus the eventual path of circulating cancer cells to distant organs is via the general circulation, to illustrate the eventual common pathway. Although this discussion will focus on breast and other cancers as clinical models of lymphatic and distant organ metastases generally, conclusions can be applied to all lymphatic and other distant metastases based on extensive animal and clinical research.

THE EVOLUTION AND PHYSIOLOGY OF THE LYMPHATIC SYSTEM

It is critical to understand the anatomy and physiology of the lymphatic system and lymph nodes in order to have a basic understanding of the meaning of lymph node metastases (7). The lodging of circulating lymphocytes in the reticular stroma of lymph nodes is a much later evolutionary development than the origin of the lymphatic vessels themselves, whose only purpose was to return interstitial fluid and intestinal nutrients to the circulation (7, 12, 13). In this later evolutionary sophistication in development of the mammalian immunological defense system, lymphocytes, which were first noted as lymphocyte aggregates in the mucosa of the respiratory and gastrointestinal tract in immediate contact with foreign antigens (12), later evolved into larger collections of lymphocytes in lymph node stroma interposed in lymph flow through lymphatic channels to further facilitate identification of foreign antigens, with subsequent production of both humeral antibodies in the innate immune system ("B" lymphocytes) or cytokine-mediated cytotoxicity in the adaptive immune system ("T" lymphocytes) in an integrated immunological response. Lymph nodes are located largely in drainage areas of body sites most exposed to the external environment, i.e., limbs, gastrointestinal tract, lungs, and oral cavity. These regional lymph node lymphocytes constitute dynamic organs: lymphocytes enter largely via the lymph node artery, lodge within the lymph node reticular stroma for periods of time, and then leave via the lymph node efferent lymphatic vessel or vein to recirculate. This trafficking of lymphocytes between blood and lymph and lymph nodes is extraordinarily complex as recently summarized in a review by Miyasaka and Tanaka (14). Lymphocytes, in the service of host immunocompetence, are exquisitely sensitive to localization in specific lymph node areas; B and T lymphocytes in circulation "home" to different respective "B" and "T" lymph node areas after passage through the lymph node high endothelial venule (HEV) cell interstases, a process governed by a variety of chemokines, cytokines, addressins, integrins, specific genetic arrangements, and ligands, claudins, and occludens (14).

Lymph nodes are also porous organs that allow passage of cells and antigens to prevent obstruction (7, 13, 15). They are not millipore filters, which would rapidly fill, obstruct lymph flow, and cause edema in tissues or limbs. When radiolabeled tumor cells are injected into the afferent nodal lymphatic vessel, they rapidly appear in the efferent lymphatic vessel and in the thoracic duct (15). Thoracic duct cannulation with selective removal of lymphocytes and return of lymph produces immunoincompetence, and in the past permitted successful human organ transplantation. Currently, this elimination of lymphocyte immunological function in organ transplantation is replicated by use of anti-lymphocyte globulin, Thymoglobulin®, Campath®, or a host of lymphocyte depleting or inactivating drugs, or interruption of the dendritic cell antigen delivery system (16, 17). It may be well that some cancers utilize "immune escape" mechanisms by cytokine interaction to avoid lymphatic trapping and antibody production.

Thus, while the original evolutionary purpose of the lymphatic system was to return interstitial fluids and nutrients to the circulation, the insertion of lymph node lymphocytes into the lymph flow completed a system of analyzing antigens (viral, bacterial, parasitic, chemical) from the hostile external environment, enabling a multilayered immunologic defensive response. Lymph nodes do not have, as a basic evolutionary function, the capturing and immunologic response to cancer cells, which in general are not originally "foreign" in the sense of representing an external nonhost substance, with some exceptions where immunological responses can be elicited, i.e., melanoma, renal cell carcinoma. Altered cancer cell antigens produced by viral infection or BCG inoculation, for instance, are manipulations or alterations of usual "self"-cancer cell antigens that, in turn, may elicit immunological responses. Indeed, as described later, deliberate immunosuppression may allow apparently dormant cancer cells to proliferate rapidly, and cause death after transplantation; when such immunosuppression is withdrawn, complete metastatic cancer regression may occur, preventing death. These examples indicate potential immunologic responses to cancer cells, as yet incompletely understood. In addition, since cancer is largely a phenomenon of an aging organism, we can be assured that lymph node metastases have little basic meaning in Darwinian evolutionary, or developmental embryological terms.

LYMPHATIC ANATOMY AND SENTINEL NODE BIOPSY

Anatomic studies of sentinel lymph nodes, particularly in breast cancer and melanoma, have indicated that there is a rational and coherent flow of lymph from the organ or limb tumor site into the regional lymphatic basin with one or two, or occasionally more, sentinel nodes initially encountered (18). This lymph flow to lymph nodes is thus not a random event, but a highly structured, anatomically defined, lymphatic vessel and lymph node pattern. The first lymph node was called the "sentinel node" by Cabanas (19), studying penile cancer, who defined the concept of the sentinel node being the doorway to the regional node basin. This assumption has now been firmly established in breast cancer, melanoma, and other cutaneous sites such as vulvar and Merkel cell cancers but is less well defined in thyroid, head and neck, gastric, colorectal, cervical, and endometrial cancers. Multiple lymph node metastases from cancers may occur as cells traverse the sentinel nodes to appear and perhaps grow in sequential echelons of nodes. In some situations, a lymph node metastasis in a sentinel node grows to block lymphatic flow, thus directing lymph and cells to other, possibly not ordinarily sequential, nodes also.

The false-negative rate (finding node metastases in the regional nodal dissection carried out after an initial negative sentinel node) is remarkably low in breast cancer, usually less than 5%, as quality guide lines suggest, and in more recent studies probably not more than 1–2% (20). This confirms the assumption of rational and sequential flow to regional nodes through lymph vessels from superficial cancers. When positive sentinel nodes do occur in breast cancer patients, there is a clear relationship between the size and prognostic features of the primary cancer and the size and number of nodal metastases probably representing the dose of metastatic cells. Thus, when patients with T1a (>1–5 mm) and T1b (>5–10 mm) breast cancers have a sentinel node metastasis, the vast majority (>70%) are found to have only one or two node metastases and these are frequently micrometastases (< 2 mm) or even smaller (<0.2 mm) and in the latter case defined as N_0(IHC+) (21). Subsequent axillary dissection, particularly when the nodes have micrometastases, seldom reveals other nodal metastases. Contrariwise, when T2 cancers are found to have a sentinel lymph node metastasis, even a micrometastasis, the chance of finding other nodal metastases in the regional node basin at later axillary dissection may exceed 50%, and these are usually macrometastases (>2 mm).

An extensive literature review, however, indicates no survival advantage for removing lymph node metastases from any organ site cancer (7, 13, 22). Admittedly, criticisms have been made of these conclusions because of wide confidence intervals on the basis of less than adequate numbers of cases in individual trials, nevertheless, the overall generalization looking over the many trials of lymphatic resections in cancers of the esophagus, lung, stomach, colon and rectum, breast, head and neck, and melanoma is clear (7, 9). Lymph node metastases, while providing a staging or prognostic role, probably have no governing or controlling role in developing later distant vital organ metastases, which in turn are what control survival.

ORGAN-SPECIFIC METASTATIC PATTERNS

Organ-specific clinical metastases are derived from cells that escape the primary cancer and previously lodged but then later grew in the liver, lung, lymph node, or other organs. The metastatic cascade of cells escaping from the primary cancer by entering either the vascular or lymphatic system (intravasation), circulating, lodging in a distant organ vascular system, or lymph node lymphatic vessel (HEV), leaving this vascular space by adhering to or traversing the endothelial lining (extravasation), and either dying, becoming viable but dormant cells growing to 1–2 mm^3 to survive by diffusion, or undergoing progressive growth by acquisition of new blood vessels (angiogenesis), is an extremely complicated and inefficient process (23). This multistep metastatic process has been well outlined, and is based on extensive laboratory and animal experiments. There is no reason to assume that these basic concepts elaborated for blood vessels in distant organs are different than lymphatics in the lymph nodes. Interesting research in recent years demonstrated that human breast cancer lymph node metastatic cells, when injected systemically in animal models specifically, lodged in lymph node stromal sites (1). This preferential selectivity of lymph node metastatic cells to lymph node stroma could be blocked, experimentally, by specific cytokines (24), thus exemplifying the highly focused metastatic pattern and the important function of the host environment (25). Research indicates that insulin-like growth factor 1 (IGF-1) (26), vascular endothelial growth factor C (VEGF-C) (27), and other features such as specific gene overexpressions can be lymph node metastases controlling substances (28). Other research demonstrates that liver and lung metastatic cells sequentially developed in animal models can be exquisitely cell and organ specific in later metastatic distribution (23, 29–31). Thus, cells from liver metastases derived from sequential generations of experimental liver metastases, when injected intravenously, caused only liver metastases. Similarly, recent genetic profiling of lung (5), bone (6), and even adrenal gland (6) metastases from human breast cancer metastatic cell lines injected in animal models had selective propensity to lodge in those same organs with a similar genetic profile indicating highly complex selective metastatic site behavior. Such a lung-specific metastatic pattern could be selectively inhibited by the transcription factor Twist. "Suppression of Twist expression in highly metastatic mammary carcinoma cells specifically inhibits their ability to metastasize from the mammary gland to the lung. Ectopic expression of Twist results in loss of E-cadherin-mediated cell–cell adhesion, activation of mesenchymal markers, and induction of cell motility, suggesting that Twist contributes to metastasis by promoting an epithelial–mesenchymal transition (EMT)" (3). These organ site specificity phenomena have been linked to a "zip-code" concept where biochemical, electrical, physical, genetic, or protein features of the cancer cell surface must interdigitate or interrelate with matched susceptible features of the organ vascular, capillary, or lymphatic endothelium (HEV) or lymph node stroma (32). A recent review (33) highlights this dendritic cell, lymphocyte, and lymph node specificity in inflammation, undoubtedly with correlates in oncology: "The signatures are imprinted on lymphocytes in draining lymph nodes, in which antigen-presenting cells direct lymphocytes to return to the organs in which they first encountered antigen. Each major organ system probably has a unique area code' that consists of lymphocyte surface molecules and counter receptors on endothelial beds. Indeed, initial indicators of distinct leukocyte-homing determinants for the lungs, joints, and the brain have been found, but much work remains to be done, including the identification of chemokine receptors on the cells that home to these various organs" (33).

Similar metastatic specificity also exists clinically in humans; for instance, resection of selected hepatic (34) or pulmonary metastases from patients with colorectal carcinoma, or pulmonary metastases from patients with sarcomas (35), can result in substantial long-term disease-free survival rates (25–30%), despite the presumed flooding of the host systemic circulation with huge numbers of circulating tumor cells over long periods of time. Another classical clinical example of such selective metastases is the high rate of liver metastases following liver transplantation for hepatocellular cancers (HCC) (36). These HCC cells, presumably circulating in the recipient after excision of the diseased liver, may lodge exclusively in the new normal donated liver to produce liver metastatic HCC, and are a major cause of failure of liver transplantation for HCC. Widespread peritoneal metastases with ascites rich with metastatic cells from ovarian cancer does not produce pulmonary metastases following peritoneovenous shunting to relieve the ascites, despite the direct shunting of malignant peritoneal metastatic cells into the central venous confluence, and thereby the pulmonary arteries and lungs (37). Clearly, the exact mechanism of such organ-specific "homing," or controlling features of metastatic cells, is at this time being elaborated (1, 2, 32), but extensive research into the metastatic cascade and microenvironmental control of extravasated metastatic cancer cell growth or dormancy bears on such a complicated interrelationship.

As a human clinical model of such a highly selective organ-specific lymph node metastatic pattern, papillary thyroid carcinoma in young "low-risk" patients is very pertinent. These young patients have a pattern of frequent regional nodal metastases (up to 75%) when routine nodal resections are performed but uncommon (<3%) distant metastases (entirely confined to lung), and a 99% disease-free survival at 20 years (38). Two-thirds of recurrences after initial surgery are lymph node metastases, which even when delayed in clinical appearance have no adverse effect on survival. This selective nodal metastatic pattern is mimicked in carcinoid and islet cell tumors of the foregut and midgut organs such as stomach, duodenum, pancreas, and intestine (39). Nodal metastases are required to even define carcinoma in many pancreatic islet cell tumors, since histological criteria alone do not clearly differentiate malignant from benign. Lymph node metastases are common, but are not controlling influences on survival, since that is determined entirely by distant vital organ metastases, particularly the liver in carcinoid tumors or islet cell cancers, or lung in low-risk thyroid cancers. This pattern of specific "lymph node only" metastases without the poor prognosis arising from vital organ metastases (liver, lung, brain) mimics the animal research studies mentioned (1, 16, 24, 26–31) that elaborate organ-specific metastatic patterns.

Despite the very frequent differentiated thyroid cancer lymph node metastases detected histologically, few low-risk group patients actually develop palpable clinical regional nodal metastases. However, 25% of young patients with clinical papillary thyroid cancer present because of palpable cervical metastases that may arise from even very small (1–3 mm) occult primary thyroid cancers (38). This presentation because of the clinical lymph node metastases from miniscule primary cancers also occurs with small intestine carcinoid tumors, where the marked desmoplastic reaction to and the bulk of the lymph node metastases is the usual cause of the clinical bowel obstruction, even when the primary carcinoid tumor is very small (<1 cm) and itself asymptomatic. Jejunal carcinoid primary tumors 5 mm or less in diameter have a node metastatic rate of 70%, and when between 5 and 10 mm in diameter have lymph node metastases in 94%. Duodenal carcinoid tumors from 8 mm to 1.5 cm in diameter have a high lymph node metastatic rate yet rarely die of disease, even when bulky, or multiple, or recurrent in lymph nodes (40). These midgut and foregut carcinoid cancer patients uncommonly die of distant liver metastases despite common nodal metastases. The organ specificity of nodal metastases is here again uniquely displayed clinically. These dramatic examples of the lymph node organ specificity of metastatic cancer cells provide insight into the general metastatic pattern, for it illustrates why many nonvital organ metastatic sites (lymph nodes especially, but also bone, subcutaneous, or cutaneous) may seem more "benign" in behavior, in terms of reduced survival duration, while in reality they are vividly demonstrating a key aspect of the metastatic process – highly specific metastatic cell to organ site behavior for separate clones of cancer cells that escape the primary tumor and complete the metastatic cascade (23). Since lymph nodes are not vital organs, unlike liver, lung, or brain, their localized involvement, or even destruction, by metastatic involvement causes, by itself, no loss of overall vital function or death. If all lymph node lymphocytes in the body are eliminated, however, immunoincompetence and death from infection may occur, but this clearly does not apply to regional lymph node metastases.

A corollary of lymphatic or other organ specificity may be the presumed sequential node to node (or liver to liver, or lung to lung) spread when multiple lymph node (or liver or lung) metastases appear. Whether these sequential regional nodal metastases arise from further shedding of specific primary cancer cells or, alternatively, from the first node-specific focus to the next and subsequent sequential regional nodes is unclear and open to debate. However, the success, by long-term disease-free survival, of liver or lung (or node) resection of a few such distant organ metastases (oligometastases) without later other liver or lung (or nodal) metastases indicates that such a cascade of organ-specific cells is not universal, and may even be uncommon.

This selective metastatic process relies on highly sophisticated and complex interactions between the metastatic cell surface and the capillary endothelium in various recipient organs (32, 41) or the stroma or HEV of the lymph node (42). A reasonable hypothesis to explain why many patients with lymph node metastases survive long-term free of vital organ metastases is that metastatic cells having the ability to lodge and grow in lymph nodes may have no capacity to lodge in, extravasate, and grow progressively in other organs, although retaining the ability to sequentially involve lymph nodes. Contrarywise, many patients with cancers in a variety of organs with negative lymph nodes still die of systemic vital organ metastases, indicating the disassociation of direct cause and effect between lymph node metastases and distant vital organ metastases that govern survival. Sarcomas have frequent pulmonary metastases, but few lymph node metastases. The vast majority (>90%) of long-term survivors in lung, gastric, colorectal, or breast cancers who had lymph node metastases at their original surgery had only one, two, or occasionally three positive lymph nodes (43). Patients who have more than five lymph node metastases at the time of the original surgical procedure in a variety of human cancers (larynx, oral cavity, stomach, esophagus, lung, colorectal, breast, and melanoma) who survive long-term disease free are the exception (<5%, usually only 1 or 2%) (43). Between 80 and 93% of 10-year disease-free survivors in these various primary cancer sites had either negative nodes or only one nodal macrometastasis detected by a single histological section through the multiple lymph nodes in the regional nodal basin. Another 4–6% had only two and another 0–4% had three nodal metastases (43). Interestingly, almost all of the cures from resection of liver or lung metastases in colorectal cancers or sarcomas have only one or two, or occasionally three, separate metastatic nodules, perhaps indicating a more universal relationship between survival after resection and the number of clinical metastatic sites (34, 44). When more than a few lymph node metastases occur in breast, gastric, colorectal, lung or other cancers, or melanoma, this is likely associated with a high rate of other clones of metastatic cells escaping the primary cancer with liver, lung, brain, or other vital organ selectivity and specificity, and/or a systemic effect that alters the distant organ microenvironment (trauma, immunosuppression, fever, etc.), that enable such selective cells to complete the metastatic cascade and become clinical metastases.

MICROMETASTASES, AND METASTATIC TUMOR CELL CLUSTERS AND TUMOR CELLS

In recent years with the advent of sentinel node biopsy, especially in breast cancer and melanoma, where extensive experience has accumulated, many sections of each sentinel lymph node (median 2) utilizing hematoxylin and eosin staining but also immunohistochemical (IHC) staining, and even reverse transcriptase polymerase chain reaction (RT-PCR) has frequently been performed. These exquisitely sophisticated techniques of lymph node analysis may detect a few metastatic cells, or even single metastatic cells, frequently in the subcapsular sinus of the lymph node. The relationship of these few metastatic cells, tumor cell clusters, or lymph node micrometastases detected only by IHC or RT-PCR to survival prognosis is at the present time uncertain (45, 46). A recent report documents circulating tumor cells in a high proportion (>33%) of patients surviving "disease free" for many years ("7–22 years after mastectomy") and on more than one occasion, indicating viable continuing, but clinically dormant, sites of ongoing metastatic disease with cancer cell shedding even in patients apparently free of clinical disease (47). Such tumor dormancy undoubtedly occurs as single cells, tumor cell clusters, or the 1–2 mm foci of cancer cells surviving by diffusion only of nutrients and waste products. Only when angiogenesis occurs with its efficiency in oxygenation and metabolic byproduct elimination does progressive growth occur to escape from dormancy.

The biological meaning of such scattered clusters or single metastatic cells or even small micrometastases is currently widely studied in clinical cancer research but is put into perspective by the results of bone marrow aspiration to detect disseminated cancer cells. The long-term outcome of patients with IHC-stained bone marrow aspirates that reveal metastatic cancer cells in breast cancer patients as reported by Diel et al. (48) and Braun et al. (49) and recently summarized by Braun et al. (50) bear on the relationship between cells in sites distant from the primary cancer and survival. Patients who had neither lymph node nor bone marrow metastatic cells had an excellent disease-free prognosis (over 95% at 4 years), while patients with both bone marrow and lymph node metastatic cells had an extremely poor prognosis (50% with clinical distant vital organ metastases at 4 years). Most interesting in their original reports, however, is the fact that patients with either bone marrow or lymph node metastatic cells have an exactly similar survival curve of about 85% disease free at 4 years, suggesting that metastatic cells detected by highly sophisticated histological techniques wherever they lodge (lymph node, bone marrow) are indicators, in a statistical sense, of the metastatic cell load, risk of later clinical metastases, and death from disease, but are not necessarily predictors of particular selective distant metastatic sites. For instance, 25% of T1a and 35% of T1b breast cancers have metastatic bone marrow cells, yet have 20-year disease-free survival rates of over 95 and 90%, respectively. Ten to fifteen percent of esophageal cancers have iliac crest marrow metastatic cells by IHC staining of aspirations; however, ribs, removed to enable esophageal resection, when flushed with fluid, revealed that the rib marrow contained metastatic cells in 80–90% of those patients (51, 52). Rib flushing is a much more extensive marrow sampling than a needle aspiration and indicates that such bone marrow metastatic cells may be much more common than ever suspected.

The implications of bone marrow or regional lymph node micrometastatic cells in early cancers are expanded by appreciation of the transplantation literature, which demonstrates the not-uncommon phenomena of donor organ dormant metastatic cells from previous "cured" donor cancers becoming clinical metastases in immuno-suppressed recipients (53). Thoracic organ donors (heart and/or lung) who previously have had cured cancer from a variety of primary sites may transmit that cancer to almost 50% of recipients (54). Of necessity these transplanted cancers arose from viable but dormant cancer cells, tumor cell clusters, or micrometastases, harbored in the transplanted donor organ. These organ donors had had cancers of a variety of organ sites including the cervix, prostate, lung, liver, kidney, or angiosarcoma, chori-ocarcinoma, and even glioblastoma of the brain, a malignancy assumed to never escape the cranium. Renal transplantation from a patient 16 years after cured early melanoma resulted in melanoma transplantation to both recipients in a recent report (55). Thus, cells from primary cancers may be shed not only to regional lymph nodes, or bone marrow, but also to distant organs, such as lung, heart, or liver, and lie dormant for decades before the microenvironment is altered (immunosuppression, trauma) and progressive rapid growth occurs (47). These disseminated cancer cells in various organs of the donor after cancers "cured" for many years bring into question what constitutes a metastases (56) and emphasizes the host factors that enable scattered but dormant metastatic cells to grow, since such cells are far more frequent than ever imagined (47, 57, 58).

This phenomenon of discovering a few metastatic cells is accentuated in regional sentinel node biopsy because this tissue is easily available, routinely removed, and extensively analyzed utilizing multiple thin sections and contemporary detailed his-tologic IHC or molecular techniques. If distant organs were inspected as carefully as regional lymph nodes in cancer patients, micrometastatic cells would undoubt-edly be discovered in the same frequency in the liver, lung, heart, or other organs, as displayed by transplanted cancers from donor organs.

METASTATIC INEFFICIENCY AND BIOLOGICAL MODELS OF CANCER DEVELOPMENT AND SPREAD

Viable metastatic cells lodging without growth in organs transplanted from "cured" cancer patients belies assumptions of metastatic efficiency; the process of the evo-lution of cells shed from primary cancers via either the lymphatics or blood vessels to clinical metastases is obviously very inefficient (23, 25). This inefficient process of progression from circulating cancer cells, to adherence on distant organ endothe-lium, to vessel wall penetration, to dormant but viable cells, to initial growth to only 2 mm limited by nutrition through diffusion, to further subsequent progressive growth after acquisition of a blood supply with oxygenation and nutrition via angiogenesis to become a clinical metastases has been elaborated and appreciated by researchers utilizing animal models (59). The development of clinical metastases may be heavily impacted by the "dose" of cancer cells shed from primary cancers, which likely is directly related to the volume and perhaps duration of the primary cancer, as well as specific poor prognostic features. This progressive behavior of cancers is postulated in the "spectrum" clinical biological model proposed by Hellman (60), which could only be elaborated through the study of the earliest and smallest cancers discovered by screening. The "spectrum" biological model of cancer development evident in breast cancer (USA and Europe) and gastric cancer (Japan) (61) detected by screening elaborated the progression from small cancers of lower grade and high curability, to later, larger cancers of higher grade and significant fatality, and postulates an increase in virulence, metastatic cell load, and metastagenicity over time, with increasing size and increasing dedifferentiation. A similar pattern has been elaborated in cervix cancer screening and is currently being demonstrated in colorectal cancer as more widespread screening is being achieved.

The entire clinical pattern of frequent cell dissemination and infrequent clinical vital organ metastases that causes death is entirely concordant with the large body of basic research in the in vitro laboratory and in vivo animal studies. This multistep metastatic processes has been summarized by Chambers et al. (59), Fidler (23, 25), Stetler-Stevenson (62), and others, and reflects decades of research activity by many authors and laboratories. Fidler has emphasized the current relationship of understanding all aspects of the metastatic process to Paget's description in 1889 of both the "seed and soil," the cancer cell and the microenvironment of the metastatic cell lodging site (23). This voluminous contemporary research bears extensive review and comprehension for it so predicts and explains clinical scenarios, which frequently seem illogical, contradictory, or unreasonable to the clinician. While animal and laboratory studies have elaborated each of the many steps in the metastatic process from intravasation to lodgment to extravasation, to dormancy, to angiogenesis, recent research has been particularly noteworthy in emphasizing features of the host metastatic cell microenvironment. These studies indicate a symbiotic relationship between the extravasated metastatic cells and their surrounding tissue, such that host defense factors can be modified by the metastatic cells, and the metastatic cells can respond to and be modified by host features. This cancer cell–host microenvironment "crosstalk" occurs with hormonal, genetic, protein, extracellular fluid, and physical environment effects (23). Metastatic cells may have paracrine effects that overwhelm local control factors to promote growth, and host tissue cells may decrease the metastatic potential of cancer cells by similar mechanisms. Highly metastatic cells from a primary cancer such as colon or skin, when grown in a subcutaneous site, may lose metastatic potential. Metastatic cell lines grown together with skin epithelium may lose metastatic ability. Different animal cancer cell lines may produce different growth and organ metastatic patterns when injected via the same route. Specific cytokines or growth factors may cause different growth patterns, and blocking of these factors may completely prevent metastatic potential, while not preventing local progressive growth. All these scenarios portray an extraordinarily complex system of cell dissemination, host function, and metastatic growth (23, 25). Cancer cell progression may be highly inefficient in some aspects, and overall, but very efficient in specific steps or in other aspects of dissemination and growth. Appreciating this complex array, however, provides insights that suggest the development of a variety of mechanisms that lead to clinical metastases, but a commonality regarding the site of metastatic growth, whether that be lymph node, liver, lung, or other sites.

CLINICAL ASPECTS OF LYMPH NODE METASTASES

Substantial data exist that indicate no survival difference in cancer patients subjected to radical regional node dissection compared to those with lesser dissections or even without dissection, in melanoma, and in head and neck, gastric, colorectal cancers, and particularly breast cancers (7). These clinical studies all confirm the indicator function, or statistical relationship, but question the outcome governing role of lymph node metastases (7). Thus, the purpose of a sentinel node biopsy or regional node dissection is not to improve survival, since that has not been clearly demonstrated, but to collect diagnostic and prognostic information for aid in systemic therapy selection to improve prognosis. Since patients do not die of regional nodal disease, but from systemic metastases in vital organs, prognosis can only be improved by preventing distant micrometastases from occurring or from developing into the clinical vital organ metastases that cause death. When clinically node negative breast cancer patients do not have axillary dissection with breast conservation and radiation therapy, the clinical risk of axillary recurrence may be 2% or less (63–66). Thus, we not only do not jeopardize patient's lives by not dissecting the axilla in breast cancer, but also we do not jeopardize them regionally because of a very low clinical regional recurrence rate. Even with sentinel lymph node biopsy that reveals metastases, failure to perform a subsequent axillary dissection is not accompanied by frequent regional nodal recurrences ($\pm$ 2%) but the patient's survival is also not jeopardized (61–67).

In breast cancer patients at extremely low risk of axillary nodal metastases, such as mammographically discovered, low grade T1a or T1b cancers or cancers with special low-risk features without lymph vessel invasion or poor nuclear grade, even sentinel node evaluation can be avoided (22, 67). Sentinel node biopsy may be useful in patients with a modest incidence of lymph node metastases (5% or more) and where the primary tumor features alone would not allow decisions about systemic therapy. Finally, traditional regional nodal dissection may be appropriate in primary breast or thyroid cancers or melanoma with clinical metastases to remove a palpable lesion that might undergo progressive growth and create local palliative problems. In a clinically positive axilla, when confirmed by fine-needle aspiration cytology, one might argue that axillary dissection has therapeutic benefit in breast cancer since it removes a palpable lesion and results in extremely low rates of axillary recurrence. Similar implications regarding lymph node metastases also occur in lung, esophagus, gastric, pancreatic, colorectal, and other cancers, but in these other situations, adjacent regional lymph nodes are removed as part of the primary surgery. Only in breast and cutaneous cancers can the option of removing or not removing regional lymph nodes be applied.

CONTEMPORARY DISEASE PRESENTATION

In recent years, there has been a dramatic decrease in the size, grade, lymph node metastases rate and, as a result, the stage of breast cancer under the impact of extensive mammographic screening (68). Melanoma patients, gastric cancer patients in Japan, and colorectal cancers are also seen at much earlier presentations as a result of screening.

The current median maximum diameter of all breast cancer in the State of Rhode Island is only 1.5 cm and the lymph node metastatic rate is only 26% (68). In invasive breast cancer discovered only mammographically, the median maximum diameter is about 1 cm and the positive node rate less than 20% and few are of high grade (69–71). Eighty percent of breast cancer sentinel node biopsy programs in the United States utilize routine IHC staining of multiple sections of the sentinel nodes without, at present, understanding the meaning of such special technique discovered micrometastases. As an example, the results of one report are biologically implausible, since a single IHC discovered micrometastasis in a single lymph node in a retrospective subset analysis 10 years later of about 10% of patients out of almost 1,000 in a randomized trial, decreased the survival rate by as much as 50% (72). Such a dramatic survival decrement associated with a few metastatic cells is greater than that seen when patients have one to three lymph node macrometastases in traditional nodal analysis. This particular study, while originally a randomized controlled trial, was subject to this retrospective selective subset analysis by pathological redefinition of axillary lymph nodes and thus cannot be taken at face value.

The current most appropriate clinical biologic model (spectrum model) (60) supplants the previous "Fisherian" model, which assumed that all breast cancers were systemic from onset, which in turn had displaced the "Halstedian" lymphatic system dominant model (8) that controlled thinking until the 1970s and is still widely accepted. In the time of Halsted (8) and Moynihan (9), it was assumed that lymph nodes were filters and only when the filter was filled with cancer cells did further cells "spillover" into the distant lymphatic vessels, which led directly to distant organs (8). In the contemporary "spectrum" model (60), the size and evolving features of the genetically unstable primary cancer undergo continued alteration, and result in greater virulence, increased likelihood of metastatic spread, a greater dose of metastatic cancer cells, and increasing risks of death. The vast majority (>75%) of current breast cancers, and in all likelihood other cancers, correspond to this model in which the ability to metastasize increases as size and resultant biological potential increases. Very small cancers with few exceptions have little ability to develop clinical metastases (73–75), or even recur locally (76) despite the documented dissemination of cells. How the "Fisherian" biological model of "systemic from origin" will eventually relate to the new information regarding the frequency of disseminated cells rather than clinical metastases as elaborated in this chapter is yet to be understood.

SUMMARY

The multistep complex metastatic cascade in cancer has been extensively studied in recent years. In addition, the concept of metastatic organ specificity has been elaborated. Histological studies in clinical situations have become far more sophisticated, enabling the frequent discovery of minor collections of cells in bone marrow and lymph nodes. Pertinent clinical evidence of the selective nodal metastatic pattern exists in differentiated thyroid cancer in younger, low-risk patients (38), yet none of the published risk group definitions indicate that lymph node metastases have a relationship to thyroid cancer survival (38). This unique clinical situation with very frequent nodal metastases but excellent survival is replicated in carcinoid cancers of the gastrointestinal tract (39, 40). The lymph node metastatic frequency without distant organ metastases in these two human cancers help cement the understanding gained from laboratory and animal research regarding metastatic specificity and hopefully will help place the role of lymph node metastases generally and their surgical removal on a more scientifically and logically based understanding. More broadly, the elaboration of the frequency of metastatic cell dissemination to distant organs as well as lymph nodes, and comprehension of the metastatic cascade with metastatic specificity may reorient our understanding of the evolution from metastatic cells to clinical metastatic disease. Additionally, these concepts reemphasize that lymph node metastases are indicators, not governors, of distant metastases and survival, and add the assumption that metastatic tumor cells and tumor cell clusters, and perhaps even micrometastases in other organs, are themselves only indicators and not governors of distant metastases and survival in human cancers since they represent dormant metastases prior to their host microenvironmental changes that, on rare occasions, lead to angiogenesis and clinical metastases.

Thus, the future may allow us to abandon some aspects of our surgical or systemic attack on clinical cancer metastases, such as lymph node removal or use of toxic chemotherapy, but open the door to more physiological and hopefully less traumatic approaches to the highly manipulable multistep genetic and physiological process of metastatic development.

The future biological models of clinical cancer behavior will have to incorporate aspects of understanding the intricate metastatic cascade, and particularly the host microenvironmental factors that permit or prevent progressive growth of dormant cells or cell clusters to clinical metastases.

ACKNOWLEDGMENT

Reprinted with kind permission of Springer Science and Business Media, Ann Surg, March 2007; Volume 14, issue 6, pp. 1790–1800.

REFERENCES

1. Irjala H, Alanen K, Grenman R, et al. Mannose receptor (MR) and common lymphatic endothelial and vascular endothelial receptor (CLEVER)-1 direct the binding of cancer cells to the lymph vessel endothelium. Cancer Res 2003; 63(15):4671-6
2. Solomayer E, Diel I, Meyberg G, et al. Metastatic breast cancer: clinical course, prognosis and therapy related to the first site of metastases. Br Cancer Res Treat 2000; 59:271-278
3. Yang J, Mani S, Donaher J, et al. Twist, A Master Regulator of Morphogenesis, Plays an Essential Role in Tumor Metastasis. Cell 2004; 117:927-939
4. Clark E, Golub T, Lander E, Hynes R. Genomic analysis of metastasis reveals an essential role for RhoC. Nature 2000; 406:532-535
5. Minn A, Gupta G, Siegel P, et al. Genes that mediate breast cancer metastasis to lung. Nature 2005; 436:518-524
6. Kang Y, Siegel P, Shu W, et al. A multigene program mediating breast cancer metastasis to bone. Cancer Cell 2003; 3:537-549
7. Gervasoni JE, Jr., Taneja C, Chung MA, Cady B. Biologic and clinical significance of lymphadenectomy. Surg Clin North Am 2000; 80(6):1631-73

8. Halsted W. The results of radical operations for the cure of carcinoma of the breast. Ann Surg 1907; 46:1-9
9. Moynihan G. The surgical treatment of cancer of the sigmoid flexure and rectum. Surg Gynecol Obstet 1908; 6:463-6
10. Neuhaus S, Clark M, Thomas J. Dr. Herbert Lumley Snow, MD MRCS (1847-1930): The Original Champion of Elective Lymph Node Dissection in Melanoma. Annals of Surgical Oncology 2004; 11(9):875-878
11. Taneja C, Cady B. Decreasing role of lymphatic system surgery in surgical oncology. J Surg Oncol 2005; 89(2):61-6
12. Kampmeier O. Evolution and Comparative Morphology of the Lymphatic System: Charles C. Thomas, 1969
13. Cady B. Is axillary lymph node dissection necessary in routine management of breast cancer? No. Principles and Practice of Oncology 1998; 12:1-12
14. Miyasaka M, Tanaka T. Lymphocyte Trafficking Across High Endothelial Venules: Dogmas and Enigmas. Nature Rev 2004; 4:360-370
15. Fisher B, Fisher E. Transmigration of Lymph Nodes by Tumor Cells. Science 1966; 152(3727):1397-1398
16. Huang RR, Wen DR, Guo J, et al. Selective Modulation of Paracortical Dendritic Cells and T-Lymphocytes in Breast Cancer Sentinel Lymph Nodes. Breast J 2000; 6(4):225-232
17. Clarke J, Cha J, Walsh M, et al. Dendritic cells as therapeutic adjuncts in surgical disease. Surgery 2005; 138(5):844-50
18. Tanis PJ, Nieweg OE, Valdes Olmos RA, Kroon BB. Anatomy and physiology of lymphatic drainage of the breast from the perspective of sentinel node biopsy. J Am Coll Surg 2001; 192(3):399-409
19. Cabanas R. An approach for the treatment of penile carcinoma. Cancer 1977; 39:456-466
20. Chao C, Wong SL, Tuttle TM, et al. Sentinel lymph node biopsy for breast cancer: improvement in results over time. Breast J 2004; 10(4):337-44
21. Cady B. Fundamentals of Contemporary Surgical Oncology: Biologic Principles and the Threshold Concept Govern Treatment and Outcomes. J Am Coll Surg 2001; 192(6):777-792
22. Cady B. Simplification of Breast Cancer Surgery. Annals of Surgical Oncology 2005; 12(1):6-8
23. Fidler I. The pathogenesis of cancer metastasis: the 'seed and soil' hypothesis revisited. Nature Reviews 2003; 3:1-6
24. Tang Y, Zhang D, Fallavollita L, Brodt P. Vascular endothelial growth factor C expression and lymph node metastasis are regulated by the type I insulin-like growth factor receptor. Cancer Res 2003; 63(6):1166-71
25. Fidler IJ. The organ microenvironment and cancer metastasis. Differentiation 2002; 70(9-10):498-505
26. LeBedis C, Chen K, Fallavollita L, et al. Peripheral lymph node stromal cells can promote growth and tumorigenicity of breast carcinoma cells through the release of IGF-I and EGF. Int J Cancer 2002; 100:2-8
27. Skobe M, Hawighorst T, Jackson DG, et al. Induction of tumor lymphangiogenesis by VEGF-C promotes breast cancer metastasis. Nat Med 2001; 7(2):192-8
28. Espana L, Fernandez Y, Rubio N, et al. Overexpression of Bcl-xL in human breast cancer cells enhances organ-selective lymph node metastasis. Breast Cancer Res Treat 2004; 87(1):33-44
29. Brodt P, Fallavollita L, Khatib AM, et al. Cooperative regulation of the invasive and metastatic phenotypes by different domains of the type I insulin-like growth factor receptor beta subunit. J Biol Chem 2001; 276(36):33608-15
30. Khatib AM, Fallavollita L, Wancewicz EV, et al. Inhibition of hepatic endothelial E-selectin expression by C-raf antisense oligonucleotides blocks colorectal carcinoma liver metastasis. Cancer Res 2002; 62(19):5393-8
31. Onn A, Isobe T, Itasaka S, et al. Development of an orthotopic model to study the biology and therapy of primary human lung cancer in nude mice. Clin Cancer Res 2003; 9(15):5532-9
32. Arap W, Kolonin M, Trepel M, et al. Steps toward mapping the human vasculature by phage display. Nat Med 2002; 8(2):121-127
33. Charo I, Ransohoff R. The Many Roles of Chemokines and Chemokine Receptors in Inflammation. N Engl J Med 2006; 354(6):610-621
34. Cady B, Jenkins RL, Steele GD, Jr., et al. Surgical margin in hepatic resection for colorectal metastasis: a critical and improvable determinant of outcome. Ann Surg 1998; 227(4):566-71
35. Vezeridis M, Moore R, Karakousis C. Metastatic patterns in soft-tissue sarcomas. Arch Surg 1983; 118:915
36. Roayaie S, Frischer JS, Emre SH, et al. Long-term results with multimodal adjuvant therapy and liver transplantation for the treatment of hepatocellular carcinomas larger than 5 centimeters. Ann Surg 2002; 235(4):533-9
37. Tarin D, Price JE, Kettlewell MG, et al. Clinicopathological observations on metastasis in man studied in patients treated with peritoneovenous shunts. Br Med J (Clin Res Ed) 1984; 288(6419):749-51

38. Cady B. Presidential address: Beyond risk groups-A new look at differentiated thyroid cancer. Surgery 1998; 124(6):947-957
39. Modlin I, Lye K, Kidd M. A 5-decade Analysis of 13,715 carcinoid tumors. Cancer 2003; 97(4):934-959
40. Mullen JT, Wang H, Yao JC, et al. Carcinoid Tumors of the Duodenum. Surgery Dec. 2005, 138(6): 971-978
41. Samani AA, Brodt P. The Receptor for the Type I Insulin-Like Growth Factor and its Ligands Regulate Multiple Cellular Functions that Impact on Metastasis. Surg Clin North Am 2001; 10(2):289-312
42. Nathanson S. Insights into the Mechanisms of Lymph Node Metastasis. Cancer 2003; 98(2):413-423
43. Cady B. Basic principles in surgical oncology. Arch Surg 1997; 132(4):338-46
44. Elias D, Liberale G, Vernerey D, et al. Hepatic and Extrahepatic Colorectal Metastases: When Resectable, Their Localization Does Not Matter, But Their Total Number Has a Prognostic Effect. Ann Surg Oncol 2005; 12(11):900-909
45. Chagpar A, Middleton LP, Sahin AA, et al. Clinical outcome of patients with lymph node-negative breast carcinoma who have sentinel lymph node micrometastases detected by immunohistochemistry. Cancer 2005; 103(8):1581-6
46. Wieder R. Insurgent micrometastases: sleeper cells and harboring the enemy. J Surg Oncol 2005; 89(4):207-10
47. Meng S, D. T, Frenkel EP, et al. Circulating Tumor Cells in Patients with Breast Cancer Dormancy. Clin Cancer Res 2004; 10:8152-8162
48. Diel I, Kaufmann M, Costa S. Micrometastatic breast cancer cells in bone marrow at primary surgery: prognostic value in comparison with nodal status. J Natl Cancer Inst 1996; 8:1652-58
49. Braun S, Pantel K, Muller P, et al. Cytokeratin-positive cells in the bone marrow and survival of patients with stage I, II, or III breast cancer. N Engl J Med 2000; 342(8):525-33
50. Braun S, FD V, BN, et al. A Pooled Analysis of Bone Marrow Micrometastasis in Breast Cancer. N Engl J Med 2005; 353:793-802
51. Bonavina L, Soligo D, Quirici N, et al. Bone marrow-disseminated tumor cells in patients with carcinoma of the esophagus or cardia. Surgery 2001; 129(1):15-22
52. O'Sullivan G, Sheehan D, Clarke A, et al. Micrometastases in esophagogastric cancer: high detection rate in resected rib segments. Gastroenterology 1999; 116(3):543-8
53. Kauffman HM, McBride MA, Delmonico FL. First report of the United Network for Organ Sharing Transplant Tumor Registry: donors with a history of cancer. Transplantation 2000; 70(12):1747-51
54. Buell JF, Trofe J, Hanaway MJ, et al. Transmission of donor cancer into cardiothoracic transplant recipients. Surgery 2001; 130(4):660-6; discussion 666-8
55. MacKie RM, Reid R, Junor B. Fatal melanoma transferred in a donated kidney 16 years after melanoma surgery. N Engl J Med 2003; 348(6):567-8
56. Page DL, Anderson TJ, Carter BA. Minimal solid tumor involvement of regional and distant sites: when is a metastasis not a metastasis? Cancer 1999; 86(12):2589-92
57. Naumov GN, MacDonald IC, Weinmeister PM, et al. Persistence of solitary mammary carcinoma cells in a secondary site: a possible contributor to dormancy. Cancer Res 2002; 62(7):2162-8
58. Fisher B, Fisher ER. Experimental evidence in support of the dormant tumor cell. Science 1959; 130:918-9
59. Chambers AF, Naumov GN, Varghese HJ, et al. Critical steps in hematogenous metastasis: an overview. Surg Oncol Clin N Am 2001; 10(2):243-55, vii
60. Hellman S. Karnofsky Memorial Lecture. Natural history of small breast cancers. J Clin Oncol 1994; 12(10):2229-34
61. Soga W, Ohyama S, K M. A statistical evaluation of advancement in gastric cancer surgery with special reference to the significance of lymphadenectomy for cure. World J Surg 1988; 12:398
62. Stetler-Stevenson W. Invasion and Metastases. 7th ed. Philadelphia: Lippincott Williams & Wilkins, 2005
63. Zurrida S, Orecchia R, Galimberti V, et al. Axillary radiotherapy instead of axillary dissection: a randomized trial. Italian Oncological Senology Group. Ann Surg Oncol 2002; 9(2):156-60
64. Louis-Sylvestre C, Clough K, Asselain B, et al. Axillary treatment in conservative management of operable breast cancer: dissection or radiotherapy? Results of a randomized study with 15 years of follow-up. J Clin Oncol 2004; 22(1):97-101
65. Naik AM, Fey J, Gemignani M, et al. The risk of axillary relapse after sentinel lymph node biopsy for breast cancer is comparable with that of axillary lymph node dissection: a follow-up study of 4008 procedures. Ann Surg 2004; 240(3):462-8; discussion 468-71
66. Cady B. A Randomized Trial Comparing Axillary Dissection to No Axillary Dissection in Elderly Patients with T1N0 Breast Cancer - Results After Long-term Follow-up. Ann Surg 2005; 242(1):7-9
67. Mendez J, Fey J, Cody H, et al. Can sentinel lymph node biopsy be omitted in patients with favorable breast cancer histology? Ann Surg Oncol 2005; 12(1):24-28

68. Coburn NG, Chung MA, Fulton J, Cady B. Decreased breast cancer tumor size, stage, and mortality in rhode island: an example of a well-screened population. Cancer Control 2004; 11(4):222-30
69. Heimann R, Munsell M, McBride R. Mammographically detected breast cancers and the risk of axillary lymph node involvement: is it just the tumor size? Cancer J 2002; 8(3):276-81
70. Norden T, Thurfjell E, Hasselgren M, et al. Mammographic screening for breast cancer. What cancers do we find? Eur J Cancer 1997; 33(4):624-8
71. Bucchi L, Barchielli A, Ravaioli A, et al. Screen-detected vs clinical breast cancer: the advantage in the relative risk of lymph node metastases decreases with increasing tumour size. Br J Cancer 2005; 92(1):156-61
72. Cote RJ, Peterson HF, Chaiwun B, et al. Role of immunohistochemical detection of lymph-node metastases in management of breast cancer. International Breast Cancer Study Group. Lancet, Vol. 354, 1999. pp. 896-900
73. Group TSOSSE. Reduction in Breast Cancer Mortality from Organised Service Screening with Mammography: Further confirmation with Extended Data and New Analytic Methods. Cancer Epidemiology, Biomarkers and Prevention In press
74. Tabar L, Yen MF, Vitak B, et al. Mammography service screening and mortality in breast cancer patients: 20-year follow-up before and after introduction of screening. Lancet 2003; 361(9367):1405-10
75. Tabar L, Chen HH, Yen MF, et al. Mammographic Tumor Features Can Predict Long-term Outcomes Reliably in Women with 1-14-mm Invasive Breast Carcinoma. Cancer 2004; 101(8):1745-1759
76. Cabioglu N, Hunt KK, Buchholz TA, et al. Improving Local Control in Breast-Conserving Therapy - A 27-Year Single-Institution Experience. Cancer 2005; 104(1):20-29

15. PATTERNS OF METASTASIS IN HEAD AND NECK CANCER

JOCHEN A. WERNER

Department of Otolaryngology, Head and Neck Surgery, Philipps-University Marburg, Marbug, Germany

INTRODUCTION

The knowledge of the lymphatic system draining the upper aerodigestive tract is much less precise than the one of the blood vessel system of the mentioned region. Discussions around the tendency of lymphogenic metastatsis are increasingly led on a molecular biologic level than on morphologic facts like the distribution and also the tightness of the regional lymph vessels. The latter aspect is of great significance because the tendency of lymphogenic metastatic spread is directly influenced by the density of the lymph vessels in the area of the primary tumor. The analysis of the lymphatic system, which is based on different examination methods, allows a nearly constant description of the architecture of the lymphatic network (1-4). In connection with the controversial discussion about optimized therapy for cases with no clinical evidence of lymphogenic metastasis, lymphatic distribution and density is of fundamental interest with regard to the value of sentinel node identification in HNSCC.

Prognosis of patients suffering from squamous cell carcinoma of the upper aerodigestive tract is defined to a lesser extent through the size of the primary tumor. It is rather the extent of metastatic disease, which in squamous cell carcinoma predominantly occurs in a lymphogenous pattern that predicts the course of the disease. In the discussion that is increasingly led on a molecular biologic level concerning the tendency of lymphogenic metastatic spread, the morphologic facts like the distribution and also the tightness of the regional lymph vessels become less important, an aspect that is of great significance because the tendency of lymphogenic metastatic spread is directly influenced by the density of the lymph vessels in the area of the primary tumor.

Adding the technique of the indirect lymphography, performed with dye or with a radioactive tracer, it is possible to integrate the lymphatic system of the upper aerodigestive tract in the cervical lymph node system. Proven regional differences concerning the density and also the orientation of the lymphatics of the upper aerodigestive tract are not only important regarding the direction and frequency of lymph node metastases, but are also significant considering the aspect of the type of neck dissection required to treat patients with squamous cell carcinomas of the head and neck (HNSCC). In connection with the controversial discussion about optimized therapy for cases with no clinical evidence of lymphogenic metastasis, lymphatic distribution and density is of fundamental interest with regard to the value of sentinel node identification in HNSCC.

MAIN DIRECTION OF LYMPHATIC DRAINAGE

The lymph fluid of the oral cavity is directed mainly in its anterior part to the lymph nodes of level I (5). From the edge of tongue and the posterior part of the floor of the mouth the lymph fluid is drained also in level II. An aspect that is possibly not well known refers to the metastatic spread in lingual lymph nodes (6, 7), which can be divided into a lateral and a median group (8). The lymph nodes of the lateral group are located either laterally to the genioglossal muscle or on the hypopharyngeal muscle alongside the lingual artery and vein. The lymph nodes of the median group are located alongside the central lymph vessels in direction of the floor of the mouth. Even though this might be rarely seen, these lymph nodes could be discussed as starting point of local recurrences (7). Ozeki et al. (6) were able to determine in carcinomas of the tongue three cases of metastases in the lingual lymph nodes (one metastasis in median and two in the lateral group). The possibility of metastatic spread in lingual lymph nodes induced the mentioned authors to indicate the necessity of an en bloc resection because the lingual lymph nodes located beyond the omohyoid muscle are normally not resected in the course of a classic neck dissection.

The physiologic lymphatic drainage of the nasopharynx flows from the nasal fornix first in dorsolateral then in dorsolaterocaudal direction (9). Furthermore, there is a lymphatic drainage parallel to the posterior midline that corresponds to the findings of Rouvière (8). According to his investigations, the lymph fluid drains from the fornix and from the posterior nasopharyngeal wall via 8–12 collectors parallel to the posterior midline. The collectors draw to the retropharyngeal lymph nodes as well as to the lymph nodes of level II and especially level V. Based on this nasopharyngeal carcinomas metastasize mainly into the mentioned groups of lymph nodes (10).

The lymphatic drainage of the palatine tonsil and of the base of the tongue is directed mainly to the lymph nodes of level II, sometimes also via collectors that drain to the retropharyngeal lymph nodes and to the lymph nodes in level III (11). The lymphatic drainage of the posterior pharyngeal wall is directed into the retropharyngeal lymph nodes of which the lymph fluid is conducted via collectors to the lymph nodes in levels II and III. Thus, the high metastatic rate of oropharyngeal carcinomas in retropharyngeal lymph nodes can be explained (12). Furthermore, there is also a direct lymphatic drainage from the posterior pharyngeal wall into levels II and III.

At this point, the hint to another phenomenon should not be omitted. Occult oropharyngeal carcinomas may present via a large, necrotic lymph node metastasis predominantly located in level II. This lymph node metastasis is often misdiagnosed as so-called *branchiogenic carcinoma* (13).

From the hypopharynx the lymph fluid is drained via collectors mostly to the lymph nodes in levels III and IV. A direct connection to level I could not be detected. Of course also lymphatic drainage to the lymph nodes of level II can be observed, even if they occur more rarely than to the levels III and IV. This concerns especially the cranial hypopharyngeal part (10).

The lymph fluid of the supraglottic and mainly also of the glottic region flows to the lymph nodes of levels II and III. From the subglottic space, the lymph fluid is conducted ventrally through the cricothyroid ligament and dorsally through the cricotracheal ligament. The subglottic lymph fluid flows to the lymph nodes of levels III and VI. The presence of a prelaryngeal lymph node located in level VI (so-called *Delphi lymph node*) depends on the age of the patient. Whereas this lymph node can be regularly observed in children up to the age of 10, only half of the examined adults between 40 and 75 are in its possession.

In summary, the direction of metastatic spread in laryngeal carcinomas corresponds in most of the cases to the above-described lymphatic drainage in the levels II and III (14).

According to the described mean lymphatic drainage of the upper aerodigestive tract, lymphatic metastatic spread into several lymph groups is depending on the location of the primary (Table 1), which directly influences surgical treatment concepts.

BYPASS OR CONTRALATERAL LYMPHATIC DRAINAGE

The direction and extent of lymphatic drainage and related lymphogenic metastatic spread are also influenced by tumor growth, accompanying inflammations, surgical measures, and radiotherapy.

The significance of these factors is also critically important in the metastatic process in contralateral cervical lymph nodes for which Ossof and Sission (15) consider three mechanisms as being responsible. The first pathway of metastatic spread occurs via afferent lymph vessels crossing to the contralateral side. This is especially true when ispilateral lymph vessels are interrupted (16). The second pathway of

Table 1. Mean metastatic spread according to the primary side

Lymph node	Level according to Robbins et al. (18)	Primary
Submental and submandibular group	I	Oral cavity Buccal mucosa Mobile tongue
Craniojugular group	II	Tonsil Soft and hard palate Base of the tongue Supraglottis Glottic
Mediojugular group	III	Larynx (glottic, supra- and subglottis) Hypopharynx Caudal part of the base of the tongue
Caudojugular group	IV	Hypopharynx Subglottis
Group containing the posterior triangle	V	Epipharynx Skin of the head
Group of the anterior compartment	VI	Thyroid gland Subglottic

contralateral metastatic spread occurs in areas that are not divided by a midline. The third pathway of metastatic spread occurs via retrograde metastatic spread along crossing, efferent lymph vessels; this is observed in cases of extended regional lymph node involvement (17).

Another example of altered lymphatic drainage direction and related lymph node metastases in unusual locations is the development of metastases at the base of a myocutaneous pedicle of a flap placed after previous extirpation of a carcinoma of the oral cavity or the pharynx. In such cases, lymphogenic metastatic spread can occur through the myocutaneous flap in levels where usually no metastases develop (1).

CONCLUSION

The lymphatic drainage directions of the different primary tumor sites of the upper aerodigestive can be summarized as follows:

- The dominating metastatic region of pharyngeal and laryngeal carcinomas is mainly level II and less commonly level III.
- Carcinomas of the anterior oral cavity drain mostly into level I and less commonly into level II (18).

Accordingly, selective neck dissection of these lymph node levels can be expected to include the majority of clinically occult metastases.

With this background, it must still be clarified whether the intraoperative identification of the radiolabeled sentinel lymph node is appropriate to reduce the extent of selective neck dissection in the suspected N0 neck, or whether neck dissection can be completely avoided in the case of histologically proven tumor-free sentinel lymph node. Opponents of such a procedure argue that selective neck dissection of one or two neck levels is much more precise and standardized than any identification of several lymph nodes encompassing the low morbidity for selective neck dissection that must not be considered. Supporters of sentinel lymphadenectomy stress both protecting the intact, i.e., nonmetastastic, cervical lymph node systems, and reducing the extent of surgery. Scarring contractures, paresthesia, and persisting lymph edemas are supposed to be reduced by a selective sentinel lymph node dissection.

REFERENCES

1. Werner JA. Untersuchungen zum Lymphgefäßsystem der oberen Luft- und Speise-wege. Shaker, Aachen, pp 1-152
2. Werner JA, Schünke M, Rudert H, Tillmann B. Description and clinical importance of lymphatics of the vocal fold. Otolaryngol Head Neck Surg 1990; 102:13-19
3. Werner JA. Untersuchungen zum Lymphgefäßsystem von Mundhöhle und Rachen. Laryngorhinootol 1995; 74:622-628
4. Werner JA. Morphologie und Histochemie von Lymphgefäßen der oberen Luft- und Speisewege: Eine klinisch orientierte Untersuchung. Laryngorhinootol 1995; 74:568-576
5. DiNardo LJ. Lymphatics of the submandibular space: an anatomic, clinical, and pathologic study with applications to floor-of-mouth carcinoma. Laryngoscope 1998; 108:206-214
6. Ozeki S, Tashiro H, Okamoto M, Matsushima T. Metastasis to the lingual lymph node in carcinoma of the tongue. J Max Fac Surg 1985; 13:277-281
7. Woolgar JA. Histological distribution of cervical lymph node metastases from intraoral/ oropharyngeal squamous cell carcinomas. Br J Oral Maxillofac Surg 1999; 37:175-180
8. Rouvière H. Anatomie des lymphatiques de l'homme. Masson et cie, Paris, 1932
9. Jung H. Intravitale Lymphabflußuntersuchungen vom Nasenrachendach beim Menschen. Laryngo Rhino Otol 1974; 53:769-773
10. Werner JA. Aktueller Stand der Versorgung des Lymphabflusses maligner Kopf-Hals Tumoren. Eur Arch Otorhinolaryng (Suppl.) 1998:1-85
11. Belz GT, Heath TJ. Lymphatic drainage from the tonsil of the soft palate in pigs. J Anat 1995; 187: 491-495
12. Vikram B. Changing patterns for failure in advanced head and neck cancer. Arch Otolaryngol Head Neck Surg 1984; 110:564-575
13. Soh KB. Branchiogenic carcinomas: do they exist? J R Coll Surg Edinb 1998; 43:1-5
14. Werner JA, Dunne AA, Myers JN. Functional anatomy of the lymphatic drain age system of the upper aerodigestive tract and its role in metastasis of squamous cell carcinoma. Head Neck. 2003; 25:322-332
15. Ossof RH, Sission GA. Lymphatics of the floor of the mouth and neck: anatomical studies related to contralateral drainage pathways. Laryngoscope 1981; 91:1847-1850
16. Larson DL, Lewis SR, Rapperport AS, Coers CR, Blocker TG. Lymphatics of the mouth and neck. Am J Surg 1965; 110:625-630
17. Werner JA, Davis RK. Metastases in Head and Neck Cancer. Springer, New York, 2004
18. Robbins KT, Clayman G, Levine PA, Medina J, Sessions R, Shaha A, Som P, Wolf GT; American Head and Neck Society; American Academy of Otolaryngology—Head and Neck Surgery. Neck dissection classification update: revisions proposed by the American Head and Neck Society and the American Academy of Otolaryngology-Head and Neck Surgery. Arch Otolaryngol Head Neck Surg. 2002; 128:751-758

16. PATTERNS OF METASTASIS IN HUMAN SOLID CANCERS

STANLEY P. L. LEONG[1], BLAKE CADY[2], DAVID M. JABLONS[1],
JULIO GARCIA-AGUILAR[1], DOUGLAS REINTGEN[3], J. A. WERNER[4],
AND YUKO KITAGAWA[5]

[1]Department of Surgery, University of California San Francisco, California, USA, [2]Comprehensive Breast Center, Rhode Island Hospital, Providence, Rhode Island, USA, [3]Lakeland Regional Cancer Center, Lakeland, Florida, USA, [4]Dept of Otolaryngology, Head & Neck Surgery, Philipps-University Marburg, Germany, [5]Department of Surgery, Keio University School of Medicine, Tokyo, Japan

INTRODUCTION

To date, lymph node status is the most important predictor for clinical outcome. Clinical models of cancer metastasis have evolved from Halsted's lymphatic dominant model in which the regional lymph nodes served as filters for cancer cells. When the filter was filled, the cancer cells would move to the other lymph nodes and distant sites. The Halsted's model (1) was then replaced by Fisher's model in which all breast cancers were considered to be systemic from their onset (2). Recently, the Fisher's model has been supplemented by the spectrum model of Hellman, in which early cancer is locally aggressive. In the process of progression, cancer cells acquire the ability to metastasize to the lymph nodes and then to the systemic sites (3, 4). Recent advances in the sentinel lymph node (SLN) concept and technology have allowed us to further study the clinical significance of micrometastasis in the SLNs and the mechanism of cancer metastasis through the lymphovascular system. Evidence from the SLN era indicate that most solid cancers progress in an orderly fashion from the primary sites to the regional lymph nodes or the SLNs in the majority of cases with subsequent dissemination to the systemic sites.

PATTERNS OF METASTASIS IN SOLID CANCER IN THE PRE-SLN ERA

Melanoma

Melanoma frequently starts from an in situ to a radial growth phase. Then it expands into a vertical growth phase, which is associated with increased risk of metastasis. Nodal status is the most reliable predictor of clinical outcome (5, 6). In the pre-SLN era, several retrospective studies noted that the regional nodal basin was the most frequent site of metastasis. Incidence of nodal metastasis is increased with thicker Breslow lesions, which may also be associated with higher frequency of systemic metastasis (7). In general, during the early phase of melanoma proliferation, the pattern of metastasis to the regional nodal basin is the predominant one in about 60% in patients with primary melanoma of 1.5–4 mm, but a minority of the patients will develop systemic disease, about 15%. From an autopsy series of 216 melanoma patients, the lymph nodes and lungs were the most frequent sites of metastasis (8). In the late stages of the disease, dissemination was widespread with involvement of multiple organs. Survival for patients with extensive dissemination was usually short. When dissemination was limited, survival was longer. Such isolated metastases could potentially be resected, resulting in longer survival.

Breast Cancer

Based on autopsy studies, women dying of breast cancer suggest that widespread metastatic disease with bones (70%), lungs (66%), and liver (61%) are the most common sites of spread. On the other hand, with early-stage, the most common site for metastatic involvement is the regional nodal basin (9). Based on an analysis of an extensive breast cancer database, Nemoto et al. demonstrated that the nodal involvement with breast cancer was the most important predictor of the clinical outcome (10). On the other hand, in early breast cancer, the appropriate treatment results in excellent outcome (11, 12). The recent decrease in mortality rate for breast cancer (13) while the incidence of breast cancer has increased by 0.5% per year between 1987 and 1998 may be explained by treatment of early breast cancer detected by screening mammography (14). Most of the early breast cancers (>75%) are in occurrence with the spectrum model in which metastatic potential increases as the tumor grows in size. Early small cancers with few exceptions have little ability to develop clinical metastases (11, 12). Survival was significantly decreased in patients with systemic dissemination of breast cancer. Overall, in stage I to II patients the 5-year survival was at least over 70% with regional lymph node involvement (Stage III) the survival dropped to 20–60%. When systemic disease was found (Stage IV) the survival dropped down to 5% (15).

Head and Neck Cancer

The lymphatic drainage pattern of the head and neck is complicated (16–20), draining to about 300 regional cervical lymph nodes, which are clarified by Robbins (21) into nine lymph node levels (level I–VI). As regional lymph node status is a significant predictor for clinical outcome in squamous cell carcinoma of the upper aerodigestive tract, detection of clinically occult lymph node metastases is an integral step in the management of the clinical N0 neck. Nodal metastasis depends on the location of the primary tumor, ranging from 12 to over 50% (median, 33%) (22–24). Numerous authors favor elective neck dissection if occult lymph node metastasis carries a probability of 20% or more. Although some authors prefer a "wait and see" strategy, this approach requires both great patient compliance and expertise on the part of the responsible physician to detect metastasis early. Another argument in favor of elective neck dissection against a "wait-and-see" approach is that the survival rate drops significantly when neck dissection is performed after clinical disease is discovered (25–27). Elective neck dissection is preferred to the "wait and see" approach. The nodal basin can be electively treated either by neck dissection or radiotherapy. An advantage of the former over the latter is that histological examination of the neck dissection specimen may provide important information for deciding adjuvant therapy, as well as about the prognosis (28).

Upper GI Cancer

Although distant metastasis is associated with hematogenous dissemination, some organ metastases are due to lymphatic spread. Lymphatic skip metastases were found in 50–60% of esophageal cancers and 20–30% of gastric cancers in a retrospective analysis of the location of solitary metastases (29, 30). Based on a retrospective analysis of gastric cancer with solitary metastasis, Sano et al. (31) reported that the perigastric nodal area close to the primary tumor was the first site of metastasis in 62% of the cases. Therefore, extended radical procedures such as esophagectomy with three-field lymph node dissection and gastrectomy with D2 lymphadenectomy have been developed to become standard procedures in Japan, even for clinically node negative cases (32, 33). The disadvantage is that such extensive dissection is associated with significant morbidity and mortality as being reported in randomized trials (34, 35). It is interesting to note that lymphatic spread from Barrett's cancer is different than that from squamous cell carcinoma in the same location with relatively lower incidence of anatomical skip metastases (36). Autopsy reports showed that both hematogenous and lymphatic metastasis is common in esophogeal carcinoma (37, 38). Intramural metastasis is characteristic of esophageal squamous cell carcinoma and is associated with poor prognosis (39). Other poor prognostic features include gastric metastasis, location of the primary lesion (middle thoracic location), size of tumor (>7 cm), histologic type (undifferentiated), and depth of invasion (T4) (40). Hematogenous spread from esophageal cancer is related to the location of primary lesions as lung metastases are associated with cervical nodal metastases from upper esophageal cancer, and liver metastases are associated with thoracic metastases from lower esophageal cancer (41). These findings suggest that the lymphatic metastasis exists in some of the patients with esophageal cancer. Lymphogenous liver metastasis by lymphaticovenous communication has been described in an animal model (42). This phenomenon was clinically supported by Kumagai et al.'s demonstration that liver metastasis was correlated with lymphatic activity in gastric cancer (43). Peritoneal dissemination is observed as an initial recurrence in 20–30% of patients undergoing curative surgery for gastric adenocaricinoma and is related to the diffuse type of the distal tumors (44). Distant recurrence is related to the proximal tumors (44). The overall recurrence rate after curative surgery for early gastric cancer is generally low (1.9%) and differentiated tumors showed a 2.3% rate of hematogenous metastasis (45). Only node-positive patients showed a relatively high rate of recurrence (10.7%).

Colorectal Cancer

Almost 50% of patients with colorectal cancer have metastasis at the time of their diagnosis with the most common sites consisting of the regional lymph nodes, the liver, the lung, and the peritoneal cavity (46). Again, like melanoma and breast cancer, nodal status is the most important prognostic factor for patients without disseminated disease. The incidence of nodal metastasis increases with the depth of tumor penetration in the bowel wall; 10% in the submucosa; 22% in the muscularis propria, and 56% reaching the pericolonic fat. Other high risk factors include tumor grade, lymphatic, and vascular invasion. Carcinoma of the colon and rectum shows different patterns of nodal metastasis. For colon cancer, the regional lymph nodes include four groups: the epicolic nodes, along the vasa recta in the wall of the colon and epiploic appendices; the pericolic nodes along the marginal vessels; the intermediate nodes along the vessels, such as the sigmoidal, left colic, middle colic, and ileocolic; and the central or apical nodes along the inferior mesenteric and superior mesenteric vessels. In 97% of patients, lymph node metastasis in colon cancer occurs to the pericolic nodes, 27% have metastasis to the intermediate nodes, and 11% with central nodal involvement (47, 48). Metastasis to the pericolic nodes occurs mostly within 7 cm from the primary tumor. Metastases occurring 10 cm from the primary tumor are unusual (48) and metastasis to the central nodes is rare. In rectal cancer, the main lymphatic spread is cephalad (80%) to the mesorectal lymph nodes along the superior rectal vessels (49). In about 75% of the rectal cancer patients, nodal metastasis is found within the mesorectum, 3 cm or less from the primary tumor. In the rest of the patient population, nodal metastasis occurs near the bifurcation of the superior rectal vessels (50). Nodal metastasis to the mesorectum distal to the primary tumor occurs in up to 20% of patients, primarily located within 2 cm from the lower margin of the primary tumor; nodal metastases beyond 4 cm are infrequent (51–53). Tumors in the lower third of the rectum may spread along the middle rectal vessels toward the internal iliac nodes. About 12% of the patients with rectal cancer undergoing curative surgery may have internal iliac nodal metastasis (54). Tumors in the anal canal may metastasize to the inguinal lymph nodes. The number of lymph nodes retrieved from surgical specimens depends primarily on the size of the tumor, the extent of surgery, and the thoroughness of the pathological exam (55). Staging of colorectal cancer depends on the number of nodes being harvested. The higher the number of nodes retrieved, the more accurate the staging is (56). Several studies show that a minimum of 12 nodes should be analyzed for adequate staging (57) and the total number of nodes retrieved had a significant impact on patient survival (58, 59). Unfortunately, only 37% of patients undergoing curative surgery for colorectal cancer in the United States had adequate lymph node evaluation (60). A cascade hypothesis has been developed from the autopsy series that metastatic disease to the visceral organs develops in discrete steps, first to the liver, then to the lung, and finally to other sites. In a series of 1,541 autopsies from multicenter databases, Weis et al. (61) found that only 15% of patients without liver involvement had metastasis to the lung or other organs, compared to 52% of patients with liver metastasis. With respect to distant organs other than the lung, 7% of patients had no liver metastasis, 27% had liver metastasis, and 55% had disease in both the liver and lung. In rectal cancer patients, the incidence of metastasis to the liver is similar to that of the lung. The high frequency of lung metastasis may be explained by the potential hematogenous spread of distal rectal cancer through the inferior iliac veins and the inferior vena cava. This streamlined flow may potentially cause the preferential location of the liver metastasis within the liver with respect to the site of the tumor in various segments of the large bowel (62). The right lobe of the liver derives its blood flow from the superior mesenteric vein and the left lobe from the splenic and inferior mesenteric veins.

Nonsmall Cell Lung Cancer

About 85% of all newly diagnosed lung cancers in the United States are nonsmall cell lung cancer (NSCLC). Lung cancer has recently exceeded hepatocellular carcinoma as the dominant cancer killer worldwide, with an estimated 1.2 million lives lost annually. In the United States, lung cancer kills more people than colorectal, prostate, and breast cancers combined. In 2004, approximately 168,000 people were diagnosed and approximately 155,000 patients died of lung cancer for an average 14.5% survival rate. Due to late stage at diagnosis, comparatively ineffective systemic control agents and lack of better understanding of the molecular pathogenesis of the disease survival for lung cancer remains comparatively abysmal (63). Spiral CT screening for at-risk populations has been applied to a large randomized prospective trial comparing spiral CT to chest X-ray. Fifty-thousand patients have been enrolled countrywide within the past year and half. This new focus on early detection has resulted in earlier stage at diagnosis and higher chance of cure (64). Regional and mediastinal nodal involvement in lung cancer predicts a worse survival. Intraoperative determination of mediastinal nodal disease (N2 stage IIIa) in the late 1980s to early 1990s was found to have less than 15% long term survival despite "complete" resection. Thus, several investigators proposed the use of induction chemotherapy and chemoradiotherapy for locally advanced, stage IIIa disease, which has become the accepted new standard of care in most centers (65–67). Despite neoadjuvant treatment and successful complete resections, positive long-term outcomes are still difficult due to the innate aggressive biology of most NSCLCs (in particular, adenocarcinomas) associated with early dissemination. As a result, newer techniques for accurate preoperative and intraoperative staging are being developed. PET scanning and CT/PET in lung cancer, like in many solid organ cancers, has become an important tool for accurate preoperative staging. In most cases of NSCLC, PET upstages at least 20–25% of patients, thereby preventing unnecessary thoracotomies. Intraoperative SLN staging may be used as an adjunct to preoperative PET/CT to identify patients with regional (hilar N1) and locally advanced (ipsilateral mediastinal N2) prior to more radical resection to achieve more accurate staging and allow the use of combined modality therapies (68).

VALIDATION OF SENTINEL LYMPH NODE (SLN) CONCEPT IN SOLID CANCERS

As mentioned above, the pre-SLN literature has established the fact that regional nodal status is the most significant predictor for clinical outcome. Gould et al. first coined the term SLN for the first lymph node in the parotid nodal basin to predict the involvement of additional lymph nodes in the parotid gland in 1960. Using penile carcinoma as a model and based on radiological identification, Cabanas advanced the concept that SLN in penile cancer could predict the route of metastasis to the inguinal nodal basin on each side of for penile carcinoma (69). Using a feline model with a blue dye technique to identify the SLN, Wong et al. were able to show that the primary anatomical site of the tumor determines the location of the SLN physiologically (70). The clinical trial to demonstrate that melanoma progressed in an orderly fashion from the primary site to the SLN in the nodal basin first and then to other lymph nodes in the same nodal basin by Morton et. al. in 1992 (71) established the practical utility of this method to define the SLN in the nodal basin with the blue dye technique. This approach was further developed in breast cancer with success to identify SLNs for breast caner in the ipsilateral axilla (72). Radiotracer to detect SLNs being developed by Alex and Krag in 1993 using a hand–held gamma probe to identify the SLNs following lymphosentigraphy has resulted in an increased sensitivity of harvesting the SLNs over the blue dye technique (73). To date, the technique has been established as a standard for the staging of melanoma (74) and breast cancer (75, 76) without the need initially to perform a more morbid radical regional lymph node dissection. About 20% of the patients will need a subsequent completion lymph node dissection when the SLNs are positive. This concept has quickly been applied to other solid cancers including the colorectal, upper gastrointestinal cancer, lung cancer, and gynecological cancer (77).

PATTERNS OF METASTASIS IN SOLID CANCER IN THE SLN ERA

Extensive literature is available to validate the concept and the application of SLN in the staging of melanoma (78) breast cancer (79). In general, the incidence of micrometastasis to the SLNs is linearly correlated with the Breslow thickness of the primary melanoma and the size of the primary breast cancer (80). Further more, micrometastasis to the SLNs and the number of SLNs being involved are associated with a poorer prognosis both in melanoma (81) and breast cancer (82). The definition of micrometastasis in the SLNs with respect to immunohistochemistry and molecular detection using RT-PCR is still yet to be defined. In general, the group that enjoys the most survival benefit in melanoma is the group with negative H&E negative immunohistochemistry and negative for RT-PCR findings (83). One of the reasons for the study to demonstrate these differences in melanoma is because melanoma is a more aggressive cancer and that 5-year follow-up has reached a significant level of maturity to predict the outcome of these patients. On the other hand, immunohistotochemical and RT-PCR positive SLNs in breast cancer in SLNs still remain to be defined. Perhaps more follow-up time is required to adequately assess the outcome for breast cancer. A recent study by Morton et al. (84) showed no therapeutic difference from the multicenter sentinel lymphadenectomy trial I (MSLTI), in which melanoma patients were randomized to wide local excision of the primary melanoma only and wide local excision plus selective sentinel lymphadenectomy. Perhaps, this can be explained by the fact that the substantial number of patients being selected were relatively low risk including patients with 1 mm Breslow thickness and also the follow-up may have to be extended longer in order to see more events with respect to recurrence and death. However, the study showed that when patients had completion lymph node dissection with microscopic metastasis to the SLN, they did much better than patients who developed macroscopic disease prior to lymph node dissection. Future studies to compare patients with positive SLNs whether they need completion lymph node dissection or not i.e., the therapeutic usage of lymph node dissection for positive SLNs will be studied in another randomized trial, so called the MSLT II. With respect to the breast carcinoma, originally planned trial of Z0011 by the American College of Surgeons Surgical Oncology Group (http://www.acosog.org), to randomize patients to have lymph node dissections vs. no lymph node dissections when the SLN was positive was prematurely terminated because of a lack of accrual. Despite some controversy still existing, the clear evidence is that positive SLNs predict a poorer prognosis for both melanoma (81) and breast cancer (82). The patients with a negative SLN following a minimally invasive selective lymphadenectomy will do much better and certainly, these patients would be spared a more extensive radical lymph node dissection.

The head and neck trial indicated that the SLN techniques may be reliable and that a positive SLN also predicted a poorer prognosis (Chap. 15). A more expanded discussion of the utility of SLN procedure for head and neck cancer is presented in Chap. 15.

In the colorectal cancer, it has been established from a retrospective analysis based on patients undergoing SLN procedures followed by the standard colectomy with regional lymph node dissection showed that the patients can be upstaged much better and more accurately with identification of SLNs than just examining the regional lymph nodes being resected from the surgical specimen. Of course, in the colorectal situation, the standard is still a resection of the colon along with the removal of the regional pericolec lymph nodes. The most important benefit is the upstaging of patients in about 30% of patients (85). In view of the current indication that at least over a 12 lymph nodes should be obtained to have an accurate analysis of the lymph node status (86, 87), the application of the SLN techniques should therefore be encouraged in the colorectal cancer. Clinical trials are ongoing to further determine the role of the SLN procedure in the staging and the management of colon cancer.

In the upper GI cancer, with the much higher incidence of upper GI cancer in Asia, the pioneering work has been developed mainly in Japan. Kitagawa et al. has reported experiences in the esophageal and gastric carcinoma (88–90). In the late stages, the identification of SLNs may not be as accurate because of increased rate of metastasis. On the other hand, in early esophageal and gastric cancer, SLN identification of micrometastasis in the SLNs during surgery, may predict the remainder of the nodal basins. Therefore, the Japanese group proposed that it should be used in early esophageal and gastric cancer to avoid a more extended esophogectomy and gastrectomy if indeed the SLNs are negative. Currently, clinical trials are ongoing in Japan to prospectively determine the role of SLNs in esophageal and gastric cancer.

In lung cancer, it has been demonstrated to be feasible in the identification of SLNs (91, 92). Clinical trials are also underway to assess the role of SLNs in lung cancer. While the techniques are being perfected in the identification of SLNs in lung cancer, the ability to select a few SLNs for further study in search of micrometastasis from an average 20–30 nodes allow the pathologist to focus their efforts on the most relevant lymph nodes and perhaps this way upstage the patients in a more reliable fashion (91). Intraoperative SLN staging may be used in addition to preoperative PET and PET/CT to identify patients with regional (hilar N1) and locally advanced (ipsilateral mediastinal N2) prior to resection to allow more accurate staging and use of combined modality therapies (68).

WHY IS PAPILLARY THYROID CANCER TO THE REGIONAL NODES RELATIVELY "BENIGN"?

Papillary thyroid carcinoma in young "low risk" patients shows a pattern of frequent regional nodal metastases (75%) when routine nodal resections are performed but distant metastases are uncommon (<3%) confining only to the lungs. A 99% disease-free survival rate at 20 years may be achieved after treatment (93). This selective nodal patterns of metastasis is similar to carcinoid and islet cell tumors of the foregut and midgut organs such as the stomach, duodenum, pancreas, and intestine (94). Since histological criteria alone do not clearly differentiate malignant from benign, nodal involvement indicated that the tumor is malignant. Therefore, in these tumors, although lymph node metastases are common, there is no impact on survival, since that is determined only by distant vital organ metastases, particularly the liver in carcinoid tumors or islet cell cancers and the lung in low-risk thyroid cancers. This pattern of specific lymph node metastases without the poor prognosis associated with vital organ metastases (liver, lung, brain) is uniquely displayed in these tumors. Why such tumors with relatively "benign" nodal metastasis remains unanswered.

WHY DOES SARCOMA METASTASIZE VIA THE VASCULAR SYSTEM RATHER THAN THE LYMPHATIC SYSTEM?

Staging of sarcoma is different from other types of solid cancer in that its prognosis depends on its grade rather than its specific histological type except for epitheloid sarcoma and angiosarcoma, which may spread to regional lymph nodes (95). Most of the sarcoma, including rhabdomyosarcoma, leiomyosarcoma, chondrosarcoma, liposarcoma, synovial sarcoma, fibrosarcoma, lymphangiosarcoma, and fibrous hystiocytoma, spread via the vascular system to the lungs most of the time (95). Billingsley has shown that pulmonary metastasis is the predominant distant metastatic site (23%), and that metastatic cells would spread via the venous circulation and lodge in the lungs as metastatic foci (96). Genetically, sarcomas may be divided into two main categories. One category is characterized by a tumor-specific translocation that appears to be central to tumor pathogenesis, and indeed is used as diagnostic criteria. The other category is characterized by complex karyotypes that are characteristic of severe genetic and chromosomal instability. Abnormalities in most sarcomas are found in the RB or p53 gene. Specific genetic alteration leads to activation of specific tyrosine kinase growth-factor receptors. Thus, some sarcomas have been successfully treated with drugs that specifically inhibit the activated kinase receptor (97). Recent molecular studies have yielded greater insight to the biology of gastrointestinal stromal tumor (GIST), with a therapeutic target against the c-kit receptor (98). It is important to determine the molecular mechanisms of why sarcoma, unlike melanoma or carcinoma, seldom spreads through the lymphatic system.

CONCLUSION

Over the past decade, it has been established that SLN concept in melanoma and breast cancer is a viable one in that the cancer cells usually spread first to the SLN within the nodal basin and then spread to other lymph nodes or systemic sites (74, 99). This finding has been extended to other types of human solid cancer (77). The central question is what specific role does the SLN plays in the process of lymphatic metastasis. From the follow-up of patients, particularly in melanoma and breast cancer patients who have undergone selective sentinel lymphadenectomy the evidence is quite strong to indicate the spectrum hypothesis of Hellman is probably correct in the sense that during early progression of cancer, SLN in the draining nodal basin is probably the most frequent site of metastasis and over time with progression of the cancer in the SLN, additional lymph nodes within the nodal basin may be involved and subsequently vascular invasion may occur resulting in distant visceral metastasis. Thus, when cancer is in its early stage, if eradicated either by surgery or radiation therapy, potentially, the patient may be cured. Therefore, it is important to further define the process of metastasis whether the spread to the requires de novo lymphatic channels (100) or the usage of existing lymphatic channels. During lymphatic spread, is there a simultaneous route of vascular invasion resulting in hemotogeonous spread of cancer cells? Can these processes be further defined with respect to the molecular and genetic profiles of the cancer cells? Based on the histologic and the clinical information, the American Joint Committee on Cancer (AJCC) has established a very sophisticated and useful classification of staging cancer in its different stages. Perhaps in the future molecular and genetic profiles of cancer can be developed so that the type of metastasis i.e., the lymphatic, vascular, or combined mode of spread may be defined on a molecular level. With advances in the identification in the receptors on the endothelial cells of the lymphatic and the vascular channels (101), there interaction with cancer cells on a molecular level need to be further examined. In the future, when the diagnose of cancer is made, the prediction whether the cancer will metastasize may be more accurately defined using molecular and genetic markers. Therefore, the current AJCC adopting the histologic and clinical features may give way to molecular staging. Such a shift in the staging of cancer based on molecular markers will enable us to individualize treatment to a cancer patient more accurately.

REFERENCES

1. Halsted, W., *The results of operations for the cure of cancer of the breast performed at the Johns Hopkins Hospital from June, 1889 to January, 1894.* Operations for Cure of Cancer of the Breast, 1894. **4**: p. 497-553.
2. Fisher, B., et al., *Twenty-year follow-up of a randomized trial comparing total mastectomy, lumpectomy, and lumpectomy plus irradiation for the treatment of invasive breast cancer.* N Engl J Med, 2002. **347**(16): p. 1233-41.
3. Hellman, S., *Karnofsky Memorial Lecture. Natural history of small breast cancers.* J Clin Oncol, 1994. **12**(10): p. 2229-34.
4. Hellman, S. and R.R. Weichselbaum, *Oligometastases.* J Clin Oncol, 1995. **13**(1): p. 8-10.
5. Balch, C.M., et al., *Final version of the American Joint Committee on Cancer staging system for cutaneous melanoma.* J Clin Oncol, 2001. **19**(16): p. 3635-48.
6. Reintgen, D., et al., *The orderly progression of melanoma nodal metastases.* Ann Surg, 1994. **220**(6): p. 759-67.
7. Leong, S.P., et al., *Clinical patterns of metastasis.* Cancer Metastasis Rev, 2006. **25**(2): p. 221-32.
8. Patel, J.K., et al., *Metastatic pattern of malignant melanoma. A study of 216 autopsy cases.* Am J Surg, 1978. **135**(6): p. 807-10.
9. Reintgen, D., R. Giuliano, and C. Cox, *Lymphatic mapping and sentinel lymph node biopsy for breast cancer.* Cancer J, 2002. **8 Suppl 1**: p. S15-21.
10. Nemoto, T., et al., *Management and survival of female breast cancer: results of a national survey by the American College of Surgeons.* Cancer, 1980. **45**(12): p. 2917-24.
11. Arnesson, L.G., S. Smeds, and G. Fagerberg, *Recurrence-free survival in patients with small breast cancer. An analysis of cancers 10 mm or less detected clinically and by screening.* Eur J Surg, 1994. **160**(5): p. 271-6.
12. Wood, W.C., et al., *Can we select which patients with small breast cancers should receive adjuvant chemotherapy?* Ann Surg, 2002. **235**(6): p. 859-62.
13. Niederhuber, J.E., *Seeking calmer waters in a sea of controversy.* Oncologist, 2002. **7**(3): p. 172-3.
14. Von Eschenbach, A.C., *NCI remains committed to current mammography guidelines.* Oncologist, 2002. **7**(3): p. 170-1.

15. Harris, J. and H. CI, *Natural history and staging of breast cancer*. Breast Diseases, 1987: p. 233-58.
16. Fisch, U.P., *Lymphographische untersuchung uber das zervikale*. Karger (Basel), 1966.
17. Fisch, U.P., *Cervical Lymphography in Cases of Laryngo-Pharyngeal Carcinoma*. J Laryngol Otol, 1964. **78**: p. 715-26.
18. Schwab, W. and K.z. Winkel, *[The current status of scintigraphy of the cervical lymphatic system]*. Nucl Med (Stuttg), 1967. **6**(2): p. 234-49.
19. Zita, G., *[Contribution on cervical lymphoscintigraphy]*. Fortschr Geb Rontgenstr Nuklearmed, 1967. **107**(5): p. 644-54.
20. Michailov, V. and C. Mlatschkov, *[Evaluation of cervical lymph node scintigraphy]*. Radiobiol Radiother (Berl), 1969. **10**(6): p. 769-77.
21. Robbins, K.T., et al., *Neck dissection classification update: revisions proposed by the American Head and Neck Society and the American Academy of Otolaryngology-Head and Neck Surgery*. Arch Otolaryngol Head Neck Surg, 2002. **128**(7): p. 751-8.
22. Hosal, A.S., et al., *Selective neck dissection in the management of the clinically node-negative neck*. Laryngoscope, 2000. **110**(12): p. 2037-40.
23. van den Brekel, M.W., et al., *The incidence of micrometastases in neck dissection specimens obtained from elective neck dissections*. Laryngoscope, 1996. **106**(8): p. 987-91.
24. Teichgraeber, J.F. and A.A. Clairmont, *The incidence of occult metastases for cancer of the oral tongue and floor of the mouth: treatment rationale*. Head Neck Surg, 1984. **7**(1): p. 15-21.
25. Gavilan, J., C. Gavilan, and J. Herranz-Gonzalez, *The neck in supraglottic cancer*. 1994: p. 576-581.
26. DeSanto, L.W., C. Magrina, and W.M. O'Fallon, *The "second" side of the neck in supraglottic cancer*. Otolaryngol Head Neck Surg, 1990. **102**(4): p. 351-61.
27. Godden, D.R., et al., *Recurrent neck disease in oral cancer*. J Oral Maxillofac Surg, 2002. **60**(7): p. 748-53; discussion753-5.
28. Werner, J.A. and R. Davis, eds. *Metastasis in Head and Neck Cancer*. Springer, Heidelberg, in press.
29. Kosaka, T., et al., *Lymphatic routes of the stomach demonstrated by gastric carcinomas with solitary lymph node metastasis*. Surg Today, 1999. **29**(8): p. 695-700.
30. Matsubara, T., et al., *Localization of initial lymph node metastasis from carcinoma of the thoracic esophagus*. Cancer, 2000. **89**(9): p. 1869-73.
31. Sano, T., et al., *Gastric lymphography and detection of sentinel nodes*. Recent Results Cancer Res, 2000. **157**: p. 253-8.
32. Akiyama, H., et al., *Radical lymph node dissection for cancer of the thoracic esophagus*. Ann Surg, 1994. **220**(3): p. 364-72; discussion 372-3.
33. Maruyama, K., et al., *Lymph node metastases of gastric cancer. General pattern in 1931 patients*. Ann Surg, 1989. **210**(5): p. 596-602.
34. Bonenkamp, J.J., et al., *Extended lymph-node dissection for gastric cancer*. N Engl J Med, 1999. **340**(12): p. 908-14.
35. Hulscher, J.B., et al., *Extended transthoracic resection compared with limited transhiatal resection for adenocarcinoma of the esophagus*. N Engl J Med, 2002. **347**(21): p. 1662-9.
36. Feith, M., H.J. Stein, and J.R. Siewert, *Pattern of lymphatic spread of Barrett's cancer*. World J Surg, 2003. **27**(9): p. 1052-7.
37. Bhansali, M.S., et al., *Pattern of recurrence after extended radical esophagectomy with three-field lymph node dissection for squamous cell carcinoma in the thoracic esophagus*. World J Surg, 1997. **21**(3): p. 275-81.
38. Mafune, K.I., Y. Tanaka, and K. Takubo, *Autopsy findings in patients with esophageal carcinoma: comparison between resection and nonresection groups*. J Surg Oncol, 2000. **74**(3): p. 196-200.
39. Yuasa, N., et al., *Prognostic significance of the location of intramural metastasis in patients with esophageal squamous cell carcinoma*. Langenbecks Arch Surg, 2004. **389**(2): p. 122-7.
40. Saito, T., et al., *Esophageal carcinoma metastatic to the stomach. A clinicopathologic study of 35 cases*. Cancer, 1985. **56**(9): p. 2235-41.
41. Kato, H., et al., *Prediction of hematogenous recurrence in patients with esophageal carcinoma*. Jpn J Thorac Cardiovasc Surg, 2003. **51**(11): p. 599-608.
42. Yamagata, K., et al., *Gastrointestinal cancer metastasis and lymphogenous spread: viewpoint of animal models of lymphatic obstruction*. Jpn J Clin Oncol, 1998. **28**(2): p. 104-6.
43. Kumagai, K., et al., *Liver metastasis in gastric cancer with particular reference to lymphatic advancement*. Gastric Cancer, 2001. **4**(3): p. 150-5.
44. D'Angelica, M., et al., *Patterns of initial recurrence in completely resected gastric adenocarcinoma*. Ann Surg, 2004. **240**(5): p. 808-16.
45. Sano, T., et al., *Recurrence of early gastric cancer. Follow-up of 1475 patients and review of the Japanese literature*. Cancer, 1993. **72**(11): p. 3174-8.

46. Niederhuber, J.E., *Colon and rectum cancer. Patterns of spread and implications for workup.* Cancer, 1993. **71**(12 Suppl): p. 4187-92.

47. Yada, H., et al., *Analysis of vascular anatomy and lymph node metastases warrants radical segmental bowel resection for colon cancer.* World J Surg, 1997. **21**(1): p. 109-15.

48. Hida, J., et al., *The extent of lymph node dissection for colon carcinoma: the potential impact on laparoscopic surgery.* Cancer, 1997. **80**(2): p. 188-92.

49. Grinnell, R.S., *The lymphatic and venous spread of carcinoma of the rectum.* Cancer Supplement, 1942. **116**: p. 200-216.

50. Steup, W.H., Y. Moriya, and C.J. van de Velde, *Patterns of lymphatic spread in rectal cancer. A topographical analysis on lymph node metastases.* Eur J Cancer, 2002. **38**(7): p. 911-8.

51. Heald, R.J., E.M. Husband, and R.D. Ryall, *The mesorectum in rectal cancer surgery—the clue to pelvic recurrence?* Br J Surg, 1982. **69**(10): p. 613-6.

52. Wang, Z., et al., *Microscopic spread of low rectal cancer in regions of the mesorectum: detailed pathological assessment with whole-mount sections.* Int J Colorectal Dis, 2005. **20**(3): p. 231-7.

53. Koh, D.M., et al., *Distribution of mesorectal lymph nodes in rectal cancer: in vivo MR imaging compared with histopathological examination. Initial observations.* Eur Radiol, 2005. **15**(8): p. 1650-7.

54. Hida, J., et al., *Does lateral lymph node dissection improve survival in rectal carcinoma? Examination of node metastases by the clearing method.* J Am Coll Surg, 1997. **184**(5): p. 475-80.

55. Thorn, C.C., et al., *What factors affect lymph node yield in surgery for rectal cancer?* Colorectal Dis, 2004. **6**(5): p. 356-61.

56. Pheby, D.F., et al., *Lymph node harvests directly influence the staging of colorectal cancer: evidence from a regional audit.* J Clin Pathol, 2004. **57**(1): p. 43-7.

57. Law, C.H., et al., *Impact of lymph node retrieval and pathological ultra-staging on the prognosis of stage II colon cancer.* J Surg Oncol, 2003. **84**(3): p. 120-6.

58. Le Voyer, T.E., et al., *Colon cancer survival is associated with increasing number of lymph nodes analyzed: a secondary survey of intergroup trial INT-0089.* J Clin Oncol, 2003. **21**(15): p. 2912-9.

59. Gunderson, L.L., et al., *Impact of T and N stage and treatment on survival and relapse in adjuvant rectal cancer: a pooled analysis.* J Clin Oncol, 2004. **22**(10): p. 1785-96.

60. Baxter, N.N., et al., *Lymph node evaluation in colorectal cancer patients: a population-based study.* J Natl Cancer Inst, 2005. **97**(3): p. 219-25.

61. Weiss, L., et al., *Haematogenous metastatic patterns in colonic carcinoma: an analysis of 1541 necropsies.* J Pathol, 1986. **150**(3): p. 195-203.

62. Wigmore, S.J., et al., *Distribution of colorectal liver metastases in patients referred for hepatic resection.* Cancer, 2000. **89**(2): p. 285-7.

63. Edwards, B.K., et al., *Annual report to the nation on the status of cancer, 1975-2002, featuring population-based trends in cancer treatment.* J Natl Cancer Inst, 2005. **97**(19): p. 1407-27.

64. Henschke, C.I., et al., *Survival of patients with stage I lung cancer detected on CT screening.* N Engl J Med, 2006. **355**(17): p. 1763-71.

65. Burkes, R.L., et al., *Induction chemotherapy with mitomycin, vindesine, and cisplatin for stage IIIA (T1-3, N2) unresectable non-small-cell lung cancer: final results of the Toronto phase II trial.* Lung Cancer, 2005. **47**(1): p. 103-9.

66. Albain, K.S., et al., *Concurrent cisplatin/etoposide plus chest radiotherapy followed by surgery for stages IIIA (N2) and IIIB non-small-cell lung cancer: mature results of Southwest Oncology Group phase II study 8805.* J Clin Oncol, 1995. **13**(8): p. 1880-92.

67. McKenna, R.J., Jr., W. Houck, and C.B. Fuller, *Video-assisted thoracic surgery lobectomy: experience with 1,100 cases.* Ann Thorac Surg, 2006. **81**(2): p. 421-5; discussion 425-6.

68. Dietlein, M., et al., *Cost-effectiveness of FDG-PET for the management of potentially operable non-small cell lung cancer: priority for a PET-based strategy after nodal-negative CT results.* Eur J Nucl Med, 2000. **27**(11): p. 1598-609.

69. Cabanas, R.M., *An approach for the treatment of penile carcinoma.* Cancer, 1977. **39**(2): p. 456-66.

70. Wong, J.H., L.A. Cagle, and D.L. Morton, *Lymphatic drainage of skin to a sentinel lymph node in a feline model.* Ann Surg, 1991. **214**(5): p. 637-41.

71. Morton, D.L., et al., *Technical details of intraoperative lymphatic mapping for early stage melanoma.* Arch Surg, 1992. **127**(4): p. 392-9.

72. Giuliano, A.E., *Mapping a pathway for axillary staging: a personal perspective on the current status of sentinel lymph node dissection for breast cancer.* Arch Surg, 1999. **134**(2): p. 195-9.

73. Alex, J.C. and D.N. Krag, *Gamma-probe guided localization of lymph nodes.* Surg Oncol, 1993. **2**(3): p. 137-43.

74. Leong, S.P., *Sentinel lymph node mapping and selective lymphadenectomy: the standard of care for melanoma.* Curr Treat Options Oncol, 2004. **5**(3): p. 185-94.

75. Singh-Ranger, G. and K. Mokbel, *The sentinel node biopsy is a new standard of care for patients with early breast cancer.* Int J Fertil Womens Med, 2004. **49**(5): p. 225-7.
76. Edge, S.B., et al., *Emergence of sentinel node biopsy in breast cancer as standard-of-care in academic comprehensive cancer centers.* J Natl Cancer Inst, 2003. **95**(20): p. 1514-21.
77. Leong, S.P., Y. Kitagawa, and M. Kitajima, *Selective sentinel lymphadenectomy for human solid cancer.* Cancer Treat Res, ed. S.T. Rosen. 2005, New York: Springer.
78. Leong, S.P., *Selective sentinel lymphadenectomy for malignant melanoma, Merkel cell carcinoma, and squamous cell carcinoma.* Cancer Treat Res, 2005. **127**: p. 39-76.
79. Cox, C.E., et al., *Selective sentinel lymphadenectomy for breast cancer.* Cancer Treat Res, 2005. **127**: p. 77-104.
80. Leong, S.P., *Paradigm of metastasis for melanoma and breast cancer based on the sentinel lymph node experience.* Ann Surg Oncol, 2004. **11**(3 Suppl): p. 192S-7S.
81. Leong, S.P., et al., *Clinical significance of occult metastatic melanoma in sentinel lymph nodes and other high-risk factors based on long-term follow-up.* World J Surg, 2005. **29**(6): p. 683-91.
82. Naik, A.M., et al., *The risk of axillary relapse after sentinel lymph node biopsy for breast cancer is comparable with that of axillary lymph node dissection: a follow-up study of 4008 procedures.* Ann Surg, 2004. **240**(3): p. 462-8; discussion 468-71.
83. Takeuchi, H., et al., *Prognostic significance of molecular upstaging of paraffin-embedded sentinel lymph nodes in melanoma patients.* J Clin Oncol, 2004. **22**(13): p. 2671-80.
84. Morton, D.L., et al., *Sentinel-node biopsy or nodal observation in melanoma.* N Engl J Med, 2006. **355**(13): p. 1307-17.
85. Saha, S., et al., *Sentinel lymph node mapping technique in colon cancer.* Semin Oncol, 2004. **31**(3): p. 374-81.
86. Compton, C.C. and F.L. Greene, *The staging of colorectal cancer: 2004 and beyond.* CA Cancer J Clin, 2004. **54**(6): p. 295-308.
87. Wong, J.H., et al., *Impact of the number of negative nodes on disease-free survival in colorectal cancer patients.* Dis Colon Rectum, 2002. **45**(10): p. 1341-8.
88. Aikou, T., et al., *Sentinel lymph node mapping with GI cancer.* Cancer Metastasis Rev, 2006. **25**(2): p. 269-77.
89. Kitagawa, Y., et al., *The role of the sentinel lymph node in gastrointestinal cancer.* Surg Clin North Am, 2000. **80**(6): p. 1799-809.
90. Kitagawa, Y., et al., *Radio-guided sentinel node detection for gastric cancer.* Br J Surg, 2002. **89**(5): p. 604-8.
91. Liptay, M.J., et al., *Intraoperative sentinel lymph node mapping in non-small-cell lung cancer improves detection of micrometastases.* J Clin Oncol, 2002. **20**(8): p. 1984-8.
92. Faries, M.B., et al., *Lymphatic mapping and sentinel lymphadenectomy for primary and metastatic pulmonary malignant neoplasms.* Arch Surg, 2004. **139**(8): p. 870-6; discussion 876-7.
93. Cady, B., *Presidential address: beyond risk groups—a new look at differentiated thyroid cancer.* Surgery, 1998. **124**(6): p. 947-57.
94. Modlin, I.M., K.D. Lye, and M. Kidd, *A 5-decade analysis of 13,715 carcinoid tumors.* Cancer, 2003. **97**(4): p. 934-59.
95. Fong, Y., et al., *Lymph node metastasis from soft tissue sarcoma in adults. Analysis of data from a prospective database of 1772 sarcoma patients.* Ann Surg, 1993. **217**(1): p. 72-7.
96. Billingsley, K.G., et al., *Pulmonary metastases from soft tissue sarcoma: analysis of patterns of diseases and postmetastasis survival.* Ann Surg, 1999. **229**(5): p. 602-10; discussion 610-2.
97. Helman, L.J. and P. Meltzer, *Mechanisms of sarcoma development.* Nat Rev Cancer, 2003. **3**(9): p. 685-94.
98. Heinrich, M.C., et al., *Kinase mutations and imatinib response in patients with metastatic gastrointestinal stromal tumor.* J Clin Oncol, 2003. **21**(23): p. 4342-9.
99. Morton, D.L., et al., *Lymphatic mapping and sentinel lymphadenectomy for early-stage melanoma: therapeutic utility and implications of nodal microanatomy and molecular staging for improving the accuracy of detection of nodal micrometastases.* Ann Surg, 2003. **238**(4): p. 538-49; discussion 549-50.
100. Sleeman, J.P., *The relationship between tumors and the lymphatics: what more is there to know?* Lymphology, 2006. **39**(2): p. 62-8.
101. Witte MH, Jones K, Wilting J, Dictor M, Selg M, McHale N, Gershenwald JE, Jackson DG (2006) *Structure function relationships in the lymphatic system and implications for cancer biology.* Cancer Metastasis Rev 25: 159-184.

17. SIGNIFICANCE OF REGIONAL DRAINING LYMPH NODES IN THE DEVELOPMENT OF TUMOR IMMUNITY: IMPLICATIONS FOR CANCER IMMUNOTHERAPY

RONGXIU ZHENG, JORGEN KJAERGAARD*, WALTER T. LEE, PETER A. COHEN, AND SUYU SHU

Center for Surgery Research, Cleveland Clinic, Cleveland, Ohio, USA
*New England Inflammation and Tissue Protection Institute, Northeastern University, Boston, Massachusetts, USA

INTRODUCTION

For the majority of human solid cancer, regional draining lymph nodes (LNs) are the initial target of metastases and the LN status serves as the most important prognostic indicator for clinical outcome of patients. In patients with cutaneous melanoma who develop metastases, tumor most often first presents in the ipsilateral regional nodes and appears preferentially in the first LN on the direct lymphatic drainage pathway from a primary melanoma (1, 2). This LN has been referred to as the sentinel node (SN). Over the past two decades, significant progress has been achieved in understanding the functional, anatomical, cellular, and molecular aspects of the SN (3). It is evident that the susceptibility of the SN to the development of metastases is closely linked to immune dysfunction induced by invading tumor cells. Studies comparing the architecture, cytology, and cellular phenotype of SN with non-SN from the same patients revealed a reduction in the aggregate area of paracortex in its dendritic and T cell densities (4, 5). These alterations and down-regulation of immune responsiveness in the SN are not irreversible, as demonstrated in patients preoperatively treated with granulocyte-macrophage colony-stimulating factor (GM-CSF) (6). Thus, efforts to reverse tumor-induced immune down-regulation in the SN may have some capacity to reduce metastases and to facilitate the initiation of antitumor immunity. Considering the complexity of physiological and immunological roles LNs play, manipulations targeted at this site may allow the isolation of functional antitumor T cells for adoptive immunotherapy. Adoptive immunotherapy is the transfer of immune effector T cells to cancer patients for therapeutic purposes. One recent example is the use of tumor-infiltrating lympho-cytes (TILs) for the treatment of advanced metastatic melanoma (7). After nonmyeloablative conditioning regimen and T cell transfer, approximately 45% of patients demonstrated an objective response. However, adoptive immunotherapy is not the only subject discussed here. This chapter will highlight historical and recent experimental evidence that draining LNs are the site of initial immune response and LNs draining a growing tumor or a tumor vaccine contain therapeutically effective T cells. For the design of effective cancer vaccines, we have recently devel-oped an electrofusion technology with which chimeric hybrids of dendritic cells (DCs) and tumor are generated. Such fusion hybrids are highly immunogenic and therapeutic. Our studies demonstrated that a single immunization could induce a therapeutic immune response in tumor-bearing animals. However, successful induction of antitumor immunity required intranodal delivery of the vaccine, underscoring the pivotal role of LNs in tumor immunotherapy.

SIGNIFICANCE OF DRAINING LNS IN THE DEVELOPMENT OF PRIMARY IMMUNE RESPONSES

The LN itself is a complex structure with a number of functional distinct compart-ments. The afferent lymphatic vessels enter the LN on its convex surface penetrating the LN capsule and entering capsule sinus. Immediately internal to this sinus is the cortex, consisting of the B-cell-enriched follicles and the interventing T-cell-enriched paracortex area. The cortex overlies the medulla which consists of medulla sinus and medulla cords. The medulla cords contain many activated T and B cells and plasma cells that have arised in the course of an ongoing immune response (8). Thus, the secondary lymphoid tissues such as LNs provide sites where antigen-presenting cells (APCs) can efficiently cooperate with naïve T and B cells in the generation of a T-cell-dependent immune response. Lymph nodes are actually the site of great activity. It is a mistake to approach the study of cellular structure of a LN with the impression that it is a static structure. Lymphocytes, both those produced in the node and those that are constantly added to the node from bloodstream, pass into the lymph that drains through the LN. Sensitized T cells and plasma cells that secrete antibod-ies are being formed in LNs as needed from activated T and B lymphocytes. Therefore, the study of a histology section of a LN suffers from the same limitation as a snapshot of a very active and ever changing scene.

   The importance of the local draining LN to the development of systemic cellular immune responses has been experimentally demonstrated since the middle of last century. In studies on chemical contact sensitivity in inbred histocompatible strain II guinea pigs, generalized sensitivity cannot be demonstrated before 4–5 days after first contact with the antigen (9–11). In this situation, the development of systemic immunity is not affected by surgical excision of the area of skin on which chemical sensitizer has been applied after 16–24 h. However, if the draining LN was removed 3 days after sensitization, immunized animals failed to become sensitized to the antigen (Fig. 1). Further evidence for the role of local LNs in the development of delayed hypersensitivity were provided by studies of Frey and Wens, demonstrating that an intact lymphatic drainage to the local LN was necessary for sensitization to occur. In their pioneer experiments with guinea pigs, skin fragments were isolated from the surrounding and underlying tissues but kept in connection with the animal by a vascular pedicle. Such an explant was kept alive in the animal through its vascular supply but with its lymphatic connections cut off. It was found impossible to sensitize animals to DNCB by applying the chemical to this explant (12). However, if the animal was sensitized at a distant site, it was possible to show sensitivity on the explanted skin once the animal had become sensitized (Fig. 2). It can therefore be concluded that an intact lymphatic drainage is necessary for sensitization to occur.

The pivotal role of the draining LN in the development of antitumor immunity has also been demonstrated in immunization experiments using syngeneic tumors, the line-10 guinea pig hepatocellular carcinoma and the mouse MCA105 fibrosarcoma. Although both tumors are highly malignant in their normal naïve hosts, they contain tumor-specific transplantation antigens (TSTA) that, with the use of bacterial adjuvants such as Bacillus Calmette-Guerin (BCG) or *Corynebacterium parvum*, immunized animals may acquire systemic immunity to reject a lethal dose of viable tumor cell challenge. Analysis of the kinetics of the occurrence of antitumor

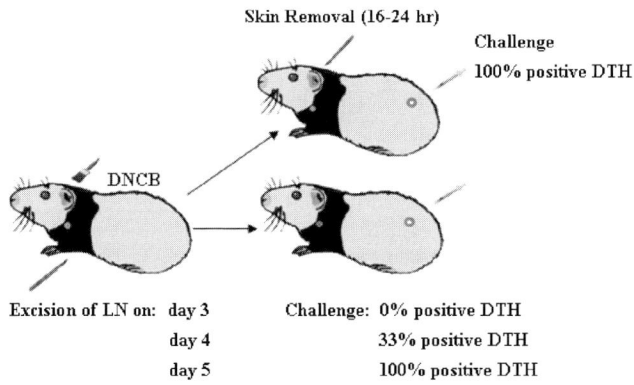

Figure 1. Development of contact sensitivity reactions requires an intact lymphatic drainage to the local LN. In inbred strain II guinea pigs, excision of the area of skin on which DNCB had been painted was only necessary for 16–24 h. Removal of draining LNs 3 days after sensitization prevented the manifestation of sensitivity (11)

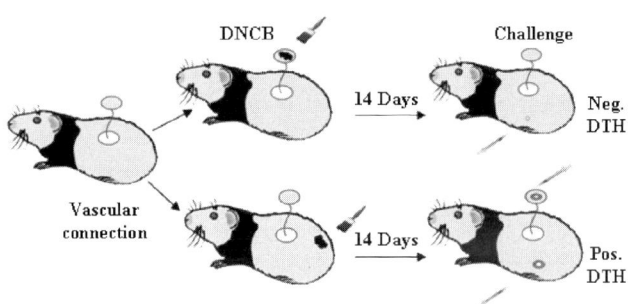

Figure 2. Significance of the local LN draining the site of primary antigenic contact. In strain II guinea pigs, skin fragments were isolated from underlying tissue but kept connected by a vascular pedicle. Application of DNCB to the explant failed to sensitize the animal. However, if the minimal was sensitized by contact with DNCB at a distant site, it was possible to show sensitivity on the explant skin once the animal had become sensitized (12)

immune response demonstrated the critical role of the draining LN. In the guinea pig line-10 hepatoma model, surgical excision of the immunization skin site within 4 days of vaccination did not impact on the eventual development of a systemic immunity (13). However, surgical removal of both the immunization skin site and the local draining LN as late as 11 days after immunization would result in the failure of developing a systemic antitumor immunity (Fig. 3).

We repeated the experiment and confirmed that greater than 90% of animals developed a systemic tumor immunity against the line-10 hepatoma if the vaccine site was allowed to be intact for 2 days. However, in guinea pigs whose vaccine sites were removed 2 days after immunization, systemic antitumor immunity could be

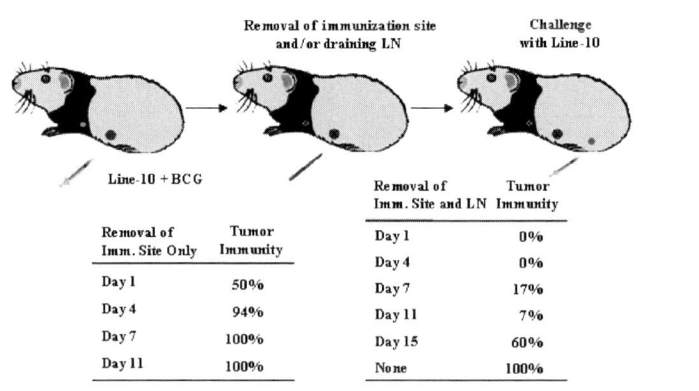

Figure 3. Development of antitumor immunity is critically dependent on intact local draining LNs. Strain II guinea pigs could be immunized to line-10 hepatoma to reject a lethal tumor challenge. While excision of immunization skin sites 4 days after immunization did not interfere with the development of a generalized antitumor immunity, removal of the draining LN as late as day 11 prevented the antitumor immune response (13)

Table 1. Significance of local draining LNs in the development of systemic immunity to the MCA 105 fibrosarcoma in C57BL/6 mice

Day of excision of immunization site[a]		Tumor immunity[b]	
2		3/18	17%
4		7/17	41%
6		16/17	94%

Day of excision of immunization site	Draining LN	Tumor immunity	
6	6	5/46	11%
6	14	27/45	60%
No	No	33/46	72%

[a]Surgically excision of skin sites at which a mixture of 1.5×10^6 live MCA 105 tumor cells and 100 μg of formalin-killed *Corynebacterium parvum* was injected.
[b]Tumor resistance was tested by challenging immunized mice with $0.2–1.0 \times 10^6$ tumor cells (14).

completely abrogated by the surgical removal of the draining LNs as late as 11 days after immunization. The significance of draining LNs in the development of antitumor immune responses was also demonstrated in the mouse. With use of the MCA105 fibrosarcoma of the C57BL/6 mouse, we found that excision of tumor immunization site on day 6 did not interfere with the development of systemic immunity to reject a tumor challenge (14). However, if both immunization site and the draining LN were excised on day 6 of immunization, the development of immunity was severely impaired (Table 1). It thus became clear that a critical period of time for an intact draining LN is necessary for the generation of a complete immune response, suggesting that the initial sensitization occurred in the draining LN rather than at the site of immunization, i.e., the skin.

TUMOR-DRAINING LNs: A SOURCE OF THERAPEUTIC T CELLS

It was possible passively to transfer contact sensitivity or tuberculin hypersensitivity to naïve animals with cells extracted from immunized donors. It is particularly noteworthy that the local draining LN contained cells capable of adoptively transferring delayed hypersensitivity as early as 4 days after sensitization (11). However, most antigens used for these studies were strongly immunogenic such as DNCB. To demonstrate a successful cell transfer against autochtonous tumors has been more challenging. In general, immune responses to malignant tumors are expected to be weaker than those to chemical sensitizers or protein antigens and the goal of cell transfer is to eradicate existing tumors rather than to confirm immunity in normal, tumor-free animals. Using the adoptive immunotherapy procedure for the treatment of 3-day established murine MCA105 tumors, we showed that freshly isolated draining LN cells prepared from mice bearing progressive tumors for various days, for the most part, failed to mediate a significant antitumor reactivity. To generate therapeutically functional T effector cells, we designed an in vitro sensitization (IVS) procedure where tumor-draining LN cells were stimulated with viable but irradiated tumor cells in the presence of the T cell growth factor, IL-2 (Fig. 4). Such a system allowed the growth of T cells in vitro, resulting in the acquisition of antitumor reactivity from otherwise nontherapeutic tumor-draining LN cells. Although the IVS system induced nonspecific T cell proliferation from LN cells of normal naïve as well as tumor-bearing mice, therapeutically functional T cells could only be generated from cultures initiated with tumor-draining LNs stimulated with specific tumor cells identical to that of stimulated LNs in vivo (Table 2). Thus, the IVS represented a secondary in vitro immune response. Tumor stimulated draining LNs must have contained tumor-sensitized but functionally immature "pre-effector" T cells.

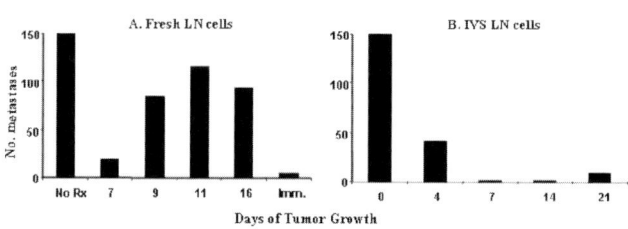

Figure 4. In vivo antitumor reactivity of freshly isolated MCA 105 tumor-draining LN cells and that of in vitro sensitized (IVS) LN cells. Popliteal LNs were obtained from mice inoculated with 5×10^5 MCA 105 tumor cells in the footpad at various stages of tumor growth. IVS cells were prepared by culture of draining LN cells with irradiated tumor cells in the presence of IL-2 for 9 days. Therapeutic efficacy of the cells was assessed by the adoptive immunotherapy of 3-day established pulmonary MCA 105 metastases. Each tumor-bearing mouse was transferred i.v. with either 5×10^7 fresh or 1.4×10^7 IVS LN cells. Mice treated with IVS cells were also given IL-2 (7, 500 U) i.p. twice daily for 3 days (15)

Table 2. Requirement for specific tumor stimulation in IVS for generating therapeutic cells from tumor-bearing mice

Tumor stimulator cells in IVS[a] (No./Well)	Adoptive immunotherapy[b]		
		Mean no. metastases (SEM)	
	IL-2	Expt. 1	Expt. 2
	−	141 (36)	126 (52)
	+	134 (51)	212 (39)
Normal spleen cell (10^6)	+	157 (46)	179 (32)
MCA 105 (4×10^5)	+	3 (1)	9 (8)
MCA 102 (2×10^5)	+	142 (49)	121 (44)
MCA 106 (2×10^5)	+	89 (29)	92 (37)

[a]Popliteal lymph node cells (2×10^5 per well) obtained from mice bearing intrafootpad MCA 105 tumor for 15 days were cultured with 2,000 R irradiated tumor stimulator cells. The IL-2 concentration was 2 U ml^{-1} for first 7 days and changed to 10 U ml^{-1} for additional 3 day culture.
[b]For adoptive immunotherapy, each animal received 4×10^6 IVS cells i.v. on day 3 and i.p. IL-2 (7,500 U, twice a day, from day 3 to day 5) (16).

The intervention by IVS allowed the differentiation as well as expansion of these pre-effector T cells to mature into fully functional antitumor effector lymphocytes.

These laboratory and preclinical observations prompted us to evaluate similarly generated tumor-sensitized T cells for the treatment of human cancer (17). Although the IVS method was theoretically attractive and technically feasible, the requirement of a large number of autologous human tumor cells from each patient has restricted its broad application in the clinic. Antigenic stimulation of pre-sensitized T cells involved the engagement of T-cell receptor (TCR), which was noncovalently associated with a cluster of low MW proteins commonly referred to as CD3. Considerable evidence suggested that the CD3 structure served to transduce the activation signals consequential to the binding of the MHC-peptide complex to the TCR. In the absence of specific antigen stimulation, monoclonal antibodies (mAbs) reactive to CD3 molecules have been shown to induce T cell proliferation by passing TCR engagement. We therefore reasoned that if the initial sensitization of T cells had already occurred in the tumor-draining LNs in vivo, the polyclonal stimulation with anti-CD3 might drive the proliferation and maturation of pre-effector cells. This was important from a practical standpoint because antigen-independent stimulation freed investigators from the constraint of needing a large number of tumor cells for IVS. In a series of experiments in the early 1990s, we tested and successfully developed a culture method in which tumor-draining LN cells were stimulated with immobilized anti-mAb for 2 days followed by culture in medium containing 4 U ml^{-1} of IL-2 (18–20). The anti-CD3/IL-2 method stimulated T cell growth with about eightfold expansion in T cell numbers and most importantly, such activated LN cells were highly efficacious in mediating the rejection of established tumors when systemically transferred into tumor-bearing mice. Again, the adoptive immunotherapy mediated by anti-CD3/IL-2 activated draining LN T cells was immunologically specific to the tumor that stimulated the draining LN in vivo (Table 3).

Table 3. Specificity of adoptive immunotherapy mediated by anti-CD3/IL-2 activated tumor-draining LN cells

Treatment		Mean no. pulmonary metastases (SEM)[b]		
Source of draining LN[a]	IL-2	MCA 106	MCA 105	MCA 102
–	–	240 (10)	250	250
–	+	216 (19)	250	250
MCA 106	+	2 (1)	250	217 (28)
MCA 105	+	246 (4)		
MCA 102	+	250		

[a]Popliteal LN cells draining the progressively growing MCA tumors in the footpad for 14 days were activated by the anti-CD3/IL-2 method.
[b]Pulmonary metastases were induced by iv injections of 3×10^5 (MCA 102), 3×10^5 (MCA 105), or 10^6 (MCA 106) tumor cells. In adoptive immunotherapy, 2×10^7 activated cells were given i.v. to each tumor-bearing mouse (20).

These laboratory results have been extrapolated for the design of several innovative clinical trials of adoptive immunotherapy for patients with recurrent and/or metastatic diseases. In these trials, surgical tumor specimens were enzymatically digested to single-cell suspensions. Some of the tumor cells were cultured in an attempt to establish tumor cell lines. Either irradiated, cultured, or fresh-frozen tumor cells were then used for inoculation of patients intradermally on the anterior upper thigh bilaterally with an adjuvant, GM-CSF (125 µg). The adjuvant was given intradermally into each inoculation site daily for 3 additional days. Inguinal LNs draining the vaccine sites were surgically excised 7–10 days after vaccination. These vaccine-draining LN cells were cultured and stimulated with 100 ng ml^{-1} of staphylococcal enterotoxin A (SEA) for 2 days. SEA strongly activates human T cells nonspecifically to induce high levels of CD25 expression. These activated cells were then expanded in culture with 10 U ml^{-1} of human recombinant IL-2 for 5–8 days. Patients received a single oral dose of cyclophosphamide (10 mg kg^{-1}) 24 h prior to adoptive transfer of activated cells. The T cells were infused through a peripheral vein over a period of 1 h. Over the past 10 years, we have used this procedure clinically to treat patients with glioblastoma multiforme (GBM) and other high grade brain tumors (21, 22), metastatic renal cell carcinoma (23) and recurrent squamous cell carcinoma of the head and neck (24). This therapy proved to be well-tolerated without discernible short- and long-term toxicity. In a few treated patients, dramatic objective clinical responses were observed. However, the majority of patients did not benefit from the immunotherapy. Upon reviewing and evaluating our approach of adoptive immunotherapy, we believe that the most vulnerable link in the procedure was the use of irradiated autologous tumor cells for in vivo stimulation of draining LNs. To improve the outcome of adoptive immunotherapy, alternative vaccine designs are needed for more effective antigen-presentation and immune stimulation in vivo.

BIOLOGICAL AND IMMUNOLOGICAL CHARACTERISTIC OF DENDRITIC-TUMOR HETEROKARYONIC HYBRIDS GENERATED BY ELECTROFUSION

As indicated previously, most tumor cells contain tumor-associated antigens (TAA) but they are poor immunogens for stimulating immune responses. Central to the induction of cellular immunity to TAA is antigen presentation by professional APCs. Among various APCs, DCs are probably the most potent initiator of immune responses (25, 26). DCs are found in many nonlymphoid tissues but can migrate via the afferent lymphatics to the T-cell-dependent areas of lymphoid organs. High levels of MHC class I and II molecules, costimulatory molecules such as CD80 and CD86 as well as several adhesion molecules such as ICAM-I and LFA-3, likely contribute to their specialized functions, soluble factors produced by DCs such as IL-12 and IL-6 also contribute to the sensitization and expansion of cytotoxic T lymphocytes (CTLs) and helper T cells. Recent advances in the in vitro generation of large numbers of monocyte-derived, nonproliferating DCs as well as that derived from CD34$^+$ progenitor cells have made it possible to explore innovative DC-based immunotherapy strategies.

In a host of preclinical experiments and clinical trials over the past decade, DCs have been used to process and present tumor antigens to the immune system. DC-based vaccines have shown promise in a number of experimental animal tumor models. This has been generally achieved by pulsing DCs with tumor peptides, lysates, or RNA derived from tumor cells (27, 28). In most studies, DC vaccine approaches have shown their effectiveness as a prophylactic vaccine and in some cases, even established murine sarcomas and carcinomas were eradicated by active immunotherapy with DCs loaded with tumor antigens. Despite a heightened immunity induced in response to vaccination, in a large number of clinical trials, objective clinical responses were disappointing (29, 30). Therefore, further improvement of the design of DC cancer vaccines and carefully executed clinical testing will be the key to the success of cancer immunotherapy.

Loading DCs with a diverse array of antigens to improve the breadth of the immune response represents an optimal choice for future development because cancer cells are much formidable to combat with limited antigen recognition. One approach is to allow DCs to phagocytose necrotic or apoptotic tumor cells or their fragments. However, optimizing this loading procedure is difficult to standardize because in most cases, loading DCs with tumor antigens is best with immature cells while mature DCs are optimal for presenting processed MHC-peptide complexes to T cells. An alternative strategy to deliver a complete set of tumor antigens to DCs is to fuse the two cell types, creating heterokaryons. A prevalent technique for fusion has been the use of polyethylene glycol (PEG). This method of fusion was not observed to produce unequivocally verifiable true heterokaryons despite the claims that such fusion hybrids were therapeutic for a mouse carcinoma tumor and induced CTLs against human breast and ovarian carcinoma cells (31–33). Particularly puzzling was the reported finding that allogeneic DCs were as effective as syngeneic DCs, suggesting most T cells would have to be primed to the autologous tumor cells rather than with DC-tumor fusion cells. Upon reviewing a large number of previously published results, one cannot help but conclude that the PEG method failed to generate a sufficient number of genuine DC-tumor hybrids. This would prove particularly egregious if prospective therapeutic trials are not successful, creating the impression that DC-tumor fusion hybrids have already received adequate clinical evaluation and optimization.

Because of the theoretical attractiveness and the technical difficulties associated with hybrid generation, we have investigated an alternative technology with which fusion hybrids could be generated by exposing cells to electric fields. The principle of this electrofusion technique is quite simple. It involves two independent but consecutive reactions (Fig. 5). The first reaction is to bring cells in close contact with one another by a process called "dielectrophoresis." When cells in suspension are exposed to an alternate electric (ac) current of low intensity, they experience an oscillating dipole effect, leading to the formation of tight membrane contacts in a pearl chain–like arrangement. Immediately following this "alignment," a direct current (dc) pulse with high intensity disrupts the bilipid layer of the cell membrane to

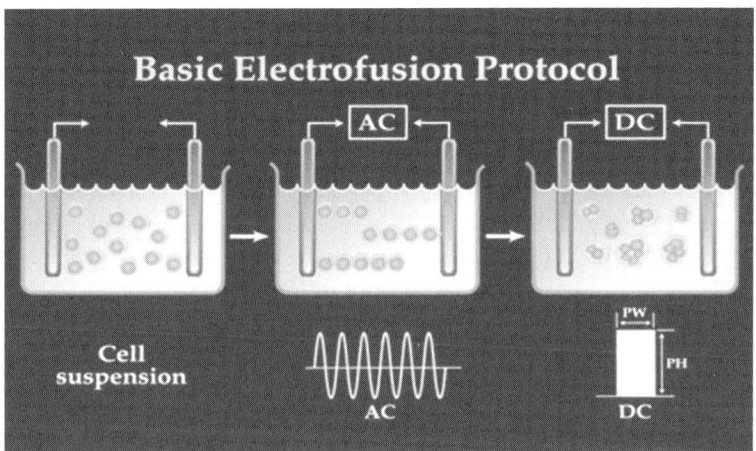

Figure 5. Principle of electrofusion. Cells in suspension (*left*) are exposed to an electric field of low intensity. The dipole effects of the electric field force cells to form pearl-chain-like alignment (*middle*). This process is often referred to as "dielectrophoresis." When cells are then subjected to a high-voltage direct current for a very short period of time, a breakdown of cell membranes occurs. Under controlled conditions, membrane breakdown is reversible. Because cells are closely adjacent to each other by force of dielectrophoresis, membrane resealing may occur between individual cells to form multicellular hybrids (*right*)

form pores. Under controlled conditions, the membrane will reseal spontaneously. Because cells are closely adjacent to each other by dielectrophoresis, membrane resealing may occur between adjacent cells to form multinucleated hybrid cells. To verify that true cell fusion had occurred, dually fluorescent cells were clearly identified using FACS analyses, confocal fluorescence microscopy, examination of stained cytospin preparations, and DNA analyses after staining with propidiumiodide.

Functionally, the electrofused DC-tumor hybrids were able to stimulate IFN-γ secretion from specific tumor immune T cells in vitro (35, 36). In the fusion experiment illustrated in Fig. 6A, GL261 tumor cells were labeled with the green fluorescence dye, CFSE before fusion. After fusion and overnight incubation, most heterologous fusion cells were found to be in the adherent cell population. To identify DC-tumor hybrids, adherent cells were stained with PE-conjugated anti-I-A mAb. I-A is a DC-associated molecule that is not present on tumor cells. Double-positive fusion cells could be easily estimated by the FACS analysis. The adherent cells could be enriched for heterokaryons from the adherent fusion mixture by magnetic anti-PE Microbead (Miltenyi Biotec, Inc., Auburn, CA). Fusion cells expressed the DC phenotype and I-A⁺, while tumor cells were I-A⁻. We used both I-A⁺ and I-A⁻ fractions to stimulate GL261 immune T cells that were derived from tumor-draining LN (35). As depicted in Fig. 6B, only I-A⁺ fusion cells were capable of stimulating T cell secretion of IFN-γ. Further analyses revealed that both CD4 and CD8 tumor immune T cells responded to the fusion cell stimulation (35, 36).

A. Purification of fusion hybrids

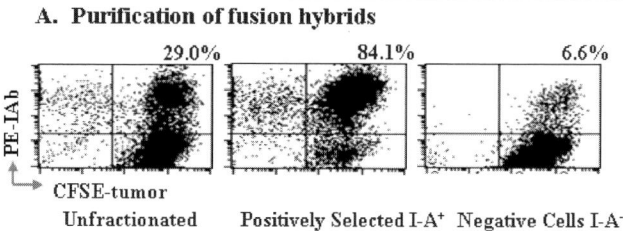

29.0%   84.1%   6.6%

PE-IAb

CFSE-tumor
Unfractionated   Positively Selected I-A⁺   Negative Cells I-A⁻

B. IFN-γ secretion

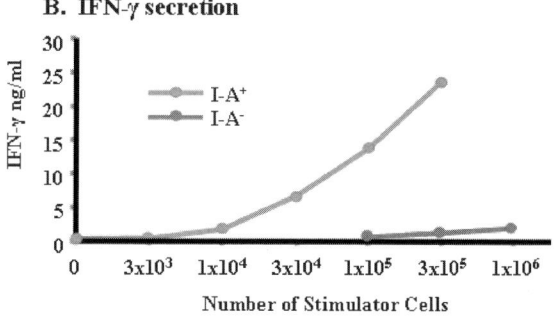

IFN-γ ng/ml

30
25 — I-A⁺
20 — I-A⁻
15
10
5
0

0   3x10³   1x10⁴   3x10⁴   1x10⁵   3x10⁵   1x10⁶

Number of Stimulator Cells

Figure 6. IFN-γ secretion by GL261 tumor-specific T cells stimulated with purified DC-GL261 fusion cells. 2×10^6 GL261 specific immune T cells were stimulated with indicated numbers of I-A⁺ or I-A⁻ DC-GL261 fusion cells. 24-h supernatants were assayed for IFN-γ concentrations by ELISA

In preclinical therapy experiments, a standard protocol of 3-day established experimental pulmonary metastases was used to evaluate the therapeutic efficacy of DC-tumor fusion hybrids. For the past 5 years, we have demonstrated the therapeutic efficacy of fusion vaccines. A single vaccination resulted in a significant antitumor response in five antigenically and histologically distinct murine tumors, including the D5Lacz melanoma, MCA 205 sarcoma, GL261 glioma, 4T1 breast cancer, and SCC VII head and neck cancer (34, 35, 37–39). We have found that effective immunotherapy with DC-tumor fusion hybrids required a co-administration of an adjuvant or a third signal reagent such as IL-12, agonistic OX-40R, and 4-1BB mAb. Also different from most other DC-based cancer vaccines, DC-tumor hybrids must be delivered directly into secondary lymphoid organs such as the LN (Fig. 7). This requirement may reflect the inability of fusion hybrids to traffic to the draining LN due to their large size and it also underscores the significance of the draining LN for initiating a therapeutic antitumor immune response.

The primary goal of developing DC-tumor fusion hybrids to improve the efficacy of immune responses was for the generation of tumor immune T cells for adoptive immunotherapy. Toward this goal, we have investigated the potential usage of DC-tumor hybrid-stimulated LNs for immune T cell generation. Seven days after intranodal inoculation of mice with DC-D5Lacz hybrids and an adjuvant (OX-40R mAb, 75 μg i.p.), an obvious hypertrophy of the draining LNs was noted. An average

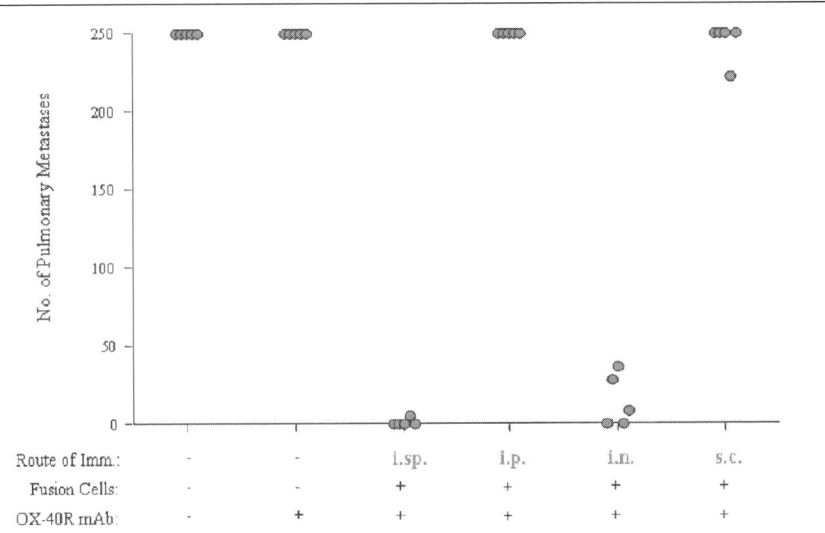

Figure 7. Effects of routes of administration on therapeutic efficacy of active immunotherapy with DC-tumor fusion hybrids. B6 mice were inoculated i.v. with MCA205 tumor cells. On day 3 of tumor growth, mice were treated with fusion cells (1×10^6) and OX-40R mAb (150 μg). On day 22, all mice were sacrificed and lungs were examined and counted for metastatic nodules. i.sp., intrasplenic; i.p., intraperitoneal; i.n., intranodule; and s.c., subcutaneous

LN cellularity of 20×10^6 per LN was ten times greater than that of a normal inguinal LN, which typically yielded approximately 2×10^6 per LN. The DC-tumor stimulated LNs contained about 40% T cells, of which, 38% CD4 and 13% CD8 T cells. The cells were activated by the anti-CD3/IL-2 method as described earlier (18, 19). Using the adoptive immunotherapy of 3-day established pulmonary D5Lacz metastasis model, we found that activated DC-tumor fusion stimulated LN cells were highly efficacious for the treatment of established metastases. As few as 20×10^6 T cells were able to eradicate all tumor nodules in the lung whereas, without the T cell transfer, all mice had greater than 250 metastases. This method of T cell generation is applicable to the clinical application because therapeutic T cells could be generated from tumor-bearing mice with equal efficiency.

In this chapter, we have summarized experimental results of nearly half a century to underscore the importance and significance of local draining LNs in response to antigenic stimulation. We also emphasized that in addition to its role in initiating a systemic immune response to tumor antigens, the draining LN is a rich source of immune T cells that may be used for cancer immunotherapy. Recent development of electrofusion technique is particularly interesting because the fusion hybrids represent the most therapeutic vaccine in preclinical studies (34–39). We are currently conducting a phase I/II clinical trial in which patients with metastatic melanoma are treated with autologous DC-tumor vaccines. Because of the difficulties associated with obtaining sufficient numbers of autologous tumor cells from individual patients, the development of fusion vaccines using allogeneic tumor cell lines that express shared common TAA becomes important future agenda if this clinical trial proves to be successful. Aside from the above discussion, several other applications can be envisioned for the use of electrofused DC-tumor hybrids as APCs. They may be useful for the identification of new TAA. If DC-tumor hybrids can stimulate tumor reactive CD4 and CD8 T lymphocytes, the antigenic specificities of those T cells could be ascertained by screening tumor-derived cDNA libraries or peptides eluted from tumor cells for recognition (40–43). Furthermore, because of the difficulty of raising therapeutic T cells in vitro with whole tumor cells, fusion hybrids may be useful for in vitro stimulation and generation of tumor reactive T lymphocytes for use in adoptive immunotherapy.

REFERENCES

1. Cochran AJ, Bhuta S, Paul E, Ribas A (2000) The shifting patterns of metastatic melanoma. Clin Lab Med 4:759-783
2. Cochran AJ, Roberts AA, Saida T (2003) The place of lymphatic mapping and sentinel node biopsy in oncology. Int J Clin Oncol 8:139-150
3. Morton DL, Wen D-R, Wong JH, Economou JS, Cagle LA, Storm FK, Foshag LJ, Cochran AJ (1992) Technical details of intraoperative lymphatic mapping for early stage melanoma. Arch Surg 127:392-399
4. Cochran AJ, Morton DL, Stern S, Lana AM, Essner R, Wen DR (2001) Sentinel lymph nodes show profound downregulation of antigen-presenting cells of the paracortex: Implications for tumor biology and treatment. Mod Pathol 14:604-608
5. Lana A-M, Wen D-R, Cochran AJ (2001) The morphology, immunophenotype and distribution of paracortical dendritic leukocytes in lymph nodes regional to cutaneous melanoma. Melanoma Res 11:1-10
6. Lee JH, Essner R, Torisu-Itakura H, Wanek L, Wang H-J, Morton DL (2004) Factors predictive of tumor-positive nonsentinel lymph nodes after tumor-positive sentinel lymph node dissection for melanoma. J Clin Oncol 22:3677-3684
7. Dudley ME, Wunderlich JR, Robbins PF, Yang JC, Hwu P, Schwartzentruber DJ, Topalian SL, Sherry R, Restifo NP, Hubicki AM, Robinson MR, Raffeld M, Duray P, Seipp CA, Rogers-Freezer L, Morton KE, Mavroukakis SA, White DE, Rosenberg SA (2002) Cancer regression and autoimmunity in patients after clonal repopulation with antitumor lymphocytes. Science 298:850-854
8. Davies AJS, Carter RL, Leuchars E, Wallis V, Koller PC (1969) The morphology of immune reactions in normal, thymectomized and reconstituted mice I. The response to sheep erythrocytes. Immunol 16: 57-69
9. Landsteiner K, Chase MW (1939) Studies on the sensitization of animals with simple chemical compounds. VI. Experiments on the sensitization of guinea pig to poison ivy. J. Exp. Med. 69:767-784
10. Sell S, Weigle WO (1959) The relationship between delayed hypersensitivity and circulating antibody induced by protein antigens in guinea pigs. J Immunol 83:257-263
11. Turk JL, Stone SH (1963) Implications of the cellular changes in lymph nodes during the development and inhibition of delayed type hypersensitivity. In: Amos B, Koprowski H (eds) "Cell-bound Antibodies". Wistar Institute Press, pp 51
12. Frey JR, Wenk P (1957) Experimental studies on the pathogenesis of contact eczema in the guinea pig. Int Arch Allergy 11:81-100
13. Hanna MG Jr, Bucana CD, Pollack VA (1980) Immunological stimulation *in situ*: the acute and chronic inflammatory responses in the induction of tumor immunity. Contemp Top Immunol 10:267-296
14. Stephenson KR, Perry-Lalley D, Griffith KD, Shu S, Chang AE (1989) Development of antitumor reactivity in regional draining lymph nodes from tumor-immunized and tumor-bearing murine hosts. Surgery 105:523-528
15. Chou T, Chang AE, Shu S (1988) Generation of therapeutic T lymphocytes from tumor-bearing mice by in vitro sensitization: culture requirements and characterization of immunologic specificity. J Immunol 140:2453-2461
16. Shu S, Chou T, Rosenberg SA (1987) Generation from tumor-bearing mice of lymphoid cells with in vivo therapeutic efficacy. J Immunol 139:295-304

17. Chang AE, Yoshizawa H, Sakai K, Cameron MJ, Sondak VK, Shu S (1993) Clinical observations on adoptive immunotherapy with vaccine-primed T lymphocytes secondarily sensitized to tumor in vitro. Cancer Res 53:1043-1050

18. Yoshizawa H, Chang AE, Shu S (1992) Cellular interactions in effector cell generation and tumor regression mediated by anti-CD3/IL-2 activated tumor-draining lymph node cells. Cancer Research 52:1129-1136

19. Kagamu H, Shu S (1998) Purification of L-selectin^{low} cells promotes the generation of highly potent CD4 antitumor or effector T lymphocytes. J Immunol 160:3444-3452

20. Yoshizawa H, Chang AE, Shu S (1991) Specific adoptive immunotherapy mediated by tumor-draining lymph node cells sequentially activated with anti-CD3 and IL-2. J Immunol 147:729-737

21. Plautz GE, Barnett GH, Miller DW, Cohen BH, Prayson RA, Krauss JC, Luciano M, Kangisser DB, Shu S (1998) Systemic T cell adoptive immunotherapy of malignant gliomas. J Neurosurg 89:42-51

22. Plautz GE, Miller DW, Barnett GH, Stevens GHJ, Maffett S, Kim J, Cohen PA, Shu S (2000) T cell immunotherapy of newly diagnosed gliomas. Clin Cancer Res 6:2209-2218

23. Plautz GE, Bukowski RM, Novick AC, Klein EA, Kursh ED, Olencki TE, Yetman RJ, Pienkny A, Sandstrom K, Shu S (1999) T cell adoptive immunotherapy of metastatic renal cell carcinoma. Urology 54:617-624

24. To WC, Wood BG, Krauss JC, Strome M, Esclamado RM, Lavertu P, Dasko D, Kim JA, Plautz GE, Leff BE, Smith V, Sandstrom-Wakeling K, Shu S (2000) Systemic adoptive T cell immunotherapy in recurrent and metastatic carcinoma of head and neck: a phase I study. Arch Otolaryngol Head Neck Surg 126:1225-1231

25. Steinman RM (1991) The dendritic cell system and its role in immunogenicity. Annu Rev Immunol 9:271-296

26. Hart DNJ (1997) Dendritic cells: unique leukocyte populations which control the primary immune response. Blood 90:3245-3287

27. Steinman RM, Dhodapkar M (2001) Active immunization against cancer with dendritic cells: the near future. Int J Cancer 94:459-473

28. Engleman EG (2003) Dendritic cell-based cancer immunotherapy. Seminars in Oncol 30:23-27

29. Ridway D (2003) The first 1000 dendritic cell vaccines. Cancer Invest 21:873-886

30. Rosenberg SA, Yang JC, Restifo NP (2004) Cancer immunotherapy: moving beyond current vaccines. Nat Med 10:909-915

31. Gong J, Chen D, Kashiwaba M, Kufe D (1997) Induction of antitumor activity by immunization with fusion of dendritic and carcinoma cells. Nat Med 3:558-561

32. Gong J, Nikrui N, Chen D, Koido S, Wu Z, Tanaka Y, Cannistra S, Avigan D, Kufe D (2000) Fusions of human ovarian carcinoma cells with autologous or allogeneic dendritic cells induce antitumor immunity. J Immunol 165:1705-1711

33. Gong J, Avigan D, Chen D, Wu Z, Koido S, Kashiwaba M, Kufe D (2000) Activation of antitumor cytotoxic T lymphocytes by fusions of human dendritic cells and breast carcinoma cells. PNAS 97:2715-2718

34. Kuriyama H, Shimizu K, Lee W, Kjaergaard J, Parkhurst MR, Cohen PA, Shu S (2004) Therapeutic vaccine generated by electrofusion of dendritic cells and tumour cells. Dev Biol (Basel) 116:157-166

35. Hayashi T, Tanaka H, Tanaka J, Wang R, Averbook BJ, Cohen PA, Shu S (2002) Immunogenicity and therapeutic efficacy of dendritic-tumor hybrid cells generated by electrofusion. Clin Immunol 104:14-20

36. Parkhurst MR, DePan C, Riley JP, Rosenberg SA, Shu S (2003) Hybrids of dendritic cells and tumor cells generated by electrofusion simultaneously present immunodominant epitopes from multiple human tumor-associated antigens in the context of MHC class I and class II molecules. J Immunol 170:5317-5325

37. Kjaergaard J, Shimizu K, Shu S (2003) Electrofusion of syngeneic dendritic cells and tumor generates potent therapeutic vaccine. Cell Immunol 225:65-74

38. Shimizu K, Kuriyama H, Kjaergaard J, Lee W, Tanaka H, Shu S (2004) Comparative analysis of antigen loading strategies of dendritic cells for tumor immunotherapy. J Immunother 27:265-272

39. Kjaergaard J, Wang L-X, Kuriyama H, Shu S, Plautz GE (2005) Active immunotherapy for advanced intracranial murine tumors by using dendritic cell-tumor cell fusion vaccines. J Neurosurg 103:156-164

40. Boon T, Coulie PG, Van den Eynde B (1997) Tumor antigens recognized by T cells. Immunol Today 18:267-268

41. Rosenberg SA (1999) A new era for cancer immunotherapy based on the genes that encode cancer antigens. Immunity 10:281-287

42. Cox AL, Skipper J, Chen Y, Henderson RA, Darrow TL, Shabanowitz J, Engelhard VH, Hunt DF, Slingluff Jr CL (1994) Identification of a peptide recognized by five melanoma-specific human cytotoxic T cells lines. Science 264:716-719
43. Hunt DF, Henderson RA, Shabanowitz J, Sakaguchi K, Michel H, Sevilir N, Cox AL, Appella E, Engelhard VH (1992) Characterization of peptides bound to the class I MHC molecule HLA-A2.1 by mass spectrometry. Science 255:1261-1263

18. TARGETING SMALL MOLECULES IN CANCER

HAROLD J. WANEBO[1,2], DAVID BERZ[3], AND ANTHONY MEGA[4]

[1]*Professor of Surgery, Boston University, Boston, MA, USA,* [2]*Adjunct Professor of Surgery, Brown University, Providence, RI, USA,* [3]*Fellow, Medical Oncology, Brown University, Providence, RI, USA,* [4]*Assistant Professor of Medicine, Medical Oncology, Brown University Providence, RI, USA*

INTRODUCTION

VEGF-Targeted Agents

The ability of tumors to induce new blood vessel formation, which potentiates tumor growth and the concept of counteracting this growth by blocking angiogenesis, has been known for multiple decades (1–3).

Most of the current angiogenic drugs target the upstream VEGF pathway (4–10). VEGF belongs to a major family of seven factors (Table 1). VEGF and its isoforms are the ligands for VEGF receptors (VEGFR)-1 and -2 (Fig. 1). Although VEGF binds to two receptor tyrosine kinases, VEGFR-1 and/or VEGFR-2, the angiogenic effects are primarily exerted through binding to VEGFR-2 (11). The binding of VEGF to these receptors on endothelial cells results in receptor dimerization and activation, which stimulates signaling cascades involving phospholipase C, protein kinase C, the Src tyrosine kinases, MAP kinase, phophatidylinositol-3-kinase (P13K), Ras GTPase-activating protein, and the Raf-Mek-Erk pathway [reviewed in (3, 5, 6)] (Fig. 1). Additionally, VEGF binds to the nontyrosine kinase neuropilin receptors (NRP-1 and NRP-2). NRP-1 can act as a co-receptor for VEGF, and as such potentiates VEGFR-2-dependent endothelial cell mitogenesis (Fig. 1).

Table 1. Expression of EGFR in human cancers (4, 7)

Tumor type	% EGFR expression
NSCLC	40–80
Head and neck	80–100
Colorectal	25–100
Gastric	33–81
Pancreatic	30–50
Ovarian	35–70
Breast	15–37
Prostate	40–90
Glioma	40–92

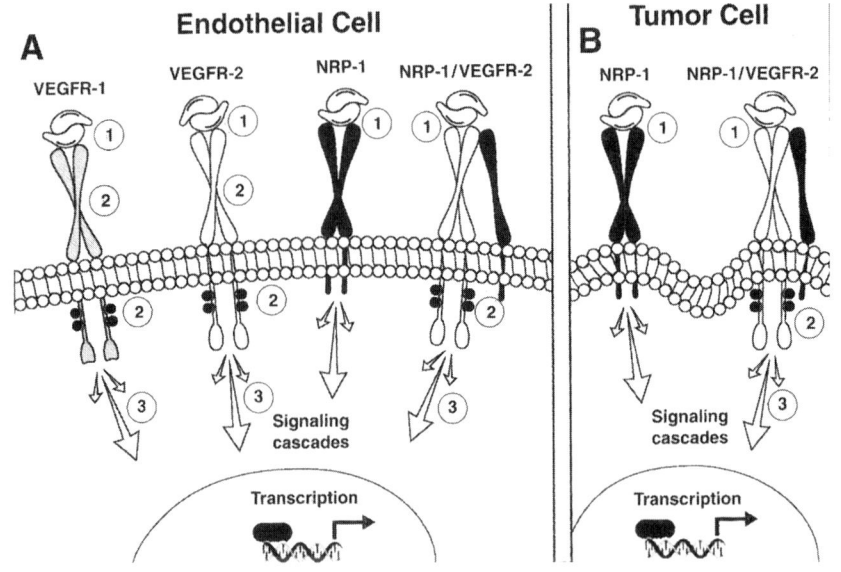

Figure 1. Anti-VEGF agents can act on endothelial and tumor cells. The sites of anti-VEGF action on (A) endothelial and (B) tumor cells are shown. (1) Blockade of VEGF ligand inhibits the interaction of VEGF with all known receptors. (2) Current anti-VEGF receptor agents target VEGFR-1 and/or VEGFR-2 by blocking VEGF binding or by inhibiting receptor phosphorylation. (3) Some agents are in development that block the signal from activated VEGF receptors to the nucleua. NPR, neuropilin; VEGF, vascular endothelial growth factor

NRP-1 is also expressed on tumor cells and often is the sole VEGF receptor on these cells. Binding of VEGF to NRP-1 has effects on tumor cell survival (12), proliferation (13), and chemotaxis. The function of NRP-2 is undefined but may be involved in lymphangiogenesis, [overviewed in (3, 6)].

Agents targeted toward VEGF may inhibit VEGF itself, block its receptors, inhibit its synthesis, or inhibit proteins in the VEGF receptor–signaling cascade. Most of these actions are targeted toward vascular endothelial cells; however, direct effects on tumor cells are possible through inhibiting interaction of VEGF with NRP-1 and with VEGFR-2 in the isolated cases in which this receptor is expressed on tumor cells (Fig. 1).

Anti-VEGF Agents

Among antibody agents which specifically antagonize VEGF, the most studied is bevacizumab, a humanized monoclonal antibody to all isoforms of VEGF. Bevacizumab has been approved for use in combination with 5-fluorouvacil (5-FU)-based chemotherapy as first-line treatment of metastatic colorectal cancer (14). The pivotal phase III clinical trial of bevacizumab in combination with irinotecan, 5-FU, and leucovorin in metastatic colorectal cancer showed greater median survival with the combination than with chemotherapy alone (20.3 vs. 15.6 month; $P < 0.0014$). This benefit occurred in the absence of few significant additional side effects relative to chemotherapy. Grade 3 hypertension was more common in bevacizumab-treated patients (11 vs. 2.3%), but was manageable (14).

Randomized studies with bevacizumab have shown clinical efficacy in other cancers as well. Response rates were higher and times to progression were longer with bevacizumab added to carboplatin and paclitaxel than with chemotherapy alone in patients with advanced or recurrent nonsmall cell lung cancer (NSCLC) (15). The overall response rates in metastatic breast cancer were higher with bevacizumab added to capecitabine than with capecitabine alone (16).

Survival was not increased in either trial. However, several clinical trials (e.g., BOND-2) are testing the effects of combining bevacizumab with agents that antagonize the epidermal growth factor receptor (EGFR) (Erbitux) (17–20) in an effort to potentiate the antitumor benefit of conventional chemotherapy (17–20).

Other anti-VEGF agents include VEGF-trap, a recombinant protein which consists of the (21) extracellular domains of human VEGFR-1 and human VEGFR-2 fused to human IgG1 Fc and antisense oligonuceotide VEGF (VEGF-AS, Veglin) (22). VEGF-trap inactivates all isoforms of VEGF-A (21), and VEGF-AS inhibits receptor binding and expression of VEGF-A, -C, and -D (22). Both have been well tolerated in phase I trials. Dose-related hypertension occurred with VEGF-trap, but no dose-limiting toxicities were apparent with VEGF-AS. Both have shown early evidence of antitumor efficacy (21, 22).

Anti-VEGF Receptor Agents

Among the agents that target VEGF receptors, the VEGF receptor tyrosine kinase inhibitors are understudy in clinical trials. These block or compete with binding of ATP, inhibiting receptor phosphorylation and the subsequent intracellular signaling casade. Two examples are PTK 787 which has activity against VEGF 1, 2, 3, and 5U 0 11 24 5 (active against VEGF2 and PDGFR). Phase II trials of PTK 787 (vatalanib) in combination with 5-FU based chemotherapy for metastatic colorectal cancer showed tolerability up to doses of 1,250 mg d^{-1}. Grades 3 and 4 adverse events included hypertension, fatigue, ataxia, neutropenia, thrombocytopenia, and dizziness (23, 24). The partial response rates ranged from 33 to 50%, and phase III trials are in process (24). The adverse events in phase I/II trials of SU011248 include fatigue and asthenia, nausea and vomiting, diarrhea, neutropenia, thrombocytopenia, lymphopenia, and decreased left ventricular ejection factor of >20% (25).

The recommended dose was 50 mg d^{-1} and major toxicity was fatigue and asthenia. A Phase II trial of SU011248 in patients with previously treated metastatic renal cell carcinoma (RCC) demonstrated partial responses in 24% of patients and stable disease in 46%.

Despite the promising results with these agents, some in this class have failed in clinical trials due to poor efficacy and safety. Semaxinib (SU5416), which was active against VEGFR-1, -2, PDGFR, Flt-4, and c-kit, was associated with a high incidence of thrombotic events, but showed no increase in 1-year event-free survival in a phase II trial in patients with RCC (26). A related molecule, SU6668, which is active against VEGF, PDGF, and fibroblast growth factor-1 receptors was under study, but phase I trials showed self-inducing clearance, which resulted in difficulty in maintaining pharmacologically active concentrations with the maximum tolerated dose (27). An other VEGF receptor-targeted agent is a raf kinase inhibitor, Sorafenib (BAY 43-90006). An early phase II trial showed a response to sorafenib in 25 (40%) of 63 evaluable, accessible patients with metastatic RCC. The most common grade 3 adverse events were hand–foot skin reaction, rash, fatigue, and hypertension (28). This promising agent will be reviewed in the next section as an important small molecule inhibitor of VEGF.

MOLECULARLY TARGETED THERAPY FOR ADVANCED RENAL CELL CANCER

Kidney cancer represents 2% of cancers worldwide with about 38,890 new cases with 12,840 deaths expected in the United States in 2006 (29). Approximately 30% of patients present with stage 4 disease, and 20–40% of resected patients will develop metastasis (30). RCC is a morphologically diverse group of neoplasms of which clear cell carcinoma is the most common form and will be the focus of this review.

Two new molecular targeted agents have been approved for RCC, sorafenib and sunitinib. Understanding the molecular pathogenesis of RCC interventional has helped identify targets (29). The pathogenesis of RCC was elucidated by the discovery of the von Hippel–Lindau (VHL) familial cancer syndrome. VHL is an autosomal dominant disease that portends an increased risk of RCC, cerebellum and spinal cord hemangioblastomas, retinal angiomas, and pheochromocytomas. RCC occurs in 40–60% patients with VHL disease and is the leading cause of death. VHL is associated with a tumor-suppressor gene found on chromosome 3p. Individuals with VHL disease carry one germline and one inactivated form of the gene. RCC occurs when the remaining wild-type allele is inactivated in the susceptible renal cell corresponding with a classic 2-Hit tumor-suppressor gene. VHL has multifaceted functions. The best characterized function in the formation of RCC is the inhibition of hypoxia-inducible factor (HIF). HIF is a heterodimeric transcription factor that, under low oxygen conditions, activates genes whose promoters contain hypoxia-response elements. These include, but are not limited to, vascular endothelial growth factor (VEGF), platelet-derived growth factor (PDFG), transforming growth factor alpha (TGFα), erythropoeitin, and matrix metalloproteinases (MMPs). These gene products have been shown to be protumorigenic in RCC through pathways involving angiogenesis, autocrine growth stimulation, apoptosis, and glucose transport.

VHL is responsible for the inactivation of HIF in normoxic condition. In this state HIF is hydroxylated allowing the binding of the VHL complex. This binding allows for polyubiquination of HIF and subsequent degradation by proteosomes. In VHL disease inactivation potential is absent due to loss of heterozygosity. In sporadic RCC, VHL inactivation is also a common event. The majority of inactivated VHLs are due to sporadic mutations leading to biallelic failure. In addition, in some cases transcription failure of VHL will occur secondary to hypermethylation. RCC lines with biallalic VHL inactivation form tumors in nude mice. Tumor formation can be abrogated by the restoration of VHL function in these cells.

The prognosis of metastatic and recurrent RCC is variable, the prognosis is poor with the median survival in the 12 month range (30, 31). Chemotherapy has limited activity. Radiotherapy may provide occasional palliative benefit to localized disease and resection of a solitary or small number of metastasis achieves occasional long term survival in selected patients (31). High dose interleukin-2 (IL-2) achieved modest (15%), objective response rates, although the median duration of response for all responders is 54 months (32). However, this therapy comes with considerable toxicity and limited assess.

In view of the limited therapeutic options for many RCC patients, there is strong interest in molecule-targeted therapies which block the VEGF receptor pathway either via targeting antibody (such as Bevacizumab) (19), or by small molecules (tyrosine kinase inhibitors) that inhibit the intracellular domain of the VEGF receptor via tyrosine kinase (6, 19, 28, 33). Sunitinib and sorafanib are two examples of tyrosine kinase inhibitors that have FDA approval for renal cancer (28, 33, 36). Thus we will focus on the two recently FDA approved drugs, sorafenib and sunitinib.

Sunitinib is an orally potent inhibitor of receptor tyrosine kinase including VEGF, PDGFR, FLT3, and c-kit. The agent is orally bioavailable. Several phase I studies identified a 50 mg daily dose given 4 weeks on and 2 weeks off as the acceptable dose for phase II studies. Subsequently antitumor activity and safety have been demonstrated in two phase II studies. Motzer et al. reported in 63 patients, a 40% objective response rate and a 27% stable disease (minimum of 3 months) rate (33). For the entire group, the median time to progression was 8.7 months and the median survival was 16.4 months. All histologic subtypes were permitted but 24 of the 25 responders had clear cell histology. A second trial restricted eligibility to clear cell histology, and reported data on 106 patients who had undergone prior nephrectomy and progressing on prior cytokine therapy as defined by RECIST-criteria. Response rates and median time to progression were similar at 39% and

8.4 months, respectively (33). A phase III trial comparing sunitinib with interferon-α has completed accrual and interim data are awaited. Fatigue (in 38%), hypertension, nausea, diarrhea, and mucositis were the most common adverse affects. Patients also experienced diminished left ventricular ejection fractions, of unclear clinical significance. Hypothyroidism can also occur and appears related to therapy duration. Hyperamalysemia has also been described (33). The FDA approved sunitinib for the treatment of metastatic RCC in January, 2006.

Sorafenib is also an orally available small molecule. Similar to sunitinib, it is an inhibitor of receptor tyrosine kinases. In addition, sorafenib inhibits serinine/threonine Raf-1 kinase, which phosphorylates raf. The Ras/Raf/MEK pathway leads to an increased production of HIF and plays a role in cell proliferation and apoptosis. Initial phase I evaluation identified 400 mg twice per day as the maximal tolerated dose for phase II trials (34–36). A phase II randomized discontinuation study subsequently established efficacy (28, 34–36).

Two hundred and two patients (mostly cytokine refractory) with RCC received sorafenib for 12 weeks. Patients who had at least 25% tumor reduction or progressive disease discontinued drug while the remaining patients ($n = 65$) were randomized to continued vs. discontinued therapy (36). Tumor reduction was seen in 71% of patients and a progression free survival (PFS) advantage of 23 vs. 6 months ($p = 0.0001$) was demonstrated in the smaller, randomized cohort. A phase III trial randomized 903 cytokine refractory, RCC patients to placebo vs. sorafenib.

PFS was 24 months in the sorafenib arm vs. 12 months with placebo ($p = 0.000001$). The objective response rate for sorafenib was only 2%; however, 78% of the patients had stable disease or minor responses (36). Primary toxicities include desquamating rash (31%), hand foot syndrome (26%), fatigue (18%), and hypertension (8%). The FDA approved sorafenib in December, 2005. The role of these two agents and others in development, portend new approaches for RCC which may supplement (or complement) high dose IL2 the only agent with a proven record of durable response.

TARGETING SMALL MOLECULES IN CANCER

EGFR Targeted Agents

EGFR is critical for growth of many epithelial malignancies. There are four members of the EGFR family receptor (or ErbB tyrosine kinase receptors) which consists of EGFR 1 (ErbB-1), EGFR 2 (ErbB-2) or HER-2, EGFR 3 (ErbB-3), and (ErbB-4) after ligand binding EGFR-4 (37–41).

EGFR dimerizes with other subfamily receptors (such as HER-2), and initiates a signaling cascade which can result in tumor proliferation, angiogenensis, survival, invasion, and metastases (1). EGFR is highly expressed in epitherlial malignancies (Table 1), and is a rationale target for inhibition (2). One can block the EGFR and initiation of its cascade by two divergent techniques. Monoclonal antibodies (MOAB) target the extracellular ligand binding domain (Table 2). Of two developed MOAB, Cetuximab has been the most studied, and has FDA approval in treatment of metastatic colorectal cancer. The other technique makes use of EGFR

Table 2. EGFR targeted therapy

Antibody	Type	Affinity-kd	Half life (h)	Dosing	Development phase
Cetuximab	lg G1 Chimeric MOAB	0.39 mm	75–95	Q1 wks (Q2 wks)	Approved
Panitumumab	lg G2 Human MOAB	50 pm	305–458	Q1 wks (Q2 wks) (Q3 wks)	Approved
Matuzumab	lg G1 Humaized MOAB	0.01 nm	94–180	Q1 wks (Q2 wks) (Q3 wks)	II (phase)
Nimotuzumab	lg G1 Humaized MOAB	1 nm	240	Q1 wks	Approved Non-USA (India, China SA)

Table 3. Small molecule-targeted agents

I. Membrane-Based Receptor Inhibition
  A. Small Molecule Type EGF (ErbB-1) Receptor Tyrosine Kinase Inhibitors
    1. Gefitinib
    2. Erlotinib
    3. EKB-569
    4. PKI-166
    5. Lapatinib
  B. Small Molecule Type (VEGF, TKI)
    1. Vatalanib (PTK787)
    2. Zactima (ZD6474)
    3. Semaxanib (SU5416)
    4. ZD4190
    5. AZD2171
    6. CEP4214
    7. CEP7055
    8. AG0137336
  C. PDGFR Inhibition and Multitargeting Drugs
    1. Imatinib
    2. Sutent (SU11248)
    3. Sorafenib(BAY43-9006)
    4. AG013736
    5. Vatalanib(PTK787)
    6. Leflunomide
II. Cytoplasmic TK Inhibition
    1. PP1
    2. PP2
    3. AZM475271
    4. siRNA
    5. AP23846
    6. SKI-606
    7. AZD05230

tyrosine kinase inhibitors (EGFR-TKs), which block the ATP binding site in the cytoplasm and will be the focus of this review (Table 3).

EGFR Tyrosine Kinases

Tyrosine Kinases are enzymes that transfer phosphate groups from ATP to the hydroxyl group of tyrosine residues on signal transduction molecules (39, 40). Phosphorylation of signal transduction molecules is a major activating event potentiating tumor growth. TKs act as relay points in a complex network of independent signaling molecules which ultimately regulate gene transcription within molecules. TK activity governs fundamental cell processes such as cell cycle, proliferation, differentiation motility, cell death, or survival (40–42). In tumor cells TKs are commonly uncontrolled, resulting in excessive phosphorylation which maintains signal transduction in a continued activated state.

Of note: EGFR-TK can autophosphorylate as well undergo phosphorylation when activated by other signaling molecules undergo such phosphotyrosine resid-ules in the EGFR-TK domain can further activate the receptor TK activity and can serve as docking sites for cytoplasmic ST molecules containing Src, or other phos-photyrosine binding motifs (39, 41, 42). Over 90 TKs are known of which 58 are transmembrane receptor type and 32 are the cytoplasm nonreceptor type (41) (Table 3). The former transduce signals from outside the cell, and the latter func-tion as relay points within the cell generally downstream of the receptor TKs.

Only a modest number of TK inhibitors have been developed as examples which target the nonreceptor cytoplasmic TKs within the cell, for example the Bcr-Ab fusion protein and C-Svc. Example of clinically targeted transmembrane receptor TKs include EGFR, HER-2 (ErbB-2NEU), PDGFR (platelet-derived growth fac-tor receptor), VEGF receptor (VEGF/ c-kit/ Stem cell factor receptor) (43, 44).

EGFR-TK in Cancer

Abnormally elevated EGF-RTK activity is associated with most of the common solid tumors including head and neck cancer, lung, breast, most of GI cancers, ovarian, cervical, and prostate cancers (Table 1) (8, 9). Multiple mechanisms of EGFR-TK activation include excess ligand expression or expression of EGFR, activating mutation, failure of inactivating mechanisms, transactivating via receptor dimerization (41, 44, 45).

The four members of EGFR family of receptor TKs include EGFR ErbB-1, ErbB-2 (HER-2), ErbB-3, ErbB-4. Ligand binding induces receptor homodimerization (41, 45, 46). ErbB-2 is the preferred binding partner for other ErbB-family members, although there is a hierachy of binding partners dictated by ligand and cell type (47). Homodimers of ErbB-3 are inactive due to impaired kinase activity, but heterodimers with ErbB-3 may activate intracellular signaling. Thus combining inhibitors of EGFR and ErbB-2 (HER-2) may synergize to inhibit certain tumor types, whereas alternative binding combinations could down regulate the effect of some inhibitors if the binding partner had an activating effect on the signaling pathway.

ErbB-1 Targeted Therapeutics

A variety of therapeutic strategies have been considered for inhibiting ErbB receptor activity. In one strategy, an antibody binds to the receptor, blocking ligand binding and/or accelerating receptor internalization and degradation. The other major strategy involves the utilization of a low-molecule-weight inhibitor of receptor thymidine kinase (RTK) activity, which blocks receptor activation.

The first ErbB receptor inhibitor to be approved by the US Food and Drug Administration (FDA) was the monoclonal antibody trastuzumab (Herceptin®; Genentech, Inc.; South San Francisco, CA). This agent is indicated for the treatment of patients with metastatic breast cancer whose tumors overexpress the ErbB-2 (HER-2/*neu*) receptor.

Other MOAB are developed to target the external domain of ErbB-1, cetux-imab (Erbitux®, IMC C-225: Imclone, Inc., New York, NY) include Panatumamab (Amgen), EMD 72000 (Merck Kgs; Darmstadt, Germany), ABX-EGF (Abgenix, Inc., Freemont, CA), and MDX-447 (Medarex Inc., Princeton, NJ). The other approach targeting the tyrosinase kinase domain of ErbB-1, is exemplified by gefi-tinib (Iressa®; AstraZeneca Pharmaceuticals, Wilmington, DE), which recently received regulatory approval in the US for the treatment of patients with NSCLC resistant to platinum agents and ocetaxel, and by erlotinib (Tarceva™; OSI Pharmaceuticals, Melville, NY).

Tyrosine Kinase Inhibitors (Overview)

Tyrosine Kinases are proteins which catalyze the phosphorylation of tyrosine residues and play an integral role in intracellular signal transduction. There are two main classes of protein tyrosine kinase (PTKs); receptor TKs and nonreceptor or cellular TKs (48). PTKs play a pivotal role in cellular signaling pathways and are involved in regulating the proliferation, migration, differentiation, angiogenesis, and antiapoptic signaling of cells.

Receptor TKs consists of an extracellular ligand binding domain, a hydrophobic transmembrane domain, and an intracellular catalytic domain. The intracellular domains of PTKs may be of two types: one which has a group of amino acids separating the kinase portion and another one in which the kinase domain is continuous (49).

The PTK receptors are activated when a ligand binds to the extracellular domain, leading to dimerization of the receptors and autophosphorylation of the tyrosine residues. The receptor TKs are selectively activated by growth factors, including EGF, VEGF, FGF, PDGF, and many others (44, 48).

Cellular PTKs are located in the cytoplasm, nucleus, or may be anchored to the inner plasma membrane of a cell. There are eight families of PTKs including: SRC, JAK, ABL, FAK, FPS, CSK, SYK, and BTK (48). It is known that many of the cellular TKs are involved in cell growth, including SRC (44).

Other functions in varied roles: FPS is involved in differentiation, ABL in growth inhibition, and FAK in cell adhesion. The interaction of specific PTKs with JAKs leads to the phosphorylation of signal transducer and activation of the transcription (STAT) family of proteins, which mediates cell division, survival, motality, invasion, and adhesion (50).

Several TKs have been found to be activated in pancreatic cancer, including EGFR (ErbB-1), HER-2/neu (ErbB-2), VEGFR-2, PDGFR-a, c-KIT, FGFR-1, and SRC (51–58). It is possible for oncogenes coding for the enzymes to be turned on, resulting in constitutively active kinases without a ligand stimulus. If TK activity is inhibited in such instances, there is an opportunity to interfere with the malignant process.

Erlotinib

Erlotinib is an orally administered quinazoline tyrosine kinase inhibitor with potent inhibitory effects on the EGFR receptor tyrosone kinases, including the mutant EGFRvIII (51). It has activity against HER-2 (52) and has no impact on the EGFR density on the cell surface (53). To exert maximal pharmacodynamic activity, relatively high concentrations of erlotinib at the receptor level are necessary (54). Erlotinib had significant in vitro activity on pancreatic cancer cell lines and in vivo on murine xenografts (55, 56) as well as potentiating the in vivo antitumor effects of paclitaxel, carboplatin (57) and gemcitabine (58).

The NCI of Canada Trial (PA.3) evaluated erlotinib and gemcitabine versus gemcitabine alone (58). In a phase III trial of 569 patients of which 25% had locally advanced disease and 75% had distant metastases. Patients were randomized to receive standard dose gencitabine 1,000 mg M^{-2} per week for 7 of 8 weeks followed by three out of every four weeks plus with either additional erlotinab or placebo (58). Erlotinab was started at 1,000 mg daily with planned escalation to 1,500 mg daily on the first prescheduled interim toxicity analysis (only 23 patients were entered at the higher dose). The addition of erlotinab to gemcitabine was associated with a small but statistically significant survival increase (1 year overall (24 vs. 17%)) and median survival (6.4 vs. 5.9 months) when compared with single agent gemcitabine. A significant improvement in performance status was also observed. The incidence of adverse events was comparable in both arms with the exception of grade I–IV rash (72 vs. 29%), diarrhea (56 vs. 41%), and stomatitis (23 vs. 14%) which were more common in the erlotinib/gemcitabine arm. Interstitial pneumonitis was also higher in the erlotinib arm (6 of 282 vs. 1 of 280) (58).

Although EGFR determination was not required for enrollment, specimens of 162 patients were centrally assessed by immunohistochemistry for EGFR expression. An EGFR positive result required ≥ 10% of the cells to show membranous staining. In this trial 53% of samples expressed EGFR. The development of an acneiform skin rash from erlotinib did predict improved survival. Patients that had improved survived compared to the group that did not (58).

This trial was the first to show a survival benefit for a combination therapy with an EGFR inhibitor with chemotherapy. In the BR21 trial reported by Shepard et al. in NSCLC, single agent erlotinib therapy was utilized (59, 60). First-line metastatic lung cancer studies such as the TRIBUTE and the TALENT trials (57, 58), which utilized a combination of erlotinib with chemotherapy did not show a survival benefit. This may be explained by tyrosine kinase inhibition induced suppression of intracellular signal transmission of cell cycle and proliferative activity. By removing cells from the cell cycle, TKs could potentially exert a functional antagonism in conjunction with chemotherapy. This suggests that erlotinib may be more effective in pancreatic cancer if investigated as a single agent. However, there has not been a phase II trial of erlotinib alone in nonsmall cell lung cancer.

EGFR inhibitors are potent radiation sensitizers (61). Although the exact mechanism for radiosensitization is not known, modification of cell cycle activity, promotion of apoptosis, and inhibition of DNA repair qualify are possible explanation (62). Erlotinib has been investigated with chemoradiation for patients with locally advanced pancreatic cancer.

The Brown University Oncology Group (ECOG) conducted a phase I trial of erlotinib in combination with gemcitabine, paclitaxel, and radiation for patients with locally advanced pancreatic cancer (63) which had demonstrated a 12-month median survival. In the Brown University trial, cohorts of three patients received escalating dosages of erlotinib with gemcitabine, 75 mg M^{-2}, and paclitaxel, 40 mg M^{-2}, weekly for 6 weeks with 50.4 radiation to the primary tumor and draining lymph nodes with a 2–3 cm margin.

Erlotinib was scheduled to be administered over three dose levels (50–100–150 mg per day) with chemoradiation, and then all patients were to receive 150 mg per day maintenance until disease progression. Seventeen patients were assessable for toxicity; 13 with locally advanced disease; and four resected patients with positive margins. Dose limiting toxicities with erlotinib $\geq$ 75 mg per day were diarrhea, dehydration, rash, myelosuppression, and small bowel stricture. The addition of erlotinib to chemoradiation appeared to produce additive diarrhea and other gastrointestinal toxicities. Erlotinib could not be increased above 50 mg per day with chemoradiation, although single agent maintenance erlotinib after chemoradiation was well tolerated at the full daily dose of 150 mg. The response rate and 14-month median survival in this small trial are promising. However, the contribution of erlotinib to this chemoradiation regimen is unclear.

A Memorial Sloan Kettering trial combined erlotinib with gemcitabine and radiotherapy in patients with locally advanced pancreatic adenocarcinoma (64). Cohorts of 3–6 patients received escalating doses of erlotinib (100 mg, 125 mg) with gemcitabine (40 mg M^{-2}, twice weekly) and RT (50.4 Gy in 28 fractions to the primary tumor and regional nodes). Four weeks following completion of chemoradiation, patients received maintenance chemotherapy with gemcitabine and erlotinib. Nine patients were enrolled. Three patients received erlotinib at 100 mg and six patients at 125 mg with radiation. Nonhemtologic toxicities included fatigue, abdominal pain, nausea/vomiting, weight loss, and rash. Grade 3/4 leucopenia ($n = 4$), and thrombocytopenia ($n = 2$) was observed only at erlotinib 125 mg Dose limiting toxicities of myelosuppression and transaminitis were observed in two patients at the 125 mg dose level.

Following the combined modality treatment, eight patients were evaluated for radiographical response. Seven patients demonstrated stable disease and one patient progressed through the treatment. Of six patients with an elevated CA19-9 at baseline, four experienced a decrease by > 50%.

Other TKI (EKB-569)

EKB-569 is a selective, irreversible EGFR tyrosine kinase inhibitor (65). Irreversible inhibitors may be partly able to overcome resistance that develops following administration of erlotinib or gefitinib. EKB-569 inhibits the growth of cancer cells that overexpress HER1 both in vitro and in vivo (66). In a phase I trial of EKB-569, the dose limiting toxicity was grade 3 diarrheas. Other toxicities include rash, nausea, and asthenia (66). EKB-569 is undergoing evaluation with gemcitabine in patients with advanced pancreatic cancer.

Nonsmall Cell Lung Cancer

The poor survival for NSCL cancer clearly calls for new treatment strategies. Cellular growth in NSCLC appears dependent on the disarrangement of membranous receptor (EGFR) triggered cellular pathways (67). Two small molecule inhibitors gefitinib and erlotinib have been widely studied in the management of NSCLC and both have obtained FDA approval for second-line therapy of NSCLC. Clinical response predictors have been evaluated from phase II data. Asian ethnicity, non- or oligosmoker status and female gender and presence of an adenocarcinomatous (particularly bronchoalveolar) histology have proven to be most valuable predictors for clinical response (68–71).

EGFR overexpression, gene amplification, and specific activating receptor mutations have been shown in preclinical models and phase II trials to predict the response to small molecule TKIs (70, 71).

However, multivariate analysis of a large phase III trial failed to show that the molecular configurations predicted or added any significant prognostic value to the above mentioned clinical predictors (72). Several other molecular predictors are under study and may be incorporated into clinical decision making in the future (73).

Erlotinib was shown in a randomized, placebo controlled phase III trial (59) to improve survival in previously treated patients with stage IIIB or VI NSCLC. Patients with an ECOG performance status of 0–3 who had received one or two prior chemotherapy regimens were stratified according to center, performance status, response to prior chemotherapy, number of prior regimens, and prior platinum-based therapy and were randomly assigned in a 2:1 ratio to receive oral erlotinib, at a dose of 150 mg daily, or placebo (59). Of 731 randomized patients, 49% had received two prior chemotherapy regimens, (93% were platinum based). The response rate was 8.9% in the erlotinib group and less than 1% in the placebo group ($P < 0.001$). Five percent of patients receiving erlotinib discontinued treatment because of toxicities. The median response was 7.9 months with erlotinib and 3.7 months in the placebo group. Progression-free survival was 2.2 months and 1.8 months, respectively, with an adjusted P-value of <0.001. Overall survival was 6.7 months in the erlotinib arm and 4.7 months in the placebo arm, what reached statistical significance. Several first-line metastatic lung cancer studies such as the TRIBUTE and the TALENT trials (57, 58) have utilized a combination of erlotinib with chemotherapy. None have shown a clear, statistically significant survival benefit.

Of note is that in a precontemplated subgroup analysis of the TRIBUTE trial oligo- and nonsmokers experienced a statistically significant survival benefit when erlotinib was added to combination chemotherapy.

The absence of a detectable survival benefit for the combination of EGFR TKIs with chemotherapeutic agents may be explained by the tyrosine kinase inhibition induced suppression of intracellular signal transmission pathways such as MAP kinase, STAT, and PI3-K and the corresponding depression of cell cycle and proliferative activity. By removing cells from the cell cycle, TKIs could potentially exert a functional antagonism in conjunction with chemotherapy.

The second FDA approved small molecule EGFR TK inhibitor, gefitinib, received approval on the base of clinical benefit detected in phase I/II trials including pretreated, symptomatic patients (75). A subsequent large scale phase III trial failed to detect a statistically significant overall survival benefit.

A planned subgroup analysis including never smokers and patients of Asian ethnicity demonstrated a statistically significant survival benefit of 8.9 vs. 6.1 and 9.5 vs. 5.5 months for the erlotinib arm. The subsequent INTACT-1/2 phase III trials failed to reveal a survival benefit for the combination of chemotherapy with gefitinib (75–77).

The combination of EGFR and VEGF inhibition has also been studied in advanced breast cancer (18, 19). Initial phase I/II studies of erlotinib and bevacizumab in renal cancer achieved response rates of 20% with a stable disease rate of 65%. ZD6474 is a small molecule TKIs with antagonistic activity on the EGFR TK as well as VEGFR TK, and is thought to show dose-related activity observed (78). A differential activity is with primarily anti-VEGFR activity at lower doses and increased EGFR antagonism at higher doses (79).

Initial phase II studies comparing ZD6474 with gefitinib (80) and the combination of ZD6474 with docetaxel vs. docetaxel alone (80) have shown encouraging results, reaching statistical significance for prolongation of TTP in the comparison of ZD6474 with gefitinib. Hence, ZD6474 has been considered for cooperative group phase III trials.

CONCLUSION

This brief review has concentrated on selected data involving the Small Molecule Inhibitors of VEGF Pathway and the ERB (EGFR family) Pathways. Limitation of space requires us to exclude data regarding the studies in the Breast and Head and Neck Cancer, and selected data in Melanoma. Some of this is quoted in the accompanying references, and some of the referred review articles.

REFERENCES

1. Folkman J: Tumor angiogenesis: Therapeutic implications. N Engl J Med 285:1182-1186, 1971
2. Greene HSN: Heterologous transplantation of mammalian tumors. I. The transfer of rabbit tumors to alien species. J Exper Med 73:461-471, 1941
3. Jain RK, PhD. Antiangiogenic therapy for cancers: Current and emerging concepts. Oncology Supplement No. 3, April 2005, p 7-16.

4. Carmeliet P, Jain RK. Angiogenesis in cancers and other diseases. Nature 407:249-257,2005.
5. Jain RK, PhD. Antiangiogenic therapy for cancers: Current and emerging concepts. Oncol April, 2005, Suppliment No.3
6. Heinz-Joseph Lenz. Antiangiogenic agents in cancer therapy. Oncol Supplement No.3, Page 17-25, 2005.
7. Kerbal R, Folkman J: Clinical translation of angiogenensis inhibitors: Nat Rev Cancer
8. Hicklin DJ, Ellis LM: Role of the vascular endolethial growth factor pathway in tumor growth and angiogenesis. J Clin Oncol 23:1011-1027, 2005.
9. Bachelder RE, Lispcomb EA, Lin X, et al. Competing autocrine pathways involving Alternative neuropilin-1 ligands regulate chemotaxis of carcinoma cells. Cancer Res 63:5230-5233, 2003.
10. Hurwitz H, Fehrenbacher L, Novotny W, et al. Bevacizumab plus irinotcan, fluorouracil, and leucovorin for metastatic colorectal cancer. N Eng J Med 350:2335-2342, 2004.
11. Gille H, Kowalski J, Li B, et al. Analysis of biological effects and signaling properties of Flt-1 (VEGF-1) and KDR (VEGF-2). A reassessment of using novel receptor-specific vascular endothelial growth factor mutants. J Biol Chem 276:3222-30, 2001.
12. Bachelder RE, Crago A, CVhung J, et al: Vascular endothelial growth factor is an autocrine survival factor for neuropilin-expressing breast carcinoma cells. Cancer res 61: 5736-5740, 2001.
13. Li M, Yang H, Chai H, et al: Pancreatic carcinoma cells express neuropilins and vascular endothelial growth factor, but not vascular endothelial growth factor receptors. Cancer 101-2341-2350, 2004.
14. Hurwitz H, Fehrenbacher L, Novotny W, et al. Bevacizumab plus irinotcan, fluorouracil, and leucovorin for metastatic colorectal cancer. N Eng J Med 350:2335-2342, 2004.
15. Johnson DH, Fehrenbacher L, Novotny W, et al. Randomized phase II trial comparing bevacizumab plus carboplatin and paclitaxel with carboplatin and paclitaxel alone in previously untreated locally advanced or metastatic non-small cell lung cancer.J Clin Oncology 22:2184-2191, 2004.
16. Miller KD, Chap LI, Holmes MA, et al. Randomized phase III trial of capecitabine compared with bevacizumab plus capecitabine in patients previously treated with breast cancer. J Clin Oncology 23: 792-799, 2005.
17. Salz LB, Lenz H, Kindler H, et al. Interim report of Randomized phase II trial of cetuxmiab/bevacizumab/irinotecan (CBI) vs. cetuximab/bevacizumab in irinotecan-refractory colorectal cancer (abstract 169b). Gastrointestinal Cancers Symposiuim, 2005.
18. Dickler M, Rugo H, Caravella, et al. Phase II trial of erlotinib (OSI – 774) an epidermal growth factor receptor tyrosine kinase inhibitor and bezacizumab a recominent Moab to VEGF in Metastatic Breast Cancer patients. Proc ASCO 23:127, 2004.
19. Hainsworth JD, Sosman JA, Spigel DR, et al. Phase II trial of bevacizumab and erlotinib in patients with metastatic renal carcinoma (RCC) (abstract 4502). Proc. Am Soc Clin Oncol 23:381, 2004.
20. Sandler AB, Blumenschein GR, Henderson T, et al. Phase I/II trial evaluating the anti-VEGF Mab bevacizumab in combination with erlotinib, a HER1/EGFR-TK inhibitor, for patients with recurrent non-small cell lung cancer (abstract 2000). Proc. Am Soc Clin Oncol 23:127, 2004.
21. Upont J, Schwartz L, Koutcher D, et al. Phase I and pharmacokinetics study of VEGF Trap administered subcutaneously (SC) to patients (Pts) with advanced solid malignancies. Abstract 3009, Proc AM Soc Clin Oncol 23:197,2004.
22. Levine AM, Quinn DI, Gorospe G, et al. Phase I trial of anti-sense oligonucleotide vascular enthelial growth factor (VEGF-AS, Veglin) in patients with relapsed and refractory malignancies (abstract 3008). Proc. Am SocClin Oncol 23:197, 2004.
23. Schleucher N, Trarbach T, Junker U, et al. Phase I/II study of PTK787/ZK 222584 (PTK/ZK), a novel, oral angiogenesis inhibitor in combination with FOLFIRI as first-line treatment for patiets with metastatic colorectal cancer (abstract 3558). Proc. Am Soc Clin Oncol 23:260, 2004.
24. Steward WP, Thomas A, Morgan B, et al. Expanded phase I/II study of PTK787/ZK 222584 (PTK/ZK), a novel, oral angiogenesis inhibitor, in combination with FOLFOX-4 as first-line treatment for patients with metastatic colorectal cancer (abstract 3556). Proc. Am Soc Clin Oncol 23:259, 2004.
25. Rosen L, Mulay M, Long J, et al. Phase I trial of SU011248, a novel tyrosine kinase Inhibitor in advanced solid tumors (abstract 765). Proc. Am Soc Clin Oncol 22:191, 2003.
26. Lara PN Jr, Quinn DI, Margolin K, et al. SU5416 plus interferon alpha in advanced renal cell carcinoma: A phase II California Cancer Consortium study with biological and imaging correlates of angiogenesis inhibition. Clin Cancer Res 9:4772-4781, 2003.
27. Brahmer JR, Kelsey S, Scigalla P, et al. A phase II study of SU6668 in patients with Refractory solid tumors (abstract 335). Proc. Am Soc Clin Oncol 21:84a, 2002.
28. Ratain MJ, Flaherty KT, Stadker WM, et al. Preliminary antitumor activity of BAY 43-9006 in metastatic renal cell carcinoma and other advanced refractory solid tumors in a phase II randomized discontinuation trial (RDT) (abstract 4501). Proc Am Soc Clin Oncol 23:381, 2004.

29. Cohen HT, McGovern FJ: Renal-cell carcinoma. N Engl J Med 353: 2477-2490, 2005.
30. Lam JS, Leppert JT, Figlin RA, et al: Surviellance following radical or partial nephrectomy for renal cell cancer. Curr Urol Rep 6: 7-18, 2005.
31. Kavolius JP, Mastorakos DP, Pavlovich C, et al: Resection of metastatic renal cell carcinoma. J Clin Oncol 16: 2261-2266, 1998.
32. Fyfe G, Fisher RI, Rosenberg SA, et al: Results of treatment of 255 patients with metastatic renal cell carcinoma who received high-dose recombinant IL-2 therapy. J Clin Oncol 13: 688-696, 1995.
33. Motzer RJ, Rini B, Bukowski RM, et al: Sunitinib in patients with metastatic renal cell carcinoma. JAMA 295: 2516-2524, 2005.
34. Awada A, Hendlisz A, gil T et al: Phase I safety and pharmacokinetics of BAY 43-9006 administered for 21 days on/7days off in patients with advanced, refractory solid tumours. Br J Cancer 92: 1855-1861, 2005.
35. Clark JW, Eder JP, Ryan D, et al: Safety and pharmacokinetics of the dual action raf kinase and VEGF receptor inhibitor, BAY 43-9006, in patients with refractory, advanced solid tumors. Clin Cancer Res 11: 5472-5480, 2005.
36. Strumberg D, Richly H, Hilger RA, et al: Phase I clinical and pharmacokinetic study of the novel Raf kinase and VEGF receptor inhibitor BAY 43-9006 in patients with advanced refractory solid tumors. J Clin Oncol 23: 965-972, 2005.
37. Mendelsohn J, Baselga J: The EGF receptor family as targets for cancer therapy. Oncogene 19 (56): 6550-6565, 2000.
38. Baselga J, Arteaga CL: Critical update and emerging trends in epidermal growth factor receptor targeting in cancer. J Clin Oncol 23 (11):2445-2459, 2005.
39. Schessinger J. Cell signaling by receptor tyrosine kinases. Cell 2000;103:211-225
40. Olayioye MA, Neve RM, Lane HA, et al. The ErbB signaling nertwork: receptor heterodimerization in development and cancer. EMBO J 2000;19:3159-3167.
41. Prenzel N, Fischer OM, Streit S, et al. The epidermal growth factor receptor family as a central element for cellular signal transduction and diversification. Endocr Relat Cancer 2001;8:11
42. Slichenmyer WJ, Fry DW. Anticancer therapy targeting the erbB family receptor tyrosine kinases. Semin Oncol 2001;28 (suppl 16):67-79.
43. Blume-Jensen P, Hunter T. Oncogenic kinase signaling. Nature 2001;411:355-365.
44. Levitzki A, Gazit A. Tyrosine kinase inhibition: an approach to drug development. Science 1995;267:1782-1788.
45. Raymond E, Faivre S, Armand JP. Epidermal growth factor receptor tyrosine kinase as a target for anticancer therapy. Drugs 2000;60 (suppl 1):15-23; discussion 41-42.
46. Moghol N, Sternberg PW. Mutiple positive and negative regulators of signaling by the EGF-receptor. Curr Opin Cell Biol 1999;11:190-196.
47. Hackel PO, Zwick E, Prenzel N et al. Epidermal growth factor receptors: critical mediators of multiplc receptor pathways. Curr Opin Cell Biol 1999;11:184-189.
48. Levitzki A, Protein tyrosine kinase inhibitors as novel therapeutic agents. Pharmacol. Ther. 1999; 82, 231-239.
49. Bender JG, Cooney EM, Kandel JJ, Yamashiro DJ. Vascular remodeling and clinical resistance to antiangiogenic cancer therapy. Drug Resist. Upgrade. 2004;7, 289-300.
50. Yarden Y. The EGFR family and its ligands in human cancer: signaling mechanisms and the therapeutic opportunities. Eur. J. Cancer. 2001; 37 (Suppl 4):S3-S8.
51. Iwata K, Provoncha K, Gibson N. Inhibition of mutant EGFRvIII transformed cells by tyrosine kinase inhibitor OSI-774 (Tarceva). Presented at the annual meeting of the American Society of Clinical Oncology, 2002. Abstract 79
52. Moyer JD, Barbacci EG, Iwata KK, et al. Induction of apoptosis and cell cycle arrest by CP-358,774, an inhibitor of epidermal growth factor receptor tyrosine kinase. Cancer Res. 1997; 57: 4838-4848.
53. Soulieres D, Senzer NN, Vokes EE, Hidalgo M, Agarwala SS, Siu LL. Multicenter phase II study of erlotinib, an oral epidermal growth factor receptor tyrosine kinase inhibitor, in patients with recurrent or metastatic squamous cell cancer of the head and neck. J Clin Oncol. 2004 Jan 1;22(1):77-85.
54. Hidalgo M. Erlotinib: preclinical investigations. Oncology (Huntingt). 2003; 17: 11-16
55. Durkin AJ, Osborne DA, Yeatman TJ, Rosemurgy AS, Armstrong C, Zervos EE EGF receptor antagonism improves survival in a murine model of pancreatic adenocarcinoma J Surg Res. 2006 Sep;135(1): 195-201
56. Ng, M.S. Tsao and T. Nicklee et al., Effects of the epidermal growth factor receptor inhibitor OSI-774, Tarceva, on downstream signaling pathways and apoptosis in human pancreatic adenocarcinoma, Mol. Cancer Ther. 1 (2002), pp. 777-783.

57. R. S. Herbst, D. Prager, R. Hermann et al. TRIBUTE – A phase III trial of erlotinib HCl (OSI-774) combined with carboplatin and paclitaxel (CP) chemotherapy in advanced non-small cell lung cancer (NSCLC); Journal of Clinical Oncology, 2004 ASCO Annual Meeting Proceedings (Post-Meeting Edition). Vol 22, No 14S (July 15 Supplement), 2004: 7011

58. U. Gatzemeier, A. Pluzanska, A. Szczesna et al. Results of a phase III trial of erlotinib (OSI-774) combined with cisplatin and gemcitabine (GC) chemotherapy in advanced non-small cell lung cancer (NSCLC); Journal of Clinical Oncology, 2004 ASCO Annual Meeting Proceedings (Post-Meeting Edition). Vol 22, No 14S (July 15 Supplement), 2004: 7010

59. Shepard FA, Rodrigues PJ, Ciuleanu T, et al. Erlotinib in previously treated non-small-cell lung cancer. N. Engl J Med 2005; 353:123-132.

60. J. Moore, Brief communication: a new combination in the treatment of Engl J Med. 2005; 353: 123-132.

61. Chinnaiyan S, Huang S, Armstrong E, et al. Radiosensitization following EGFR signaling inhibition by erlotinib (Tarceva). Int J Rad Onc Biol Phys. 2003;57(suppl 1):S294

62. Harari P, Huang SM. Combining EGFR inhibitors with radiation or chemotherapy: will preclinical studies predict clinical results? Int J Radiat Oncol Biol Phys. 2004 Mar 1;58(3):976-83.

63. D. Iannitti, T. Dipetrillo and P. Akerman et al., Erlotinib and chemoradiation followed by maintenance erlotinib for locally advanced pancreatic cancer: a Phase I study, Am. J. Clin. Oncol. 28 (2005), pp. 570–575.

64. J. S. Kortmansky, E. M. O'Reilly, B. D. Minsky et al. A phase I trial of erlotinib, gemcitabine and radiation for patients with locally-advanced, unresectable pancreatic cancer; Journal of Clinical Oncology, 2005 ASCO Annual Meeting Proceedings Vol 23, No. 16S, Part I of II (June 1 Supplement), 2005: 4107

65. Erlichman, C., Hidalgo, M., Boni et al. Phase I study of EKB-569, an irreversible inhibitor of the epidermal growth factor receptor, in patients with advanced solid tumors. J Clin Oncol. (24)115: 2225-6, 2006.

66. Cappuzzo, F, Varella-Garcia, M, Shigematsu, H, et al. Increased HER2 Gene Copy Number Is Associated With Response to Gefitinib Therapy in Epidermal Growth Factor Receptor-Positive Non-Small-Cell Lung Cancer Patients. J Clin Oncol 2005; 23:5007.

67. Perez-Soler, R, Chachoua, A, Hammond, LA, et al. Determinants of tumor response and survival with erlotinib in patients with non–small-cell lung cancer. J Clin Oncol 2004; 22:3238

68. Janne, PA, Gurubhagavatula, S, Yeap, BY, et al. Outcomes of patients with advanced non-small cell lung cancer treated with gefitinib (ZD1839, "Iressa") on an expanded access study. Lung Cancer 2004; 44:221.

69. Lynch, TJ, Bell, DW, Sordella, R, et al. Activating mutations in the epidermal growth factor receptor underlying aresponsiveness of non-small-cell lung cancer to gefitinib. N Engl J Med 2004; 350:2129.

70. Tokumo, M, Toyooka, S, Kiura, K, et al. The Relationship between Epidermal Growth Factor Receptor Mutations and Clinicopathologic Features in Non-Small Cell Lung Cancers. Clin Cancer Res 2005; 11:1167.

71. Tsao, MS, Sakurada, A, Cutz, JC, et al. Erlotinib in lung cancer - molecular and clinical predictors of outcome. N Engl J Med 2005; 353:133.

72. Aviel-Ronen, S, Fiona H, Blackhall FH, Shepherd, FA, Tsao, MS. K-ras Mutations in Non-Small-Cell Lung Carcinoma: A Review. Clin Lung Cancer 2006; 8:30.

73. Tsao, M, Zhu, C, Sakurada, A, et al. An analysis of the prognostic and predictive importance of K-ras mutation status in the National Cancer Institute of Canada Clinical Trials Group BR.21 study of erlotinib versus placebo in the treatment of non-small cell lung cancer (abstract). J Clin Oncol 2006; 24:365.

74. Fukuoka, M, Yano, S, Giaccone, G, et al. Multi-Institutional Randomized Phase II Trial of Gefitinib for Previously Treated Patients With Advanced Non-Small-Cell Lung Cancer. J Clin Oncol 2003; 21:2237.

75. Herbst, RS, Johnson, DH, Mininberg, E, et al. Phase I/II trial evaluating the anti-vascular endothelial growth factor monoclonal antibody bevacizumab in combination with the HER-1/epidermal growth factor receptor tyrosine kinase inhibitor erlotinib for patients with recurrent non-small-cell lung cancer. J Clin Oncol 2005; 23:2544.

76. Giaccone, G, Herbst, RS, Manegold, C, et al. Gefitinib in Combination With Gem citabine and Cisplatin in Advanced Non-Small-Cell Lung Cancer: A Phase III Trial–INTACT 1. J Clin Oncol 2004; 22:777.

77. Herbst, RS, Giaccone, G, Schiller, JH, et al. Gefitinib in Combination With Paclitaxel and Carboplatin in Advanced Non-Small-Cell Lung Cancer: A Phase III Trial–INTACT 2. J Clin Oncol 2004; 22:785.

78. Matsumori, Y, Yano, S, Goto, H. et al. ZD6474, an inhibitor of vascular endothelial growth factor receptor tyrosine kinase inhibits growth of experimental Lung metastasis and production of malignant pleural effusions in a non-small cell lung cancer model. Oncol Res. 2006;16(1):15-26.

79. Natale, RB, Bodkin, D, Govindan, R, et al. ZD6474 versus gefitinib in patients with advanced NSCLC: Final results from a two-part, double-blind, Randomized Phase II Trial (abstract). J Clin Oncol 2006; 24:364s.
80. Heymach JV, Johnson BE, Prager D., et al. A phase II trial of ZD6474 plus docetaxel in patients with previously treated NSCLC: Followup results (Abstract) J Clin Oncol 2006; 24:368.

19. UPDATE ON THE ROLE OF EGFR INHIBITORS IN CANCER THERAPEUTICS

MICHALIS V. KARAMOUZIS[1,2] AND ATHANASSIOS ARGIRIS[1,2]

[1]*Division of Hematology-Oncology, Department of Medicine, University of Pittsburgh, Pittsburgh, Pennsylvania, USA*
[2]*Head and Neck Cancer Program, University of Pittsburgh Cancer Institute, Pittsburgh, Pennsylvania, USA*

INTRODUCTION

The epidermal growth factor receptor (EGFR) is a type I tyrosine kinase receptor that plays a central role in signal transduction pathways that regulate key cellular functions in epithelial malignancies. After ligand binding, EGFR homo- or heterodimerizes with other members of the EGFR family of receptors, such as HER-2, and activates a signaling cascade that participates in tumor proliferation, angiogenesis, survival, and invasion/metastasis (61). Multiple studies have demonstrated that EGFR is commonly overexpressed in a variety of epithelial malignancies (Table 1) and its high expression usually correlates with worse patient outcome (4, 34).

On the basis of a strong biologic rationale, EGFR has emerged as a promising target for anticancer therapy. Multiple EGFR inhibition strategies are under intense evaluation (Table 2).

EGFR tyrosine kinase inhibitors (EGFR-TKIs) that block the ATP binding site in the cytoplasm, such as erlotinib and gefitinib, and monoclonal antibodies against the extracellular ligand-binding domain of the receptor, such as cetuximab and panitumumab, are the two most studied clinical approaches (6).

In recent years, EGFR inhibitors have been introduced in the standard management of many solid tumors. Currently, in the United States, erlotinib has obtained regulatory approval for the treatment of previously treated, advanced nonsmall cell lung cancer (NSCLC) and advanced pancreatic cancer, cetuximab has been approved

Table 1. EGFR expression in various human malignant neopmasms

Malignancy	EGFR expression (%)
NSCLC	40–80
Head and Neck	80–100
Colorectal	25–100
Stomach	33–81
Pancreas	30–50
Ovarian	35–70
Breast	15–37
Prostate	40–90
Gliomas	40–92

Table 2. Anti-EGFR treatment strategies

Category	Examples
Monoclonal antibodies	C225 (Cetuximab)
	ABX-EGF (Panitumumab)
	EMD 72000 (Matuzumab)
	h-R3
Toxic ligands	TP-38
	DAB(389) EGF
Tyrosine kinase inhibitors	
Reversible inhibitors	Quinazolines (Gefitinib, Erlotinib)
	Pyridopyrimidines (PD-158780)
	Pyrolopyrimidines (PK-166)
	Other molecules (GW-572016 - Lapatinib, AG-1478)
Irreversible inhibitors	Quinazolines (CI-1033, EKB-569, PD-183805)
Nucleic acid-based gene silencing techniques	Antisense oligonucleotides
	Ribozymes
	RNA interference

for irinotecan-refractory colorectal cancer and locally advanced head and neck carcinomas, and panitumumab has been approved for previously treated metastatic colorectal cancer. The status of selected agents that target EGFR is listed in Table 3.

As these agents are becoming widely available and are changing the standard of care in many solid tumors, it is also evident that they benefit only a fraction of patients. Therefore, the identification of predictors of efficacy, especially at the molecular level, which may optimize patient selection, has been the subject of ongoing investigation. Here, we will summarize the current status of clinical testing with EGFR inhibitors in common malignancies, such as NSCLC, and head and neck, pancreatic, colorectal, and breast cancers, highlight ongoing research regarding molecular predictive factors and consider the future perspectives of this class of agents.

Table 3. The current status of selected anti-EGFR agents for cancer therapy

	Agent	Type of inhibitor	Status in the US	Manufacturer
Monoclonal antibodies	Cetuximab (Erbitux, C225)	Chimeric antibody	Approved in metastatic colorectal cancer and head and neck cancer. Phase III studies ongoing in NSCLC, colorectal cancer and pancreatic cancer	BMS/ImClone
	Panitumumab (Vectibix, ABX-EGF)	Human antibody	Approved in metastatic colorectal cancer. Phase I/II studies ongoing in head and neck cancer, and other cancers	Amgen
	Matuzumab (EMD 72000)	Humanized antibody	Phase II studies ongoing in NSCLC, colorectal, head and neck, cervical, gastric, and ovarian cancers	EMD Pharmaceuticals
Tyrosine kinase inhibitors	Gefitinib (Iressa, ZD1839)	Aniloquinazoline; reversible	Negative data emerged in phase III trials in advanced NSCLC. Phase II/III trials ongoing in head and neck and other cancers	AstraZeneca
	Erlotinib (Tarceva, OSI-774)	Aniloquinazoline; reversible	Approved in advanced NSCLC and pancreatic cancer. Phase II/III studies ongoing in other tumor types	Genentech/OSI
	EKB-569	3-cyanoquinoline; irreversible	Phase II studies in colorectal cancer and NSCLC	Wyeth-Ayerst
	Lapatinib ditosylate (Tykerb, GW572016)	Dual EGFR and HER2 inhibitor; reversible	Positive phase III trial in metastatic HER-2(+) breast cancer. Phase II trials in head and neck, lung, and other cancers	GlaxoSmithKline

MOLECULAR ASPECTS OF ANTI-EGFR THERAPY

EGFR is a member of the ErbB (EGFR) family of receptors with intrinsic tyrosine kinase activity. This family consists of four closely related receptors: EGFR (HER-1, ErbB1), HER-2 (ErbB2 or HER-2/*neu*), HER-3 (ErbB3), and HER-4 (ErbB4). Structurally, each receptor is composed of an extracellular ligand-binding domain, a transmembrane domain, and an intracellular domain. All receptors in the EGFR family have intrinsic tyrosine kinase activity, except for HER-3. The receptors exist as inactive monomers but upon binding to ligands, such as epidermal growth factor (EGF) and transforming growth factor alpha (TGF-α), they undergo conformational changes favoring homo- or heterodimer formation (85). Although HER-2 has no known natural ligands, it is the most frequent partner for heterodimerization; EGFR and HER-2 heterodimers have been found to be more potent in vitro than EGFR homodimers (101). The process of EGFR dimerization favors intermolecular autophosphorylation of key tyrosine residues in the activation loop of catalytic tyrosine kinase domains and subsequent phosphorylation (activation) of multiple downstream molecular pathways. The most important EGFR-activated pathways are (a) Ras-Raf-MEK-ERK pathway, which is mainly responsible for cellular proliferation; (b) PI3K-PDK1-AKT pathway that is mostly involved in apoptosis modulation; and (c) Jak/Stat pathway that is important for both cellular proliferation and apoptosis control (36, 102) (Fig. 1). Alternatively, activation of EGFR pathway can be achieved through indirect crosstalk with other molecules, such as with G-protein coupled receptors, platelet derived growth factor (PDGF), and hormone receptors (37, 84). EGFR activity is governed by many levels of complexity, as it is the case with most intracellular signal transduction pathways. In particular, it seems that EGFR activity might be cell and/or tissue specific and may depend upon the binding ligand, the forming dimmer, the activating downstream signaling cascade and the crosstalk interactions with other intracellular pathways (47).

EGFR activation also increases HNSCC cell invasion. The downstream molecules that mediate EGFR ligand-induced motility are not well defined. Phospholipase C (PLC) gamma-1 is a phosphor-inositide specific phodpholipase that on activation hydrolyses phosphatidylinositol (4,5) biphosphate (PIP2) into inositol-triphosphate (IP3) and diacylglyecerol (DAG). IP3 mediates the release of Ca+2 ions from intracellular stores and DAG activates PKC. These events are followed by actin remodeling within the cell enabling HNSCC cell motility. It has been demonstrated that PLC is downstream of EGFR and involved in HNSCC invasion on EGFR ligand (EGF) stimulation (96).

The implication of EGFR in malignancy is achieved by at least four major mechanisms: overexpression of EGFR ligands, mutational activation of EGFR, amplification of EGFR, and transactivation of other membrane receptors (44, 67). At least seven common classes of mutants (vI–vVII) have been identified in gliomas, most containing a deletion of specific exons encoding part of the extracellular domain of the EGFR molecule, leading to constitutive ligand-independent

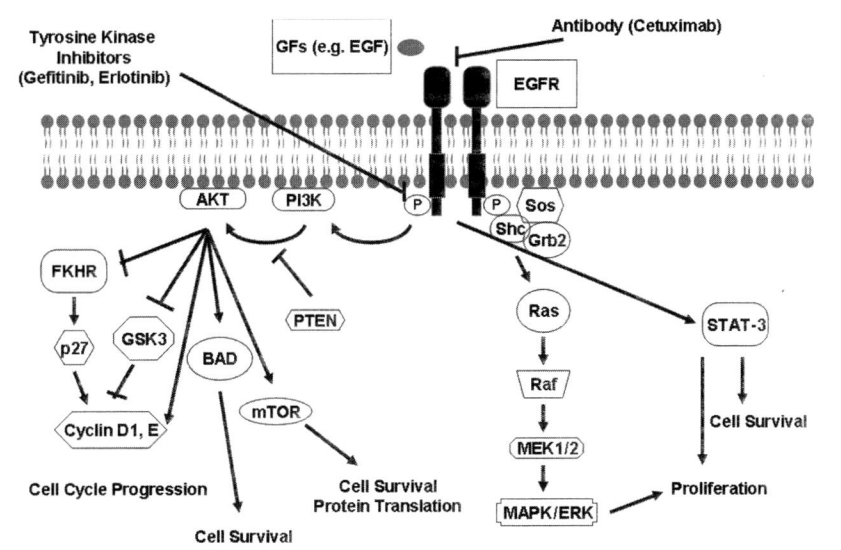

Figure 1. Overview of EGFR signaling network. EGFR (HER-1) is a member of ErbB/HER membrane receptors with intrinsic TK activity. This family comprises four closely related receptors, which exist as inactive monomers. Upon binding to ligands, such as EGF, the receptors undergo conformational changes favoring homo- or heterodimer formation. EGFR dimerization process triggers intermolecular autophosphorylation of key tyrosine residues in the activation loop of catalytic TK domains and subsequent phosphorylation (activation) of downstream signaling pathways. Notably, EGFR autophosphorylation stimulates the PI-3K and STAT pathways. The Ras/MAPK cascade, linked to cell growth and proliferation, is also activated by EGFR-TK activation and Shc protein, via interaction with Grb2/Sos. Stimulated PI-3K activates – through a series of well-characterized steps – Akt, which inhibits the activities of the FKHRs (mediators of apoptosis and cell-cycle arrest), resulting in cell proliferation and survival. The tumor-suppressor protein PTEN negatively regulates PI-3K signaling. Other components of the PI-3K signaling pathway include GSK-3, BAD (a pro-apoptotic protein of Bcl-2 family), mTOR, and other proteins. mTOR directly phosphorylates and activates ribosomal S6 kinase-1 (S6K-1), which is an important regulator of cell size. PI-3K- and Ras-directed signaling cascades interact through various downstream molecules. Alternatively, activation of the EGFR pathway can be achieved through indirect crosstalk with other molecules, such as G-protein coupled receptors, platelet-derived growth factor (PDGF), and hormone receptors.

receptor activation and altered down stream effects (55). Activating mutations of EGFR in the kinase domain have been found almost exclusively in NSCLC (9, 60, 68, 110).

EGFR INHIBITORS IN THE TREATMENT OF SOLID TUMORS

Nonsmall Cell Lung Cancer

Lung cancer is the leading cause of cancer-related death worldwide (45). The multistep natural history of lung carcinogenesis can be considered as a gradual accumulation of genetic and epigenetic aberrations resulting in the deregulation of cellular homeostasis (97). During the past few years, several new agents targeting specific and critical pathways have been evaluated for the prevention and treatment of NSCLC. Among them, agents targeting the EGFR have been shown to result in clinical benefit in patients with advanced NSCLC (30, 70).

Gefitinib and erlotinib, two agents classified as EGFR tyrosine kinase inhibitors (EGFR-TKIs), produced objective response rates of 10–20% in phase II clinical trials in patients with previously treated, advanced NSCLC (26, 53, 72). Recently, two large phase III randomized trials that compared an EGFR-TKI with placebo in patients with NSCLC have reported results. In the first study, erlotinib was compared with placebo for the second- or third-line treatment of patients with advanced NSCLC (87). This study randomized 731 patients in a 2:1 ratio to receive erlotinib 150 mg orally, once a day or placebo. Patients on placebo had a median survival of 4.7 months, whereas those on erlotinib had a median survival of 6.7 months, a difference that was statistically significant ($P = 0.001$). However, gefitinib, in a similar clinical setting, failed to improve overall survival when compared with placebo, even though survival benefit was seen in certain patient subgroups, such as the Asians and the nonsmokers (94). The discrepancy of the results of these two similarly designed clinical trials may have been due to a number of reasons. First, it is possible that gefitinib was given in a suboptimal biologically active dose. Preclinical data have shown that the concentration of EGFR-TKIs that is necessary for EGFR molecular pathway blocking is greater than the one that inhibits EGFR autophosphorylation (2). In this regard, it has been assumed that a gefitinib dose of 250 mg, once-daily, might be suboptimal, since it is far below the maximum tolerated dose (MTD), in contrast with erlotinib which is given at the MTD. However, accumulated data from phase II trials evaluating gefitinib have shown that doses of 250 and 500 mg daily are equally efficacious (94). It remains uncertain whether higher doses of gefitinib, beyond 500 mg, are likely to enhance efficacy. Secondly, it may be simply that gefitinib is inactive in this setting despite the encouraging objective response rates observed in the initial phase II studies. Thirdly, treatment arms may have been imbalanced in terms of a number of important clinical and molecular characteristics, such as smoking history and the presence of EGFR mutations.

Other clinical studies were designed to evaluate EGFR-TKIs in combination with chemotherapy. However, four phase III trials which evaluated erlotinib or gefitinib in combination with standard first-line chemotherapy for advanced NSCLC reported negative results (28, 30, 38, 39). As in the case of the gefitinib monotherapy trial in previously treated advanced NSCLC, inappropriate patient selection on the basis of clinical characteristics and/or molecular markers may partially explain the negative results. Moreover, preclinical data suggest that the optimal use of EGFR-TKIs, which result in G1 phase arrest of the cell cycle, may be sequentially following chemotherapy (108). A number of clinical trials utilizing sequential administration of chemotherapy and EGFR-TKIs are currently ongoing.

Cetuximab has also been studied in phase II trials in NSCLC, as single-agent and in combination with chemotherapy, with promising results (59, 76, 78, 95). Ongoing randomized trials are evaluating the addition of cetuximab to chemotherapy in the first-line (49, 107) and second-line treatment of NSCLC.

Head and Neck Cancer

Head and neck squamous cell carcinomas (HNSCC) are considered EGFR-dependent neoplasms since they exhibit EGFR over-expression in about 90% or more of cases (44). Therefore, anti-EGFR strategies have been extensively studied in this malignancy. Phase II trials with the EGFR-TKIs gefitinib and erlotinib have shown modest single agent activity in recurrent or metastatic HNSCC, whereas lapatinib, a dual EGFR and HER-2 inhibitor, showed no significant single-agent activity in the same setting (1, 20, 46, 89). Gefitinib at a dose of 500 mg per day resulted in an overall response rate of 11%, median time to progression 3.4 months, and median survival 8.1 months; in contrast, a study from the same group showed that gefitinib at a lower dose of 250 mg was less active (21). Erlotinib at a dose of 150 mg daily was evaluated in a study of 115 patients with recurrent and/or metastatic HNSCC (89). The overall objective response rate was 4.3%, median progression-free survival 9.6 weeks, and median overall survival 6 months. Recently, there have been reports of encouraging preliminary results with the combination of gefitinib or erlotinib with other biological agents (e.g., bevacizumab) (105) or chemoradiotherapy (22, 83). A recently completed phase III study compared gefitinib (at either a 250 or 500 mg daily dose) with methotrexate and results are pending, whereas an ongoing phase III trial is comparing docetaxel with or without gefitinib in patients with recurrent or metastatic HNSCC (ECOG 1302).

Cetuximab has been extensively studied for the treatment of HNSCC and recently obtained regulatory approval for this disease. A recent phase III randomized trial demonstrated that the addition of cetuximab to radiation improved locoregional control as well as survival compared with radiation alone in patients with locally advanced HNSCC (10). The magnitude of survival improvement of 10% at 3 years was comparable to what achieved with the addition of platinum-based regimens to radiation. Therefore, radiation plus cetuximab emerged as a standard regimen for the treatment of locally advanced HNSCC. In recurrent or metastatic HNSCC, a randomized study conducted by the Eastern Cooperative Oncology Group (ECOG 5397), compared cisplatin plus cetuximab with cisplatin alone (12). The addition of cetuximab to cisplatin increased the objective response rates from 10 to 26% and the median progression-free survival from 2.7 to 4.2 months but the latter difference did not reach statistical significance, presumably due to the relatively small sample size of the trial (117 patients total). Moreover, cetuximab has been shown to have single-agent activity in platinum-refractory HNSCC. A phase II trial that enrolled

103 patients with platinum-refractory recurrent or metastatic HNSCC, reported an objective response rate of 13%, median time to progression of 2.3 months, and median survival of 5.9 months (98). Two other phase II studies evaluated cetuximab in combination with platinum compounds in HNSCC patients who had progressed while receiving platinum-based regimens (7, 40). Efficacy parameters were comparable with the use of single-agent cetuximab that argues against the readministration of platinum in platinum-refractory patients. In locally advanced HNSCC, a phase II study evaluated the efficacy and toxicity of the combination of cetuximab with cisplatin and accelerated boost radiotherapy for patients with locoregionally advanced HNSCC. Although, the study was prematurely closed because of increased frequency of significant adverse events, including two deaths, which may have not been specifically related to the incorporation of cetuximab to chemoradiotherapy, promising preliminary efficacy was reported (73). Currently, RTOG is comparing this regimen to radiation and cisplatin alone. Moreover, multiple other groups have completed or currently studying combinations of radiation, cetuximab, and platinum agents.

Nasopharyngeal Carcinoma

The percentage of positivity and intensity of EGFR expression in nasopharyngeal carcinoma (NPC) is variable, but approximately 80–90% of cases have been reported as EGFR positive (57). EGFR expression has been shown to correlate with survival, locoregional control, and distant metastasis (18). Preclinical studies also provide a strong biologic basis for the use of EGFR inhibitors in this disease, as Epstein-Barr virus proteins have been implicated in EGFR expression and downstream signaling processes (91, 93). Activating somatic mutations in the EGFR tyrosine kinase domain may not be present in NPC (56). A number of clinical trials from Asia have reported results with the use of EGFR inhibitors. A single arm multicenter phase II trial demonstrated significant clinical activity and acceptable toxicity profile of cetuximab in combination with carboplatin in platinum-resistant patients with metastatic or locally recurrent NPC (16). Similar to a number of studies in other solid tumors, the development of rash due to cetuximab was associated with improved survival. Finally, gefitinib is being evaluated as a single agent for the treatment of previously treated recurrent or metastatic nasopharyngeal cancer (17).

Colorectal Cancer

Colorectal carcinoma is one of the leading causes of cancer death worldwide (45). Recently, several agents have been added to the list of active agents against colorectal cancer. The incorporation of irinotecan or oxaliplatin into 5-FU/LV-based regimens improved response rates and survival over FU/LV alone, achieving a median survival for patients with metastatic colorectal cancer of about 20 months (48). More recently, molecularly targeted agents have been successfully introduced in the treatment of colorectal cancer. Bevacizumab, an anti-VEGF humanized monoclonal antibody, has been shown to improve efficacy parameters, including the overall survival, when used in combination with FU/LV-based regimens in metastatic colorectal cancer (41, 43).

Anti-EGFR monoclonal antibodies have also produced significant clinical results. Cetuximab, as a single agent, resulted in an objective response rate of 9% in irinotecan-refractory, advanced colorectal cancer (81). A subsequent randomized phase II trial evaluated the combination of cetuximab and irinotecan vs. cetuximab alone in irinotecan-refractory patients (23). The combination was proven to be clearly superior in terms of response rates and progression-free survival. This study confirmed previous observations that the addition of cetuximab to irinotecan reverses irinotecan refractoriness, although the exact mechanism has not been yet elucidated. Currently, phase III trials of cetuximab plus chemotherapy and/or bevacizumab for the treatment of advanced colorectal cancer are ongoing in the first-line setting (104). Although studies in colorectal studies, as well as in most NSCLC studies, required EGFR tumor over-expression, cetuximab might be equally active in EGFR negative tumors (19). This remains to be evaluated prospectively in clinical trials.

Panitumumab (ABX-EGF) is a new fully humanized anti-EGFR IgG2 monoclonal antibody that is now available for the treatment of advanced colorectal cancer. Initial phase I/II studies evaluated the efficacy and safety of this monoclonal antibody in patients with refractory metastatic colorectal cancer (100). A phase III trial which compared panitumumab as a single agent to best supportive care in patients with previously treated metastatic colorectal cancer recently reported results. Panitumumab resulted in a 46% reduction in the risk of tumor progression and an objective response rate of 8% (32). Planned and ongoing clinical studies are evaluating panitumumab in combination with chemotherapy and bevacizumab in the first-line therapy of advanced stage colorectal cancer and in the adjuvant setting (109).

Multiple phase II studies of EGFR-TKIs have been conducted in colorectal cancer patients (5). Despite evidence of biological activity, gefitinib, erlotinib, and lapatinib have demonstrated modest clinical activity as single-agent agents in previously treated patients with metastatic colorectal cancer (25, 66, 79). Furthermore, several clinical trials are investigating EGFR-TKIs combined with chemotherapy. Preliminary results suggest that the addition of an EGFR-TKI may increase the activity of oxaliplatin-based regimens, while it may result in considerable toxicities when combined with irinotecan-containing regimens (5, 54).

Pancreatic Cancer

EGFR inhibitors were the first novel agents to show promise in pancreatic cancer. A recent phase III randomized trial showed that the addition of erlotinib 100 mg per day to standard gemcitabine chemotherapy resulted in a small but statistically significant survival benefit in advanced pancreatic cancer patients (63). The median survival was 6.4 months with the combination vs. 5.9 months with gemcitabine alone (adjusted hazard ratio, 0.81, $p = 0.025$); the 1-year survival rates were 24 vs. 17%, respectively. Progression-free survival was also improved with erlotinib (hazard ratio, 0.76). Multiple other trials are currently ongoing testing EGFR inhibitors in combination with other chemotherapeutic agents and/or radiotherapy (5, 33, 52).

Breast Cancer

Breast cancer is the most common cancer in women. The EGFR family of receptors plays a major role in promoting breast cancer cell proliferation and malignant growth. The EGFR and HER-2 are frequently overexpressed in breast cancer, and their overexpression is associated with a more aggressive clinical behavior. Cumulative evidence has also supported the importance of crossinteraction between estrogen receptor and EGFR and HER-2 signaling pathways (84). These data have generated interest in invsestigating the EGFR family of receptors as potential targets for the development of new anticancer drugs. Proof of principle for this approach was provided by the demonstration that the addition of trastuzumab, a monoclonal antibody against HER-2, to standard chemotherapy confers a survival advantage in patients whose tumors overexpress HER-2 in both the metastatic and adjuvant disease settings (35, 74, 77, 88).

The first clinical studies of EGFR-TKIs in patients with metastatic breast cancer produced disappointingly low response rates (8, 92, 106). However, preclinical and clinical data have suggested that EGFR-TKIs may restore sensitivity to antiestrogens (65). Ongoing clinical trials are evaluating the therapeutic efficacy of combining EGFR-TKIs with endocrine therapy as well as chemotherapy (27, 75).

Lapatinib is a dual tyrosine kinase inhibitor of EGFR and HER-2. Initial phase I/II studies have shown promising clinical activity in solid tumors, with the most notable results in advanced breast cancer, including tumors refractory to trastuzumab (11, 90). Preliminary results of a phase III clinical trial of capecitabine with or without lapatinib in patients with HER-2 positive, advanced breast cancer who previously failed trastuzumab showed that the addition of lapatinib significantly improved progression-free survival (8.5 vs. 4.5 months, $P = 0.00016$) (29). The toxicity profile of the combination was acceptable. Interestingly, patients who received lapatinib had a reduced risk of developing brain metastasis.

PREDICTIVE MARKERS OF ANTI-EGFR THERAPY

The identification of molecular and/or clinical predictors of outcome with EGFR-targeted therapies is being intensively investigated. Paradoxically, in most studies with EGFR inhibitors EGFR protein expression has not been found to be associated with antitumor activity, which contrasts the utility of HER-2 expression and/or amplification in selecting patients with breast cancer for treatment with trastuzumab. Of interest is that the onset and severity of skin rash, a class effect of EGFR inhibitors, has been consistently shown to correlate with patient outcome (80). An intriguing hypothesis is that the development of rash with EGFR inhibitors is associated with CA-repeat polymorphisms in intron 1 of the EGFR gene (3).

Clinical trials with EGFR-TKIs in NSCLC patients have identified a number of important clinical predictive parameters, such as gender, histologic subtype, smoking status, and ethnicity. The field of molecular predictive factors is a rapidly evolving one. In 2004, function-gaining somatic mutations in EGFR were identified that lead to exceptional clinical responses to the EGFR-TKIs in NSCLC (60, 68). These mutations are present in a relatively small fraction of NSCLC patients (approximately 10% in Caucasians), are seen in higher frequency in patients with certain clinical characteristics (e.g., nonsmokers, Asians, etc.), and can partially account for the demonstrated clinical benefit from these agents. EGFR activating mutations have only been detected in the tyrosine kinase domain, are not always present in patients responding to TKIs, and seem to be very rare in other tumor types. Moreover, a novel inhibiting EGFR mutation has also been detected (50, 69). Based on these data, clinical trials are ongoing evaluating the activity of EGFR inhibitors as single-agent treatment in chemotherapy naïve patients with advanced NSCLC and EGFR activating mutations (42, 71).

EGFR gene copy number emerged as another predictor of EGFR-TKI activity in NSCLC (14) and possibly cetuximab in colorectal cancer (64). The Ras/mitogen-activated protein kinase (MAPK) and phosphatidylinositol-3 kinase (PI-3K)/Akt molecular pathways are downstream signaling networks linking EGFR activation to cell proliferation and survival. Mutations in these downstream effectors of EGFR signaling are also being evaluated as potential predictors of outcome (13, 15). Activating mutations in EGFR and K-ras may be functionally redundant and therefore mutually exclusive (51). Accumulating preclinical and clinical evidence suggests that patients with K-ras mutant cancers may represent a separate group of patients with inherent resistance to anti-EGFR targeting (Table 4).

Table 4. Evaluation of K-Ras mutations in patients with human malignant neoplasms treated with EGFR inhibitors

Neoplasm	Study population	Primary conclusion	Reference
NSCLC	274 patients with advanced NSCLC who participated in TRIBUTE trial	Patients with K-Ras-mutant NSCLC had decreased time-to-progression and survival when treated with erlotinib and chemotherapy	(24)
NSCLC	246 patients with advanced NSCLC who participated in BR.21 trial	Patients with K-Ras mutations did not appear to derive any survival benefit from erlotinib	(99)
Bronchioalveolar cancer (BAC)	102 patients with BAC treated with erlotinib	K-Ras mutations predicted resistance to erlotinib	(62)
Colorectal cancer (CRC)	30 patients with metastatic CRC treated with cetuximab	K-Ras mutations predicted resistance to cetuximab and were associated with a worse prognosis	(58)

FUTURE PERSPECTIVES

The promise of EGFR targeting in cancer therapeutics is enormous. Small molecule TKIs and monoclonal antibodies against the extracellular domain of the receptor are the currently most promising anti-EGFR therapies. A number of challenges have emerged that will need to be addressed by clinical and basic research, including the following (1) elucidating the mechanisms governing acquired and/or inherent resistance to anti-EGFR approaches, (2) identifying accurate and easily reproducible methods to select patients who benefit the most from EGFR inhibitors, and (3) establishing the most effective combined use of EGFR inhibitors with radiotherapy and chemotherapy as well as with other molecularly targeted agents. In particular, the combination of EGFR inhibitors and anti-angiogenesis agents has attracted the interest of many investigators. It is well established that the EGFR pathway interacts with several other important growth factor cascades during carcinogenesis, including the vascular endothelial growth factor (VEGF)/VEGF-receptor pathway. In preclinical models, EGFR inhibition causes a dose-dependent inhibition of VEGF. Preclinical and clinical resistance to EGFR inhibitors has been also associated with increased VEGF levels (103). Combined blockage of the VEGF pathway and other growth factor pathways (e.g., EGFR or PDGFR) has demonstrated additive effects in vivo (86). Therefore, combined targeting of the tumor and the tumor vasculature may result in enhanced antitumor efficacy. Currently, combinations of EGFR inhibitors with angiogenesis inhibitors are being pursued in multiple solid tumors (e.g., colorectal cancer, lung cancer, and head and neck cancer) (82). The heterogeneity of malignant tumors seems to require a treatment program designed to attack a series of specific molecular targets. Tailored molecularly based anticancer treatment represents a prerequisite and a challenge for the optimal use of anti-EGFR treatment strategies in the future.

ABBREVIATIONS

NSCLC; Nonsmall cell lung cancer
HNSCC; Head and neck squamous cell carcinomas
NPC; Nasopharyngeal carcinoma
EGF; Epidermal growth factor
TGF-α; Transforming growth factor α
PDGF; Platelet derived growth factor
VEGF; Vascular endothelial growth factor
EGFR; Epidermal growth factor receptor
TK; Tyrosine kinase domain
TKIs; Tyrosine kinase inhibitors
5FU; 5-fluorouracil
LV; Leucovorin
FKHR; Forkhead transcription factor
Grb2; Growth factor receptor-binding protein 2
GSK-3; Glycogen synthase kinase-3

MAPK; Mitogen-activated protein kinase

MEK; MAPK/Extracellular signal-regulated kinase (Erk) kinase

mTOR; Mammalian target of rapamycin

PI-3K; Phosphatidylinositol-3 kinase

PTEN; Phosphatase and tensin homologue deleted on chromosome 10

Sos; Son of sevenless

TAT-3; signal transducer and activator of transcription-3.

REFERENCES

1. Abidoye OO, Cohen EE, Wong SJ, Kozloff MF, Nattam SR, Stenson KM, Blair EA, Day, Dancey JE, Vokes EE. (2006) A phase II study of lapatinib (GW572016) in recurrent/metastatic (R/M) squamous cell carcinoma of the head and neck (SCCHN). J Clin Oncol 24: 5568A
2. Akita RW, Sliwkowski MX. (2003) Preclinical studies with Erlotinib (Tarceva). Semin Oncol 30(3 Suppl 7): 15-24
3. Amador ML, Oppenheimer D, Perea S, Maitra A, Cusati G, Iacobuzio-Donahue C, Baker SD, Ashfaq R, Takimoto C, Forastiere A, Hidalgo M. (2004) An epidermal growth factor receptor intron 1 polymorphism mediates response to epidermal growth factor receptor inhibitors. Cancer Res 64: 9139-9143
4. Ang KK, Berkey BA, Tu X, Zhang HZ, Katz R, Hammond EH, Fu KK, Milas L. (2002) Impact of epidermal growth factor receptor expression on survival and pattern of relapse in patients with advanced head and neck carcinoma. Cancer Res 62: 7350-7356
5. Arnold D, Peinert S, Voigst W, Schmoll HJ. (2006) Epidermal growth factor receptor tyrosine kinase inhibitors: present and future role in gastrointestinal cancer treatment: a review. Oncologist 11: 602-611
6. Baselga J, Arteaga CL. (2005) Critical update and emerging trends in epidermal growth factor receptor targeting in cancer. J Clin Oncol 23: 2445-2459
7. Baselga J, Trigo JM, Bourhis J, Tortochaux J, Cortés-Funes H, Hitt R, Gascón P, Amellal N, Harstrick A, Eckardt A. (2005) Phase II multicenter study of the antiepidermal growth factor receptor monoclonal antibody cetuximab in combination with platinum-based chemotherapy in patients with platinum-refractory metastatic and/or recurrent squamous cell carcinoma of the head and neck. J Clin Oncol 23: 5568-5577
8. Baselga J, Albanell J, Ruiz A, Lluch A, Gascón P, Guillém V, González S, Sauleda S, Marimón I, Tabernero JM, Koehler MT, Rojo F. (2005) Phase II and tumor pharmacodynamic study of gefitinib in patients with advanced breast cancer. J Clin Oncol 23: 5323-5333
9. Blehm KN, Spiess PE, Bondaruk JE, Dujka ME, Villares GJ, Zhao YJ, Bogler O, Aldape KD, Grossman HB, Adam L, McConkey DJ, Czerniak BA, Dinney CP, Bar-Eli M. (2006) Mutations within the kinase domain and truncations of the epidermal growth factor receptor are rare events in bladder cancer: implications for therapy. Clin Cancer Res 12: 4671-4677
10. Bonner JA, Harari PM, Giralt J, Azarnia N, Shin DM, Cohen RB, Jones CU, Sur R, Raben D, Jassem J, Ove R, Kies MS, Baselga J, Youssoufian H, Amellal N, Rowinsky EK, Ang KK. (2006) Radiotherapy plus cetuximab for squamous-cell carcinoma of the head and neck. N Engl J Med 354: 567-578
11. Burris HA 3rd, Hurwitz HI, Dees EC, Dowlati A, Blackwell KL, O'Neil B, Marcom PK, Ellis MJ, Overmoyer B, Jones SF, Harris JL, Smith DA, Koch KM, Stead A, Mangum S, Spector NL. (2005) Phase I safety, pharmacokinetics, and clinical activity study of lapatinib (GW572016), a reversible dual inhibitor of epidermal growth factor receptor tyrosine kinases, in heavily pretreated patients with metastatic carcinomas. J Clin Oncol 23: 5305-5312
12. Burtness B, Goldwasser MA, Flood W, Mattar B, Forastiere AA. (2005) Phase III randomized trial of ciplatin plus placebo compared with cisplatin plus cetuximab in metastatic/recurrent head and neck cancer: An Eastern Cooperative Oncology Group study. J Clin Oncol 23: 8646-8654
13. Cappuzzo F, Magrini E, Ceresoli GL, Bartolini S, Rossi E, Ludovini V, Gregorc V, Ligorio C, Cancellieri A, Damiani S, Spreafico A, Paties CT, Lombardo L, Calandri C, Bellezza G, Tonato M, Crinò L. (2004) Akt phosphorylation and gefitinib efficacy in patients with advanced non-small-cell lung cancer. J Natl Cancer Inst 96: 1133-1141
14. Cappuzzo F, Hirsch FR, Rossi E, Bartolini S, Ceresoli GL, Bemis L, Haney J, Witta S, Danenberg K, Domenichini I, Ludovini V, Magrini E, Gregorc V, Doglioni C, Sidoni A, Tonato M, Franklin WA, Crino L, Bunn PA Jr, Varella-Garcia M. (2005) Epidermal growth factor receptor gene and protein and gefitinib sensitivity in non-small-cell lung cancer. J Natl Cancer Inst 97: 643-655

15. Cappuzzo F, Toschi L, Tallini G, Ceresoli GL, Domenichini I, Bartolini S, Finocchiaro G, Magrini E, Metro G, Cancellieri A, Trisolini R, Crino L, Bunn PA Jr, Santoro A, Franklin WA, Varella-Garcia M, Hirsch FR. (2006) Insulin-like growth factor receptor 1 (IGFR-1) is significantly associated with longer survival in non-small-cell lung cancer patients treated with gefitinib. Ann Oncol 17: 1120-1127

16. Chan AT, Hsu MM, Goh BC, Hui EP, Liu TW, Millward MJ, Hong RL, Whang-Peng J, Ma BB, To KF, Mueser M, Amellal N, Lin X, Chang AY. (2005) Multicenter, phase II study of cetuximab in combination with carboplatin in patients with recurrent or metastatic nasopharyngeal carcinoma. J Clin Oncol 23: 3568-3576

17. Chan AT, Ma B, Hui EP. (2006) Phase II study of gefitinib in metastatic or locoregionally recurrent nasopharyngeal carcinoma (NPC). J Clin Oncol 24: 15509A.

18. Chua DT, Nicholls JM, Sham JS, Au GK. (2004) Prognostic value of epidermal growth factor receptor expression in patients with advanced stage nasopharyngeal carcinoma treated with induction chemotherapy and radiotherapy. Int J Radiat Oncol Biol Phys 59: 11-20

19. Chung KY, Shia J, Kemeny NE, Shah M, Schwartz GK, Tse A, Hamilton A, Pan D, Schrag D, Schwartz L, Klimstra DS, Fridman D, Kelsen DP, Saltz LB. (2005) Cetuximab shows activity in colorectal cancer patients with tumors that do not express the epidermal growth factor receptor by immunohistochemistry. J Clin Oncol 23: 1803-1810

20. Cohen EE, Rosen F, Stadler WM, Recant W, Stenson K, Huo D, Vokes EE. (2003) Phase II trial of ZD1839 in recurrent or metastatic squamous cell carcinoma of the head and neck. J Clin Oncol 21: 1980-1987

21. Cohen EE, Kane MA, List MA, Brockstein BE, Mehrotra B, Huo D, Mauer AM, Pierce C, Dekker A, Vokes EE. (2005) Phase II trial of gefitinib 250 mg daily in patients with recurrent and/or metastatic squamous cell carcinoma of the head and neck. Clin Cancer Res 11: 8418-8424

22. Cohen EE. (2006) Role of epidermal growth factor receptor pathway-targeted therapy in patients with recurrent and/or metastatic squamous cell carcinoma of the head and neck. J Clin Oncol 24: 2659-2665

23. Cunningham D, Humblet Y, Siena S, Khayat D, Bleiberg H, Santoro A, Bets D, Mueser M, Harstrick A, Verslype C, Chau I, Van Cutsem E. (2004) Cetuximab monotherapy and cetuximab plus irinotecan in irinotecan-refractory metastatic colorectal cancer. N Engl J Med 351: 337-345

24. Eberhard DA, Johnson BE, Amler LC, Goddard AD, Heldens SL, Herbst RS, Ince WL, Jänne PA, Januario T, Johnson DH, Klein P, Miller VA, Ostland MA, Ramies DA, Sebisanovic D, Stinson JA, Zhang YR, Seshagiri S, Hillan KJ. (2005) Mutations in the epidermal growth factor receptor and in KRAS are predictive and prognostic indicators in patients with non-smal-cell lung cancer treated with chemotherapy alone and in combination with erlotinib. J Clin Oncol 23: 5900-5909

25. Fields ALA, Rinaldi DA, Henderson CA, Germond CJ, Chu L, Brill KJ, Leopold LH, Berger MS. (2005) An open-label multicenter phase II study of oral lapatinib (GW572016) as single-agent, second-line therapy in patients with metastatic colorectal cancer. A phase II, open-label, multucenter study of GW572016 in patients with metastatic colorectal cancer refractory to 5-FU in combination with irinotecan and/or oxaliplatin. J Clin Oncol 23: 3583A.

26. Fukuoka M, Yano S, Giaccone G, Tamura T, Nakagawa K, Douillard JY, Nishiwaki Y, Vansteenkiste J, Kudoh S, Rischin D, Eek R, Horai T, Noda K, Takata I, Smit E, Averbuch S, Macleod A, Feyereislova A, Dong RP, Baselga J. (2003) Multi-institutional randomized phase II trial of gefitinib for previously treated patients with advanced non-small cell lung cancer. J Clin Oncol 21: 2237-2246

27. Fountzilas G, Pectasides D, Kalogera-Fountzila A, Skarlos D, Kalofonos HP, Papadimitriou C, Bafaloukos D, Lambropoulos S, Papadopoulos S, Kourea H, Markopoulos C, Linardou H, Mavroudis D, Briasoulis E, Pavlidis N, Razis E, Kosmidis P, Gogas H. (2005) Paclitaxel and carboplatin as first-line chemotherapy combined with gefitinib (IRESSA) in patients with advanced breast cancer: a phase I/II study conducted by the Hellenic Cooperative Oncology Group. Breast Cancer Res Treat 92: 1-9

28. Gatzemeier U, Pluzanska A, Szczesna A, Kaukel E, Roubec J, Brennscheidt U, De Rosa F, Mueller B, Von Pawel J. (2004) Results of a phase III trial of erlotinib (OSI-774) combined with cisplatin and gemcitabine (GC) chemotherapy in advanced non-small cell lung cancer (NSCLC). J Clin Oncol 22: 619A.

29. Geyer CE, Forster JK, Cameron D, Chan S, Pienkowski T, Romieu CG, Jagiello-Gruszweld A, Crown J, Kaufman B, Chan A. (2006) A phase III randomized, open-label, international study comparing lapatinib and capecitabine versus capecitabine in women with refractory advanced or metastatic breast cancer (EGF100151). Proc Am Soc Clin Oncol 2006.

30. Giaccone G, Herbst RS, Manegold C, Scagliotti G, Rosell R, Miller V, Natale RB, Schiller JH, von Pawel J, Pluzanska A, Gatzemeier U, Grous J, Ochs JS, Averbuch SD, Wolf MK, Rennie P, Fandi A, Johnson DH. (2004) Gefitinib in combination with gemcitabine and cisplatin in advanced non-small-cell lung cancer: A phase III trial – INTACT 1. J Clin Oncol 22: 777-784

31. Giaccone G. (2005) Epidermal growth factor receptor inhibitors in the treatment of non-small cell lung cancer. J Clin Oncol 23: 3235-3242
32. Gibson TB, Ranganathan A, Grothey A. (2006) Randomized phase III trial results of panitumumab, a fully human anti-epidermal growth factor receptor monoclonal antibody, in metastatic colorectal cancer. Clin Colorectal Cancer 6: 29-31
33. Graeven U, Kremer B, Sudhoff T, Killing B, Rojo F, Weber D, Tillner J, Unal C, Schmiegel W.(2006) Phase I study of the humanised anti-EGFR monoclonal antibody matuzumab (EMD 72000) combined with gemcitabine in advanced pancreatic cancer. Br J Cancer 94: 1293-1299
34. Grandis J, Melhem MF, Gooding WE, Day R, Holst VA, Wagener MM, Drenning SD, Tweardy DJ. (1998) Levels of TGF-alpha and EGFR protein in head and neck squamous cell carcinoma and patient survival. J Natl Cancer Inst 90: 824-832
35. Joensuu H, Kellokumpu-Lehtinen PL, Bono P, Alanko T, Kataja V, Asola R, Utriainen T, Kokko R, Hemminki A, Tarkkanen M, Turpeenniemi-Hujanen T, Jyrkkiö S, Flander M, Helle L, Ingalsuo S, Johansson K, Jääskeläinen AS, Pajunen M, Rauhala M, Kaleva-Kerola J, Salminen T, Leinonen M, Elomaa I, Isola J. (2006) Adjuvant docetaxel or vinorelbine with or without trastuzumab for breast cancer. N Engl J Med 354: 809-820
36. Jorissen RN, Walker F, Pouliot N, Garrett TP, Ward CW, Burgess AW. (2003) Epidermal growth factor receptor: mechanisms of activation and signaling. Exp Cell Res 284: 31-53
37. He H, Levitzki A, Zhou HJ, Walker F, Burgess A, Maruta H. (2001) Platelet-derived growth factor requires epidermal growth factor receptor to activate p21-activated kinase family kinases. J Biol Chem 276: 26741-26744
38. Herbst RS, Giaccone G, Schiller JH, Natale RB, Miller V, Manegold C, Scagliotti G, Rosell R, Oliff I, Reeves JA, Wolf MK, Krebs AD, Averbuch SD, Ochs JS, Grous J, Fandi A, Johnson DH. (2004) Gefitinib in combination with paclitaxel and carboplatin in advanced non-small-cell lung cancer: A phase III trial-INTACT 2. J Clin Oncol 22: 785-794
39. Herbst RS, Prager D, Hermann R, Fehrenbacher L, Johnson BE, Sandler A, Kris MG, Tran HT, Klein P, Li X, Ramies D, Johnson DH, Miller VA. (2005) TRIBUTE: a phase III trial of erlotinib hydrochloride (OSI-774) combined with carboplatin and paclitaxel chemotherapy in advanced non-small-cell lung cancer. J Clin Oncol 23: 5892-5899
40. Herbst RS, Arquette M, Shin DM, Dicke K, Vokes EE, Azarnia N, Hong WK, Kies MS. (2005) Phase II multicenter study of the epidermal growth factor receptor antibody cetuximab and cisplatin for recurrent and refractory squamous cell carcinoma of the head and neck. J Clin Oncol 23: 5578-5587
41. Hurwitz H, Febrenbacher L, Novotny W, Cartwright T, Hainsworth J, Heim W, Berlin J, Baron A, Griffing S, Holmgren E, Ferrara N, Fyfe G, Rogers B, Ross R, Kabbinavar F. (2004) Bevacizumab plus irinotecan, fluorouracil, and leucovorin for metastatic colorectal cancer. N Engl J Med 350: 2335-2342
42. Inoue A, Suzuki T, Fukuhara T, Maemondo M, Kimura Y, Morikawa N, Watanabe H, Saijo Y, Nukiwa T. (2006) Prospective phase II study of gefitinib for chemotherapy naive patients with advanced non-small-cell lung cancer with epidermal growth factor receptor gene mutations. J Clin Oncol 24: 3340-3346
43. Kabbinavar FF, Hambleton J, Mass RD, Hurwitz HI, Bergsland E, Sarkar S. (2005) Combined analysis of efficacy: the addition of bevacizumab to fluorouracil/leucovorin improves survival for patients with metastatic colorectal cancer. J Clin Oncol 23: 3706-3712
44. Kalyankrishna S, Grandis JR. (2006) Epidermal growth factor receptor biology in head and neck cancer. J Clin Oncol 24: 2666-2672
45. Kamangar F, Dores GM, Anderson WF. (2006) Patterns of cancer incidence, mortality, and prevalence across five continents: defining priorities to reduce cancer disparities in different geographic regions of the world. J Clin Oncol 24: 2137-2150
46. Kane MA, Cohen E, List M, Mehrotra B, Gustin D, Mauer A, Cella D, Vokes E. (2004) Phase II study of 250 mg gefitinib in advanced squamous cell carcinoma of the head and neck (SCCHN). J Clin Oncol 22: 5586A
47. Karamouzis MV, Gorgoulis VG, Papavassiliou AG. (2002) Transcription factors and neoplasia: vistas in novel drug design. Clin Cancer Res 8: 949-961
48. Kelly H, Goldberg RM. Systemic (2005) Therapy for Metastatic Colorectal Cancer: Current Options, Current Evidence. J Clin Oncol 23:C4553-4560
49. Kelly K, Herbst RS, Crowley JJ, McCoy J, Atkins JN, Lara PN, Dakhil SR, Albain KS, Kim ES, Gandara DR. (2006) Concurrent chemotherapy plus cetuximab or chemotherapy followed by cetuximab in advanced non-small cell lung cancer (NSCLC): A Randomized Phase II study selectional trial SWOG 0342. J Clin Oncol 24: 7015A

50. Kobayashi S, Boggon TJ, Dayaram T, Janne PA, Kocher O, Meyerson M, Johnson BE, Eck MJ, Tenen DG, Halmos B. (2005) EGFR mutation and resistance of non-small-cell lung cancer to gefitinib. N Engl J Med 352: 786-792

51. Kosaka T, Yatabe Y, Endoh H, Kuwano H, Takahashi T, Mitsudomi T. (2004) Mutations of the epidermal growth factor receptor gene in lung cancer: biological and clinical implications. Cancer Res 64: 8919-8923

52. Krempien R, Muenter MW, Huber PE, Nill S, Friess H, Timke C, Didinger B, Buechler P, Heeger S, Herfarth KK, Abdollahi A, Buchler MW, Debus J. (2005) Randomized phase II study evaluating EGFR targeting therapy with cetuximab in combination with radiotherapy and chemotherapy for patients with locally advanced pancreatic cancer—PARC: study protocol [ISRCTN56652283]. BMC Cancer 5: 131

53. Kris MG, Natale RB, Herbst RS, Lynch TJ Jr, Prager D, Belani CP, Schiller JH, Kelly K, Spiridonidis H, Sandler A, Albain KS, Cella D, Wolf MK, Averbuch SD, Ochs JJ, Kay AC. (2003) Efficacy of gefitinib, an inhibitor of the epidermal growth factor receptor tyrosine kinase, in asymptomatic patients with non-small cell lung cancer: a randomized trial. JAMA 290: 2149-2158

54. Kuo T, Cho C, Halsey J, Wakelee HA, Advani RH, Ford JM, Fisher GA, Sikic BI. (2005) Phase II study of gefitinib, fluorouracil, leucovorin, and oxaliplatin therapy in previously treated patients with metastatic colorectal cancer. J Clin Oncol 23: 5613-5619

55. Lal A, Glazer CA, Martinson HM, Friedman HS, Archer GE, Sampson JH, Riggins GJ. (2002) Mutant epidermal growth factor receptor up-regulates molecular effectors of tumor invasion. Cancer Res 62: 3335-3339

56. Lee SC, Lim SG, Soo R, Hsieh WS, Guo JY, Putti T, Tao Q, Soong R, Goh BC. (2006) Lack of somatic mutations in EGFR tyrosine kinase domain in hepatocellular and nasopharyngeal carcinoma. Pharmacogenet Genomics 16: 73-74

57. Leong JL, Loh KS, Putti TC, Goh BC, Tan LK. (2004) Epidermal growth factor receptor in undifferentiated carcinoma of the nasopharynx. Laryngoscope 114: 153-157

58. Lievre A, Bachet JB, Le Corre D, Boige V, Landi B, Emile JF, Côté JF, Tomasic G, Penna C, Ducreux M, Rougier P, Penault-Llorca F, Pierre Laurent-Puig P. (2006) KRAS mutation status is predictive of response to cetuximab therapy in colorectal cancer. Cancer Res 66: 3992-3995

59. Lilenbaum R, Bonomi P, Ansari R, Lynch T, Govindan R, Janne P, Hanna N. (2005) A phase II trial of cetuximab as therapy for recurrent non-small cell lung cancer (NSCLC): Final results. J Clin Oncol 23: 7036A

60. Lynch TJ, Bell DW, Sordella R, Gurubhagavatula S, Okimoto RA, Brannigan BW, Harris PL, Haserlat SM, Supko JG, Haluska FG, Louis DN, Christiani DC, Settleman J, Haber DA. (2004) Activating mutations in the epidermal growth factor receptor underlying responsiveness of non-small-cell lung cancer to gefitinib. N Engl J Med 350: 2129-2139

61. Mendelsohn J, Baselga J. (2000) The EGF receptor family as targets for cancer therapy. Oncogene 19: 6550-6555

62. Miller VA, Zakowski M, Riely GJ, Pao W, Ladanyi M, Tsao AS, Sandler A, Herbst R, Kris MG, Johnson DG. (2006) EGFR mutations and copy number, EGFR expression and KRAS mutation as predictors of outcome with erlotinib in bronchioalveolar cell carcinoma (BAC). Results of a prospective study. J Clin Oncol 24: 364A

63. Moore MJ, Goldstein D, Hamm J, Figer A, Hecht J, Gallinger S, Au H, Ding K, Christy-Bittel J, Parulekar W. (2005) Erlotinib plus gemcitabine compared to gemcitabine alone in patients with advanced pancreatic cancer. A phase III trial of the National Cancer Institute of Canada Clinical Trials Group [NCIC-CTG]. J Clin Oncol 23: 1A

64. Moroni M, Veronese S, Benvenuti S, Marrapese G, Sartore-Bianchi A, Di Nicolantonio F, Gambacorta M, Siena S, Bardelli A. (2005) Gene copy number for epidermal growth factor receptor (EGFR) and clinical response to antiEGFR treatment in colorectal cancer: a cohort study. Lancet Oncol 6: 279-286

65. Nicholson RI, Hutcheson IR, Knowlden JM. (2004) Non-endocrine pathways and endocrine resistance: Observations with antiestrogens and signal transduction inhibitors in combination. Clin Cancer Res 10: 346S-354S

66. Niederle N, Freier W, Porschen R. (2005) Erlotinib as single agent in 2nd and 3rd line treatment in patients with metastatic colorectal cancer. Results of a two-cohort multicenter phase II study. Eur J Cancer 3(suppl 3): 184

67. Oliveira S, Van Bergen en Henegouwen PM, Storm G, Schiffelers RM. (2006) Molecular biology of epidermal growth factor receptor inhibition for cancer therapy. Expert Opin Biol Ther 6: 605-617

68. Paez JG, Janne PA, Lee JC, Tracy S, Greulich H, Gabriel S, Herman P, Kaye FJ, Lindeman N, Boggon TJ, Naoki K, Sasaki H, Fujii Y, Eck MJ, Sellers WR, Johnson BE, Meyerson M. (2004) EGFR mutations in lung cancer: correlation with clinical response to gefitinb therapy. Science 304: 1497-1500

69. Pao W, Miller VA. (2005) Epidermal growth factor receptor mutations, small-molecule kinase inhibitors, and non-small-cell lung cancer: current knowledge and future directions. J Clin Oncol 23: 2556-2568
70. Patel JD, Pasche B, Argiris A. (2004) Targeting non-small cell lung cancer with epidermal growth factor tyrosine kinase inhibitors: where do we stand, where do we go. Crit Rev Oncol Hematol 50: 175-186
71. Paz-Ares L, Sanchez JM, Garcia-Velasco A, Massuti B, López-Vivanco G, Provencio M, Montes A, Isla D, Amador ML, Rosell R. (2006) A prospective phase II trial of erlotinib in advanced non-small cell lung cancer (NSCLC) patients with mutations in the tyrosine kinase (TK) domain of the epidermal growth factor receptor (EGFR). J Clin Oncol 24: 7020A
72. Perez-Soler R, Chachoua A, Hammond LA, Rowinsky EK, Huberman M, Karp D, Rigas J, Clark GM, Santabárbara P, Bonomi P. (2004) Determinants of tumor response and survival with erlotinib in patients with non—small-cell lung cancer. J Clin Oncol 22: 3238-3247
73. Pfister DG, Su YB, Kraus DH, Wolden SL, Lis E, Aliff TB, Zahalsky AJ, Lake S, Needle MN, Shaha AR, Shah JP, Zelefsky MJ. (2006) Concurrent cetuximab, cisplatin, and concomitant boost radiotherapy for locoregionally advanced, squamous cell head and neck cancer: a pilot phase II study of a new combined-modality paradigm. J Clin Oncol 24: 1072-1078
74. Piccart-Gebhart MJ, Procter M, Leyland-Jones B, Goldhirsch A, Untch M, Smith I, Gianni L, Baselga J, Bell R, Jackisch C, Cameron D, Dowsett M, Barrios CH, Steger G, Huang CS, Andersson M, Inbar M, Lichinitser M, Láng I, Nitz U, Iwata H, Thomssen C, Lohrisch C, Suter TM, Rüschoff J, Süto T, Greatorex V, Ward C, Straehle C, McFadden E, Dolci S, Gelber RD. (2005) Trastuzumab after adjuvant chemotherapy in HER2-positive breast cancer. N Engl J Med 353: 1659-1672
75. Polychronis A, Sinnett HD, Hadjiminas D, Singhal H, Mansi J, Shivapatham D, Shousha S, Jiang J, Peston D, Barrett N. (2005) Preoperative gefitinib versus gefitinib and anastrozole in postmenopausal patients with oestrogen-receptor positive and epidermal-growth-factor-receptor-positive primary breast cancer: a double-blind placebo-controlled phase II Randomised Trial. Lancet Oncol 6: 383-391
76. Robert F, Blumenschein G, Herbst RS, Fossella FV, Tseng J, Saleh MN, Needle M. (2005) Phase I/IIa study of cetuximab with gemcitabine plus carboplatin in patients with chemotherapy-naive advanced non-small-cell lung cancer. J Clin Oncol 23: 9089-9096
77. Romond EH, Perez SA, Bryant J, Suman VJ, Geyer CE Jr, Davidson NE, Tan-Chiu E, Martino S, Paik S, Kaufman PA, Swain SM, Pisansky TM, Fehrenbacher L, Kutteh LA, Vogel VG, Visscher DW, Yothers G, Jenkins RB, Brown AM, Dakhil SR, Mamounas EP, Lingle WL, Klein PM, Ingle JN, Wolmark N. (2005) Trastuzumab plus adjuvant chemotherapy for operable HER2-positive breast cancer. N Engl J Med 353: 1673-1684
78. Rosell R, Daniel C, Ramlau R, Szczesna A, Constenla M, Mennecier B, Pfeifer W, Mueser M, Montaner I, Gatzemeier U. (2004) Randomized phase II study of cetuximab in combination with cisplatin (C) and vinorelbine (V) vs. CV alone in the first-line treatment of patients (pts) with epidermal growth factor receptor (EGFR)-expressing advanced non-small-cell lung cancer (NSCLC). J Clin Oncol 22: 7012A
79. Rothenberg ML, LaFleur B, Levy DE, Washington MK, Morgan-Meadows SL, Ramanathan RK, Berlin JD, Benson AB, Coffey RJ. (2005) Randomized phase II trial of the clinical and biological effects of two dose levels of gefitinib in patients with recurrent colorectal adenocarcinoma. J Clin Oncol 23: 9265-9274
80. Saltz L, Kies M, Abbruzzese JL, Azarnia N, Needle M. (2003) The presence and intensity of the cetuximab-induced acne-like rash predicts increased survival in studies across multiple malignancies. J Clin Oncol 21: 817A
81. Saltz LB, Meropol NJ, Loehrer PJ, Needle MN, Kopitz J, Mayer RJ. (2004) Phase II trial of cetuximab in patients with refractory colorectal cancer that expresses the epidermal growth factor receptor. J Clin Oncol 22: 1201-1208
82. Saltz LB, Lenz H, Hochster H, Wadler S, Hoff P, Kemeny N, Hollywood E, Gonen M, Wetherbee S, Chen H. (2005) Randomized Phase II Trial of Cetuximab/Bevacizumab/Irinotecan (CBI) versus Cetuximab/Bevacizumab (CB) in Irinotecan-Refractory Colorectal Cancer. J Clin Oncol 23: 3508A
83. Savvides P, Argarwala SS, Greskovich J, Argiris A, Bokar J, Cooney M, Hoppel C, Stepnick DW, Lavertu P, Remick S. (2006) Phase I study of the EGFR tyrosine kinase inhibitor erlotinib in combination with docetaxel and radiation in locally advanced squamous cell cancer of the head and neck (SCCHN). J Clin Oncol 24: 5545A
84. Schiff R, Massarweh SA, Shou J, Bharwani L, Mohsin SK, Osborne CK. (2004) Cross-talk between estrogen receptor and growth factor pathways as a molecular target for overcoming endocrine resistance. Clin Cancer Res 10: 331S-336S
85. Schlessinger J. (2002) Ligand-induced, receptor-mediated dimerization and activation of EGF receptor. Cell 110: 669-672
86. Shaheen RM, Ahmad SA, Liu W, Reinmuth N, Jung YD, Tseng WW, Drazan KE, Bucana CD, Hicklin DJ, Ellis LM. (2001) Inhibited growth of colon cancer carcinomatosis by antibodies to vascular endothelial and epidermal growth factor receptors. Br J Cancer 85: 584-589

87. Shepherd FA, Pereira J, Ciuleanu TE, Tan EH, Hirsh V, Thongprasert S, Campos D, Maoleekoonpiroj S, Smylie M, Martins R, van Kooten M, Dediu M, Findlay B, Tu D, Johnston D, Bezjak A, Clark G, Santabárbara P, Seymour L. (2005) Erlotinib in previously treated non-small-cell lung cancer. N Engl J Med 353: 123-132

88. Slamon DJ, Leyland-Jones B, Shak S, Fuchs H, Paton V, Bajamonde A, Fleming T, Eiermann W, Wolter J, Pegram M, Baselga J, Norton L. (2001) Use of chemotherapy plus a monoclonal antibody against HER2 for metastatic breast cancer that overexpresses HER2. N Engl J Med 344: 783-792

89. Soulieres D, Senzer NN, Vokes EE, Hidalgo M, Agarwala SS, Siu LL. (2004) Multicenter phase II study of erlotinib, an oral epidermal growth factor receptor tyrosine kinase inhibitor, in patients with recurrent or metastatic squamous cell cancer of the head and neck. J Clin Oncol 22: 77-85.

90. Spector NL, Blackwell K, Hurley J, Harris JL, Lombardi D, Bacus S, Ahmed SB, Boussen H, Frikha M, Ayed FB. (2006) EGF103009, a phase II trial of lapatinib monotherapy in patients with relapsed/refractory inflammatory breast cancer (IBC): Clinical activity and biologic predictors of response. J Clin Oncol 24: 502A

91. Stevenson D, Charalambous C, Wilson JB. (2005) Epstein-Barr virus latent membrane protein 1 (CAO) up-regulates VEGF and TGF alpha concomitant with hyperplasia, with subsequent up-regulation of p16 and MMP9. Cancer Res 65: 8826-8835

92. Tan AR, Yang X, Hewitt SM, Berman A, Lepper ER, Sparreboom A, Parr AL, Figg WD, Chow C, Steinberg SM, Bacharach SL, Whatley M, Carrasquillo JA, Brahim JS, Ettenberg SA, Lipkowitz S, Swain SM. (2004) Evaluation of biologic end points and pharmacokinetics in patients with metastatic breast cancer after treatment with erlotinib, an epidermal growth factor receptor tyrosine kinase inhibitor. J Clin Oncol 22: 3080-3090

93. Tao Y, Song X, Deng X, Xie D, Lee LM, Liu Y, Li W, Li L, Deng L, Wu Q, Gong J, Cao Y. (2005) Nuclear accumulation of epidermal growth factor receptor and acceleration of G1/S stage by Epstein-Barr-encoded oncoprotein latent membrane protein 1. Exp Cell Res 303: 240-251

94. Thatcher N, Chang A, Parikh P, Rodrigues Pereira J, Ciuleanu T, von Pawel J, Thongprasert S, Tan E, Pemberton K, Archer V. (2005) Gefitinib plus best supportive care in previously treated patients with refractory advanced non-small-cell lung cancer: results from a randomised, placebo-controlled, multicentre study (Iressa Survival Evaluation in Lung Cancer). Lancet 366: 1527-1537

95. Thienelt CD, Bunn PA Jr, Hanna N, Rosenberg A, Needle MN, Long ME, Gustafson DL, Kelly K. (2005) Multicenter phase I/II study of cetuximab with paclitaxel and carboplatin in untreated patients with stage IV non-small-cell lung cancer. J Clin Oncol 23: 8786-8793

96. Thomas SM, Coppelli FM, Wells A, Gooding WE, Song J, Kassis J, Drenning SD, Grandis JR. (2003) Epidermal growth factor receptor-stimulated activation of phospholipase Cgamma-1 promotes invasion of head and neck squamous cell carcinoma. Cancer Res 63: 5629-5635

97. Toyooka S, Tokumo M, Shigematsu H, Matsuo K, Asano H, Tomii K, Ichihara S, Suzuki M, Aoe M, Date H, Gazdar AF, Shimizu N. (2006) Mutational and epigenetic evidence for independent pathways for lung adenocarcinomas arising in smokers and never smokers. Cancer Res 66: 1371-1375

98. Trigo J, Hitt R, Koralewski P, Diaz-Rubio E, Rolland F, Knecht R, Amellal N, Bessa EH, Baselga J, Vermorken JB. (2004) Cetuximab monotherapy is active in patients with platinum-refractory recurrent/metastatic squamous cell carcinoma of the head and neck (SCCHN): Results of a phase II study. J Clin Oncol 22: 488A

99. Tsao M, Zhu C, Sakurada A, Zhang T, Whitehead M, Kamel-Reid S, Ding K, Seymour L, Shepherd F. (2006) An analysis of the prognostic and predictive importance of K-ras mutation status in the National Cancer Institute of Canada Clinical Trials Group BR.21 study of erlotinib versus placebo in the treatment of non-small cell lung cancer. J Clin Oncol 24: 365A

100. Tyagi P. (2005) Recent results and ongoing trials with panitumumab (ABX-EGF), a fully human anti-epidermal growth factor receptor antibody, in metastatic colorectal cancer. Clin Colorectal Cancer 5: 21-23

101. Yarden Y, Sliwkowski MX. (2001) Untangling the ErbB signalling network. Nat Rev Mol Cell Biol 2: 127-137

102. Yu H, Jove R. (2004) The STATs of cancer—new molecular targets come of age. Nat Rev Cancer 4:97-105.

103. Vallbohmer D, Zhang W, Gordon M, Yang DY, Yun J, Press OA, Rhodes KE, Sherrod AE, Iqbal S, Danenberg KD, Groshen S, Lenz HJ. (2005) Molecular determinants of cetuximab efficacy. J Clin Oncol 23: 3536-3544

104. Venook A, Niedzwieski D, Hollis D, Sutherland S, Goldberg R, Alberts S, Benson A, Wade J, Schilsky R, Mayer R. (2006) Phase III study of irinotecan/5FU/LV (FOLFIRI) or oxaliplatin/5FU/LV (FOLFOX) ± cetuximab for patients with untreated metastatic adenocarcinoma of the colon or rectum: CALGB 80203 preliminary results. J Clin Oncol 24: 3509A

105. Vokes EE, Cohen EE, Mauer AM, Karrison TG, Wong SJ, Skoog-Sluman LJ, Kozloff MF, Dancey J, Dekker A. (2005) A phase I study of erlotinib and bevacizumab for recurrent or metastatic squamous cell carcinoma of the head and neck (HNC). J Clin Oncol 23: 5504A
106. von Minckwitz G, Jonat W, Fasching P, du Bois A, Kleeberg U, Lück HJ, Kettner E, Hilfrich J, Eiermann W, Torode J, Schneeweiss A. (2005) A multicentre phase II study on gefitinib in taxane- and anthracycline-pretreated metastatic breast cancer. Breast Cancer Res Treat 89: 165-172
107. von Pawel J, Park K, Pereira R, Szczesna A, Yu C, Ganul VL, Krzakowski M, Roh JK, Pilz K, Pirker R. (2006) Phase III study comparing cisplatin/vinorelbine plus cetuximab versus cisplatin/vinorelbine as first line treatment for patients with epidermal growth factor (EGFR) – expressing advanced non-small cell lung cancer (NSCLC) (FLEX). J Clin Oncol 24: 7109A
108. Xu JM, Paradiso A, McLeod HK. (2004) Evaluation of epidermal growth factor receptor tyrosine kinase inhibitors combined with chemotherapy: Is there a need for a more rational design? Eur J Cancer 40: 1807-1809
109. Wainberg Z, Hecht JR. (2006) A Phase III Randomized, open-label, controlled trial of chemotherapy and bevacizumab with or without panitumumab in the first-line treatment of patients with metastatic colorectal cancer. Clin Colorectal Cancer 5: 363-367
110. Willmore-Payne C, Holden JA, Layfield LJ. (2006) Detection of EGFR- and HER2-activating mutations in squamous cell carcinoma involving the head and neck. Mod Pathol 19: 634-640

20. NEW PROMISES IN THE ADJUVANT, AND PALLIATIVE TREATMENT OF MELANOMA

AXEL HAUSCHILD[1], DIRK SCHADENDORF[2], CLAUS GARBE[3], SELMA UGUREL[2] AND KATHARINA C. KÄHLER[1]

[1]Department of Dermatology, University of Kiel, Kiel, Germany, [2]Skin Cancer Unit, German Cancer Research Centre and University Hospital Mannheim, University of Heidelberg, Mannheim, Germany, [3]Division of Dermatooncology, Department of Dermatology, University Medical Center Tuebingen, Germany

INTRODUCTION

In the last decade the incidence of melanoma has been increasing. Malignant melanoma of the skin is the most frequent cause of mortality from skin cancer. Despite exhaustive efforts to increase early detection and in prevention campaigns, 20–25% of all melanoma patients will die due to disseminated metastases. Once melanoma has spread to regional lymph nodes, survival diminishes to approximately 30–55%. After dissemination to visceral organs, only very few patients can be cured. The median survival with stage IV (AJCC classification) disseminated melanoma is approximately 6–12 months. To date, therapy of disseminated melanoma still has failed to show a significant impact on overall survival. In the adjuvant setting interferon-α is until today the only drug which has shown beneficial effects in high-risk cutaneous melanoma patients. In addition to the development of new targeted drugs the identification of patient subgroups with anticipated benefit will be of importance.

INTERFERON-α IN ADJUVANT SYSTEMIC TREATMENT OF MELANOMA

Since the 1980s the interferons play an important role in the treatment of high risk primary and of metastatic melanoma (1, 2). Different types of interferon have been studied and applied to melanoma patients (3–5). Beneath interferon-α likewise interferon-β and interferon-γ have been examined in melanoma patients without currently any further clinical relevance. In humans, there is a variety of different interferon-α subtypes and, altogether, 21 different interferon-α genes located on chromosome 9q21 have been identified (6). It remains presently unclear if the different subtypes of interferon-α are related to different functional activities. They all have a high homology in amino acid sequence and several of the subtypes obviously activate the same genes. Two subtypes have been developed for therapeutic purposes so far which are interferon-α_{2a} (Roferon-A®) and interferon-α_{2b} (Intron-A®). These two interferons differ from each other only in two of 166 amino acids and they, obviously, are widely identical in their therapeutic and side effects and in their adverse events.

Interferons-α have first been studied in metastatic melanoma. They have been applied in high dosages with 5–20 MIU m^{-2} body surface three times weekly. Mainly 10 MIU m^{-2} body surface have been used and objective response rates of 10–15% were reported (7–9). All studies published are small and are monocenter trials in selected patients and no external reviews of imaging examinations in order to check the responses have been performed. Thus, the true response rate to interferon-α may probably be lower when evaluated in larger, multicenter trials with external review of imaging examinations.

EFFECTS OF INTERFERON-α

Interferon-α and interferon-β both belong to type I interferons and both bind to interferon type 1 receptor (6, 9). The signaling cascade which is mediated by receptor binding of interferon-α is rather well understood (10, 11). Binding of interferon-α to the receptor activates two janus kinases tyk-2 and JAK-1. Activated janus kinases recruit "STAT" factors in the cytoplasma. Six different "STAT" factors are presently known. Always two "STAT" factors form dimers which are capable to go to the nucleus. In combination with additional stabilizing molecules, they form interferon stimulated gene factors in the nucleus. These bind to interferon stimulated response elements at the DNA which are a specific DNA sequence comprising 14 base pairs (Fig. 1). There they act as transcription factors and activate a number of genes. Among these are genes responsible for virus inhibition like the MX proteins (inhibiting viral replication), 2'5'-OAS (induces mRNA degradation) and PKR (inhibiting translation). Additional genes are involved in immune regulation like the activation of IL-12, IL-15, and interferon-γ. Likewise toll-like receptors are activated by interferon-α. A third major effect of interferon-α is growth inhibition of tumor cells which is mediated viral activation of p21 and the p200 family which mediate growth arrest. Furthermore, caspases are activated which mediate cell death. Thus, the three main effects of interferons-α are inhibition of

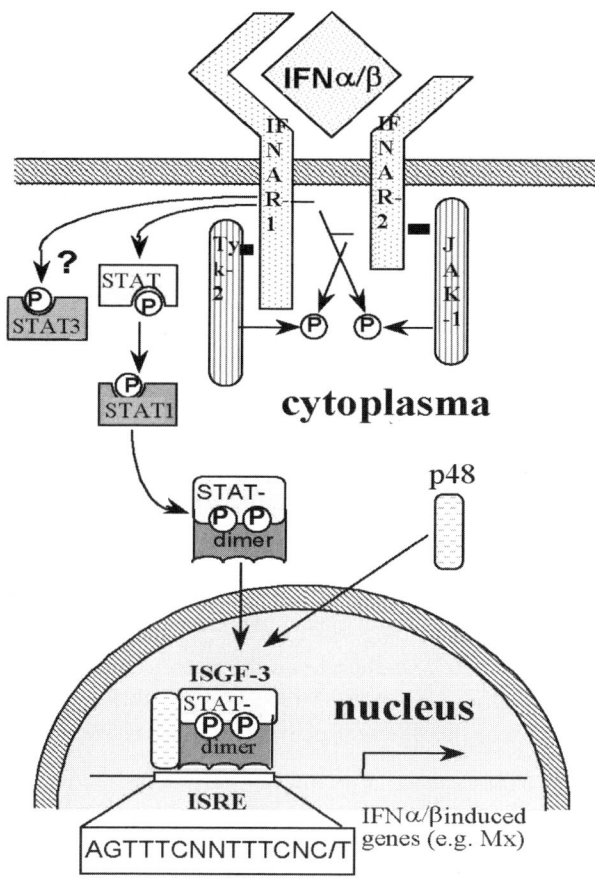

Figure 1. IFN signal transduction. The binding of IFN proteins to their specific receptor rapidly induces tyrosine phosphorylation of the receptor by JAK kinases; these phosphorylated tyrosines provide a docking site for the STAT proteins which are subsequently phosphorylated by the Jak kinases. Activated STAT proteins dimerize to one another. Dimeric STAT then translocates into the nucleus and acts by direct binding to DNA. In combination with additional stabilizing molecules, they form interferon stimulated gene factors in the nucleus. These bind to interferon stimulated response elements at the DNA which are a specific DNA sequence comprising 14 base pairs

viral growth, growth inhibition of tumor cells, and immunostimulatory effects by activation of different cytokines.

DIFFERENCES OF PEGYLATED INTERFERON-α COMPARED TO CLASSIC INTERFERON-α

Interferon-α as produced by gene technology are pure proteins without any side chains. Natural interferons-α, however, are glycosylated. This influences mainly the pharmacokinetics of these molecules. Pegylation means polyethylene glycosylation of the protein molecules and either one or several side chains bind to the protein molecule. This chemical modification likewise influences the pharmacokinetics and the half-life time of the molecules (Table 1). The half-life time in the serum is clearly lower with 3–6 h for the classic interferon-α compared to 40–60 h for the pegylated interferon-α (Table 2) (12, 13). Furthermore, also the route of excretion is changed from renal to hepatic elimination. The clearly longer half-life of pegylated interferon-α allows once weekly application instead of three times weekly application of classic interferon-α. Additionally, the efficacy of pegylated interferon-α seems to be increased, at least in its anti-viral activity. Elimination rates of the viral load in hepatitis-C and hepatitis-B are clearly more effective with the use of pegylated interferon-α as compared to classic interferon-α (14–19). Therefore, there is some hope that pegylated interferon-α may likewise be more effective in the treatment of malignancies. There are some hints from renal cell cancer and from chronic lymphatic leukemia that pegylated interferon-α is an effective agent for treating cancer (20–22). It is an important question whether the action of pegylated interferon-α parallels that of classic interferon. This question had been addressed in a skin mouse model carrying tumors of a melanoma cell line (23). It has been shown that pegylated interferon-α_{2a} has very similar growth inhibitory effects in this xenogenic tumor model like classic interferon-α. Furthermore, the pattern of gene activation and gene silencing was nearly identical for both interferon types, the pegylated interferon-α and the classic interferon-α. Therefore, the mode of action of both interferons seems to be identical and differences in their efficacy seem to be attributed to the different pharmacokinetics (24).

Table 1. Pharmacokinetics of pegylated Interferons: Comparison between pegylated Interferon-$\alpha2$ (Pegasys®) and pegylated Interferon-α_{2b} (PegIntron®)

Characteristics	Pegasys	PegIntron
PEG chain	40 kDa arborized	12 kDa linear
Molecular weight (Dalton)	60 kDa	31 kDa
Half-life (h)	50–130	27–39
$T_{max (h)}$	72–96 h	15–44 h

Table 2. Overview on new drug developments and their targets for metastatic melanoma patients

Signal transduction inhibitors	Ubiquitin–Proteasome complex inhibitors	Angiogenesis inhibitors
Sorafenib (BAY 43- 9006) [RAF, VEGF-R, PDGF-R inhibition]	Bortezomib [26S proteasome inhibitor]	Thalidomide Bevacizumab Sorafenib (BAY 43-9006) [anti-VEGF]
CCI-779 [m-TOR inhibition]	Histone deacetylase inhibitor	Revlimide (CC-5013) [anti-VEGF]
PD 0325901	MS-275	Vitaxin (MEDI-522) CNTO-95 [anti-$\alpha v \beta_3$ integrin]

ADJUVANT TREATMENT WITH INTERFERON-α

Interferon-α is until today the only drug which has shown beneficial effects in the adjuvant treatment of high-risk cutaneous melanoma patients. Interferon-α is rather well established in the adjuvant treatment in clinical stages II and III, although not all studies showed significant benefits for patients under treatment with interferon-α. Mainly two different treatment regimens have been introduced with high and low dosages of interferon-α. Significant benefits in terms of recurrence-free and overall survival have been shown for both regimens (25–29). However, some studies did not find significant beneficial effects (30–33). The best dosage and duration of treatment remains still to be defined (34–36). Currently, for adjuvant treatment with pegylated interferon-α in high-risk melanoma patients no larger trial has been completed and evaluated. There are several trials which are presently conducted and will be evaluated during the next years.

The first trial has been performed by the EORTC and 1,256 patients with microscopic and macroscopic lymph node metastasis have been recruited into this trial (37). The trial design was simple and patients were randomized into the following arms: Arm A is treated with pegylated interferon-α_{2a} (PEG-Intron®) 6.0 μg kg^{-1} per week for the first 8 weeks followed by a long-term maintenance treatment period of 5 years at 3.0 μg kg^{-1} per week vs. Arm B with observation only. Recruitment has already been completed in the year 2003 and final evaluation will be presented in June 2007.

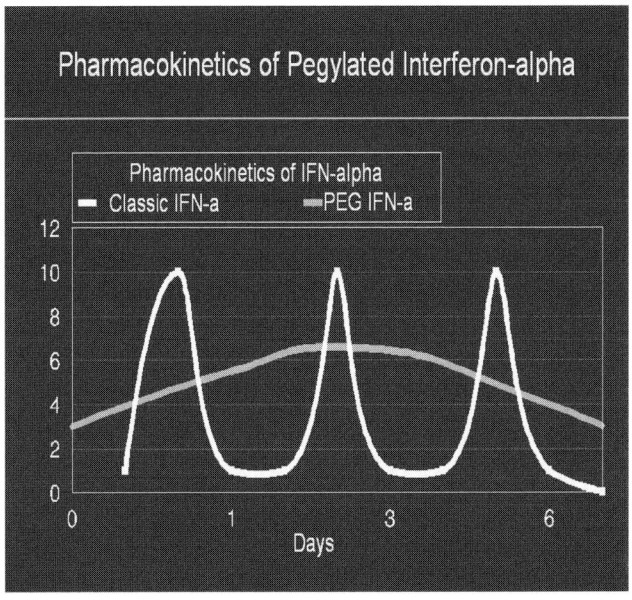

Figure 2. Pharmacokinetics of pegylated Interferon-α compared with conventional Interferon-α

Another trial has been initiated by the European Association of Dermatologic Oncology (EADO). In this trial, patients with stage II-melanoma, according to the old TNM-classification, have been recruited. This comprises patients with more than 1.5 mm tumor thickness, including those, who have been found positive for micrometastatic disease by sentinel lymph node biopsy. The trial has been planned in order to recruit 890 patients, which are randomized to the following arms: Pegylated interferon-α_{2b} 100 µg once weekly for 36 months, vs. reference treatment with interferon-α_{2b} 3 × 3 MIU per weekly for 18 months (this is an approved dosing regimen in Europe).

A third trial has been initiated by the German Dermatologic Cooperative Oncology Group (DeCOG) in which pegylated interferon-α_{2a} (Pegasys) is utilized. The trial is planned to recruit 880 patients and patients are randomized into two arms: Treatment with 180 µg pegylated interferon-α_{2a} (Pegasys) weekly for 24 months, vs. treatment with classic interferon-α_{2a}, (Roferon-A) 3 × 3 MIU weekly for 24 months.

Thus, the future will show if pegylated interferon-α is effective as an adjuvant treatment at all and if it is more effective than classic non pegylated interferons.

SYSTEMIC TREATMENT OF DISSEMINATED MELANOMA (STAGE IV, AJCC CLASSIFICATION)

Dacarbazine (DTIC) is actually considered as the standard chemotherapy regimen in stage IV melanoma, with reported response rates between 5 and 18% since bio- or polychemotherapy has not achieved any survival benefit (38, 39). This poor outcome does not rely on an impaired penetration of chemotherapeutics into the tumor, but has been proposed to be caused by chemoresistance mechanisms intrinsic to melanoma cells (40).

CHEMOSENSITIVITY TESTING AS A NEW APPROACH

A number of nonstandard antimelanoma drugs were tested in small studies to demonstrate some efficacy; these observations indicate a subgroup of patients exhibiting high sensitivity to certain anticancer drugs. Diagnostic tools are needed to identify this subgroup among the presumably high number of overall chemoresistant patients. For these purposes, various in vitro chemosensitivity assays such as the ATP bioluminescence assay (ATP-TCA) have been developed and tested in the preclinical and clinical setting (41). The ATP-TCA was shown to comprise high sensitivity, high reproducibility, and a low failure rate and prospective studies using this approach revealed a good correlation between in vitro sensitivities and in vivo tumor responses (41). The present study tested the feasibility of pretherapeutic in vitro chemosensitivity testing using the ATP-TCA method in a multicenter setting and results are published in a recent report in detail (42).

Between January 2001 and May 2004, 82 patients (ITT) were enrolled into the study from 11 participating DeCOG centers. Fifty seven patients (69.5%) received an assay-directed chemotherapy within 1 month after enrollment, 25 patients (30.5%) received other than test-directed or no chemotherapy. Four out of 57 patients treated per protocol had to be excluded from analysis due to different reasons. Of 82 patients 53 (64.6%) were evaluable for all study endpoints (PP).

Chemosensitivity test assay showed a high yield with a success rate of 97.6%. The remaining 79 evaluable chemosensitivity assays on melanoma samples revealed a heterogenous sensitivity to different chemotherapeutics and combinations. The drug combinations with the highest in vitro sensitivities were gemcitabine + treosulfan, paclitaxel + cisplatin, paclitaxel + doxorubicin, and gemcitabine + cisplatin represented by the *best sensitivity index*.

Treatment responses (ITT, PP) were low as expected from previous trials in melanoma with a progression arrest (CR, PR + SD) in only around 1/3 of patients. The median follow-up time was 19.3 months. In regard to different chemotherapy regimens, gemcitabine + treosulfan as well as paclitaxel + cisplatin showed a significantly better overall survival than gemcitabine + cisplatin and paclitaxel + doxorubicin ($p = 0.032$; Fig. 3a). Using critlevel analysis and arbitrary testing of different cut-off values, a threshold value of 100 could be determined for the best sensitivity index to differentiate between chemosensitive and resistant patients. Patients whose tumors were considered chemosensitive (best sensitivity index ≤ 100) revealed a significantly better response (CR + PR + SD 59.1 vs. 22.6%, $p = 0.01$) and overall survival (median 14.6 vs. 7.4 months, $p = 0.041$; Fig. 3b) than patients who were tested chemoresistant (best sensitivity index > 100). OR differed between both groups without reaching statistical significance (36.4 vs. 16.1%, $p = 0.114$). Multivariate analysis revealed serum LDH ($p = 0.03$) and overall performance ($p = 0.03$) as the strongest independent predictors of overall survival, followed by best sensitivity index ($p = 0.18$) and AJCC M category ($p = 0.80$). Serum LDH, overall performance status, and AJCC M category showed no significant differences between chemosensitive and chemoresistant patients. CTC grade 3/4 toxicities were experienced by 19/57 (33.3%) patients, with the majority presenting as myelosuppression. A treatment discontinuation was required in one patient only; no fatal outcome was observed. Patients who experienced grade 3/4 toxicities revealed a favorable overall survival compared to patients without (median 14.2 vs. 5.9 months; $p = 0.036$). Grade 3/4 toxicities mainly occurred in patients who received multiple treatment cycles. Eight out of 19 (42%) patients experiencing these toxicities received more than four cycles, compared to only 4/34 (12%) patients with less than four cycles.

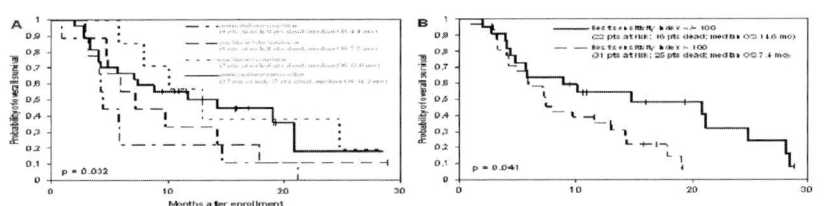

Figure 3. Kaplan Meier curves, showing the probability of overall survival of the PP population by different treatment regimens (**a**), and by best sensitivity index of in vitro chemosensitivity testing (**b**)

PERSPECTIVES OF CHEMOSENSITIVITY TESTING

Pretherapeutic chemosensitivity testing of melanoma tissue samples using the ATP-TCA was proved as a feasible method in this study and yielded interpretable results without delay in the vast majority of samples, even if applied in a multicenter setting. Melanoma tissues revealed heterogeneous chemosensitivities, with drug combinations showing higher sensitivities than single agents. The most effective combinations were gemcitabine + treosulfan, paclitaxel + cisplatin, paclitaxel + doxorubicin, and gemcitabine + cisplatin. As a second major finding of this trial, we observed good efficacy of assay-directed individualized chemotherapy. OR was 24.5% (PP), and thus was obviously superior to recent reports of OR under standard DTIC monochemotherapy (43). Median OS was 8.8 months (PP), which is comparable to the results reported under DTIC (43). Our third and most important finding was that in vitro ATP-TCA chemosensitivity testing correlated with in vivo therapy outcome of melanoma patients. Patients whose tumor tissue samples were tested sensitive to one of the investigated drugs or drug combinations revealed higher response rates and a prolonged overall survival than patients who were tested resistant. For the differentiation between "chemosensitive" and "chemoresistant," a threshold sensitivity index could be defined, which should be evaluated precisely in subsequent studies. This index was shown to predict the outcome of individual patients to chemotherapy in terms of tumor responsiveness and overall survival (Fig. 3b). This offers the possibility of future therapy decisions based on the results of in vitro chemosensitivity testing, thus enhancing treatment efficacy in sensitive patients while sparing toxicity in resistant patients, who might then be admitted to alternative treatment regimens. However, it should be noticed, that the sensitivity index was no independent predictor of overall survival, as were serum LDH and overall performance. Without an obvious correlation to chemosensitivities, distinct therapy regimens (gemcitabine + treosulfan, paclitaxel + cisplatin) showed higher response and survival rates than others (paclitaxel + doxorubicin, gemcitabine + cisplatin). This might be due to the well-known limitations inherent to drug sensitivity assays, mainly caused by the biology of the tumor, which cannot be completely imitated by in vitro test conditions. In addition, it should be mentioned, that we had to define dosing regimens for each drug or drug combination, which were chosen based on empiric data gained by small phase I/II studies and possibly might not lead to full effectiveness of the drug at the tumor site. Subsequent studies will be necessary to optimize drug dosing and treatment schedules.

In conclusion, this cooperative group study contributes to the recognition of in vitro chemosensitivity testing as a reasonable tool for the selection of individualized chemotherapy regimens. As recently controversially discussed (44–46), the ASCO Working Group on Chemotherapy Sensitivity and Resistance Assays stated, that based on the current level of evidence chemosensitivity assays should not be recommended for clinical use outside of study protocols (37). Moreover, the working group recommended a comparison of patients for whom chemotherapy was chosen based on the results of chemosensitivity testing with patients whose therapy was chosen empirically, to be the only effective study design. However, in the situation of melanoma one should consider, that currently no distinct alternative to empiric therapy, which is DTIC monochemotherapy, exists (38, 43). In fact, the present study was not designed to compare two different therapy regimens, but rather to help identify the individually most effective drugs among multiple nonstandard options. Our results demonstrate that the assay used in this study is predictive of therapy outcome, and indicate that nonstandard chemotherapeutics are effective in melanoma if they are applied selectively based on individual chemosensitivity profiles. However, these encouraging results need further evaluation by prospectively randomized trials. A subsequent phase-III study protocol comparing patients treated on the basis of chemosensitivity assay results with patients treated with DTIC standard chemotherapy is currently being developed by the DeCOG.

ADVANCES IN THE INDIVIDUALIZED TREATMENT OF MELANOMA (STAGE IV)

The current standards of care in the advanced metastatic melanoma setting (stage IV, AJCC classification) are poor. To date, randomized trials have failed to demonstrate the superiority of one regimen over another one. It is therefore crucial that patients with disseminated malignant melanoma be recruited into clinical trials. In recent years there have been impressive advances in our knowledge of the biology and nature of cancer development and the growth and progression to metastasis. The approach "from bench to bedside" is current reality in the treatment of several solid tumors and hematologic malignancies. The identification of new targets to facilitate individualized melanoma treatment is now an important issue.

There is an ongoing debate about the appropriate medical treatment for advanced metastatic melanoma patients. Single agent chemotherapy with Dacarbazine is far away from being considered as a "gold standard" but is still used as a reference and comparator in prospective-randomized clinical trials. Recently, Eigentler and coworkers published a systematic review of 41 randomized clinical studies, identified by a comprehensive search (38). They found that although some treatment regimens (especially combinations of several chemotherapeutic agents) appeared to increase response rates, none of the treatment schedules actually affected overall survival. Contemporary multinational clinical trials that utilize the RECIST criteria for response evaluation have published response rates in the range of 5–10%. It is clear that there is a dire need to improve both response rates and overall survival. Therefore, most opinion leaders believe that patients with advanced metastatic melanoma should preferentially be treated within clinical trials. To justify this, the theoretical benefit of new treatment options must be considered to be potentially at least equivalent to those of conventional treatment modalities. Authoritative guidelines for the care of melanoma patients, for instance in Germany, recommend that participation in clinical trials be implemented as a treatment of first choice (www.ado-homepage.de).

TARGETED THERAPIES

Research to increase knowledge and understanding of the cellular mechanisms precipitating and modulating neoplasia is one of the best hopes for a breakthrough in the treatment of melanoma patients. The detection of potential targets for individualized treatment modalities is therefore crucial. In a recent editorial by Cheson on individualizing therapy for hematologic malignancy, he pointed out that tumors will no longer be classified on the basis of their morphologic appearance and immunophenotype but instead by their abnormal gene expression profile, aberrant enzymatic pathways and receptor or other biologic abnormalities (47). These and other techniques such as RNA profiling (48) have the potential to facilitate future therapeutic advances via a more selective treatment approach. A number of translational research projects are being integrated into the current crop of clinical trials on melanoma. One of the main goals over the next decade is to identify and describe relevant biomarkers in order to develop targeted therapies that may offer the best potential to melanoma patients. Furthermore, they could be used to monitor the course of disease during treatment. One example under development is serum proteomic finger printing. This was shown not only to discriminate between clinical stages in melanoma patients but also to predict disease progression (49).

A broad spectrum of targeted therapeutic strategies is currently being addressed in clinical trials. These include signal transduction pathways inhibitors, proteasome inhibitors, histone deacetylation (HDAC) inhibitors, and inhibitors of tumor angiogenesis. An overview is given in Table 2.

Antisense oligonucleotides targeted against Bcl-2 mRNA (Oblimersen) were one of the first of such a targeted therapeutic approach tested in a large randomized clinical trial. In a mouse xenotransplantation model (50) and a clinical phase I/II study (51), Bcl-2 antisense oligonucleotides demonstrated efficacy. It was hypothesized that a decrease in Bcl-2 protein levels could overcome the chemoresistance of malignant melanoma caused in part by this proto-oncogene. In the clinical pilot study published by Jansen and coworkers, six out of 14 patients with advanced malignant melanoma demonstrated an antitumor response mostly in the soft tissues (51). Unfortunately, a subsequent international multicenter trial of 771 patients with advanced melanoma, randomized to receive Dacarbazine with or without Oblimersen did not confirm findings of the pilot study. Although there was a trend to a greater efficacy in terms of response rates, progression-free-survival and median survival, the combination regimen failed to demonstrate statistically significant differences which were acceptable for the FDA. It remains questionable as to whether a combination of Dacarbazine and Oblimersen can significantly overcome chemoresistance. This study did not include a translational research component to evaluate for instance the Bcl-2 levels before and after treatment. Without this data it remains unclear if a subgroup of patients exists that might benefit from this regimen.

Signal transduction pathways inhibitors are a major focus for new drug development. A number of mechanisms involved in tumor growth, progression, and metastasis are initiated by the activation of tyrosine kinases associated with cell-surface receptors. Gefitinib and Erlotinib, small molecules that selectively inhibit epidermal growth factor receptor (EGFR) tyrosine kinase activity have demonstrated high response rates amongst subgroups of patients with nonsmall cell lung cancer that have one of two known mutations of the EGFR that are sensitive to these drug. This has proven to be an excellent prototype for the development of other such targeted therapies (52). In melanoma, the importance of the Ras-MAPK signal transduction pathway has recently been highlighted by the discovery of a high frequency of activating BRAF mutations (53). Molecules that interfere with this signal transduction pathway have been introduced into clinical trials.

One of these studies examined the use of Sorafenib (BAY 43-9006) with Carboplatin and Paclitaxel in patients with stage IV melanoma mostly pretreated by chemotherapeutic agents or immunotherapy. Sorafenib is a multiple kinase inhibitor that has been shown to inhibit tumor growth and tumor angiogenesis by targeting Raf kinase, vascular endothelial growth factor receptor (VEGF-R), and platelet-derived growth factor receptor (PDGF-R). A presentation on a phase I/II trial on 105 patients given by Keith Flaherty in March 2006 demonstrated a response rate of 27%. Surprisingly, another 58% of treated patients showed stabilized disease during treatment. Of interest, the response rate was not affected by the stage of disease (M1a–M1c) nor by previous adjuvant interferon treatment. Of note, the responses were also independent of the BRAF mutation status. Similar rates of disease nonprogression were observed in patients with a mutation of this gene and patients without a mutation of the V599E gene. As expected with carboplatin and paclitaxel, many patients developed grade IV (CTC classification) myelosuppression. Sorafenib did not cause any additional toxicity despite a typical skin rash, hand–foot-syndrome, and abdominal discomfort with diarrhea.

Phase III trials are currently underway in the US, Europe, and Australia. These trials are using the same design, which is defined as Carboplatin and Paclitaxel plus either Sorafenib or an oral placebo. The US trial will be performed in patients who are treatment-naïve and suffering from advanced metastatic melanoma, whereas the patients in the European/Australian trial are receiving Sorafenib or a placebo as a second-line investigational after treatment failure with conventional chemotherapy.

Inhibitors of the PI3K/AKT signal transduction pathway, for instance the mTOR inhibitor CCI-779, have also been used in melanoma patients. The outcome of the trial on CCI-779 in 33 metastatic melanoma patients does not justify further testings in a single agent setting (54).

The ubiquitin–proteasome pathway is another integral component in tumor development and is therefore a target for interventions that modify the effects of oncogenic mutations affecting it. Bortezomib, an inhibitor of the 26S proteasome has been successfully introduced in the therapy for a number of hematological malignancies (55). Animal studies investigating different agents targeting the proteasome pathway led to Bortezomib being chosen for clinical studies as it had significant efficacy and a favorable toxicity profile. Bortezomib was also used in patients with metastatic melanoma in a phase II trial. However, this trial was discontinued after only 27 patients, because only six of the treated patients (22%) achieved disease stability and objective remissions were not observed. Furthermore, 42% of the patients demonstrated grade III toxicity including sensory neuropathy, thrombocytopenia, constipation, fatigue, and other adverse events. Bortezomib as a single agent was not considered to be an efficacious therapy for metastatic melanoma (56).

Changes in DNA methylation and histone acetylation are present in a variety of human tumors including melanoma. These findings accelerated the development and characterization of drugs that affect the so-called epigenetic silencing of tumor suppressor genes and other genes involved in the biology of cancer. Histone deacetylase (HDAC) inhibitors are therefore interesting molecules that can induce cell cycle arrest, differentiation and apoptosis in vitro, and retain other potent anti-tumor activities in vivo. Of these HDAC inhibitors, only few have been used in clinical melanoma trials. MS-275 is an orally active synthetic pyridyl carbamate. Some patients with melanoma were treated as part of a phase I study on MS-275 in patients with advanced and refractory solid tumors and lymphoma (57). Disease stabilization was observed in highly pretreated patients. In another phase I trial on MS-275, a long-lasting, almost complete response in a patient with advanced metastatic melanoma confined to the lung and lymph nodes was observed. These promising early results led to a multicentric phase II trial on 28 melanoma patients in Germany. Patients with at least one prior systemic treatment in stage IV disease without brain involvement were included into this trial. Angiogenesis is necessary for the growth of primary tumors and metastases. Drug discovery efforts have identified several potential therapeutic targets in endothelial cells and selective inhibitors capable of slowing tumor growth or producing tumor regression by blocking angiogenesis in vivo tumor models (58). More than 75 angiogenesis inhibitors have entered clinical trials. Most phase III trials have demonstrated that as single agents, antiangiogenesis drugs are not an efficacious therapy for metastatic melanoma. It appears that at least in advanced metastatic disease, combinations of antivascular antibodies with chemotherapy are more effective.

Of all the targets for potential antiangiogenic agents, vascular endothelial growth factor (VEGF) is the best characterized to date. Bevacizumab, a humanized anti-VEGF monoclonal antibody, was the first antiangiogenic drug to be approved for humans. The most striking results were observed in patients with advanced colorectal cancer in combination with chemotherapy. First results of trials examining the efficacy of Bevacizumab in patients with metastatic melanoma are eagerly awaited.

Thalidomide, a drug with also immunomodulatory properties, was studied in several melanoma trials with or without the addition of the cytotoxic agent Temozolomide. There were some promising results especially for the combination treatment published by Hwu and coworkers (59). As a derivative of Thalidomide, CC-5013 (Revlimide) is an effective blocker of VEGF. In addition it has a pronounced immunomodulatory effect, too (60). Revlimide has been examined in a large-sized phase III trial for pretreated stage IV melanoma patients. The activity of Revlimide as a single-agent treatment has been compared to an oral placebo in a double-blinded study. The results of this trial have not been published, but a statement released on the internet explained that Revlimide did not significantly improve outcomes in patients with melanoma. Data from trials examining the combination of Revlimide with other antineoplastic agents such as chemotherapy are not yet available. These disappointing results serve as another example of the failure of antiangiogenic agents when used as single agents in cancer patients.

Vitaxin is a humanized monoclonal antibody that acts by inhibiting $\alpha v\beta 3$ integrin in endothelial cells of tumor vessels. A phase II randomized, open-label study has examined the efficacy of Vitaxin in metastatic melanoma (61). This study explored the antitumor activity and safety of Vitaxin (8 mg kg^{-1} per week) with or without Dacarbazine (1,000 mg m^{-2} once every 3 weeks). Whereas Vitaxin alone showed no objective tumor response, the combination with DTIC revealed a 13% response rate. However, the median survival was longer in the group treated with Vitaxin alone. It is difficult to interpret these results without a comparative analysis a phase III trial.

In conclusion, there have been several therapeutic attempts to improve the outcome of patients with metastatic melanoma. Despite promising results from studies with the pluripotent molecule Sorafenib, no truly encouraging results for patients with melanoma are seen on the horizon. Nevertheless, individualized therapy with small molecules attacking specific tumor targets is a fascinating approach and requires our attention in the future. As it has become more obvious that single-agent approaches are not as effective as originally thought, we need to learn about combinations of agents with additive or synergistic effects. The identification of biomarkers in the tumor tissue or blood of cancer patients is crucial for the development of new agents and the design of new clinical trials. Trials must be accompanied by an extensive translational research program in order to achieve a better understanding of the mode of action to improve the treatment of metastatic melanoma in the future. As long as outcomes in the treatment of advanced metastatic melanoma remain poor, patients should be recruited into well-designed clinical trials.

REFERENCES

1. Kirkwood JM, Resnick GD, Cole BF (1997) Efficacy, safety, and risk-benefit analysis of adjuvant interferon alfa-2b in melanoma. Semin Oncol 24: S16-S23
2. Legha SS (1997) The role of interferon alfa in the treatment of metastatic melanoma. Semin Oncol 24: S24-S31
3. Garbe C, Krasagakis K, Zouboulis CC, Schroder K, Kruger S, Stadler R, Orfanos CE (1990) Antitumor activities of interferon alpha, beta, and gamma and their combinations on human melanoma cells in vitro: changes of proliferation, melanin synthesis, and immunophenotype. J Invest Dermatol 95: 231S-237S
4. Garbe C, Krasagakis K (1993) Effects of interferons and cytokines on melanoma cells. J Invest Dermatol 100: 239S-244S
5. Horikoshi T, Fukuzawa K, Hanada N, Ezoe K, Eguchi H, Hamaoka S, Tsujiya H, Tsukamoto T (1995) In vitro comparative study of the antitumor effects of human interferon-alpha, beta and gamma on the growth and invasive potential of human melanoma cells. J Dermatol 22: 631-636

6. Le Page C, Genin P, Baines MG, Hiscott J (2000) Interferon activation and innate immunity. Rev Immunogenet 2: 374-386
7. Garbe C, Kreuser ED, Zouboulis CC, Stadler R, Orfanos CE (1992) Combined treatment of metastatic melanoma with interferons and cytotoxic drugs. Semin Oncol 19: 63-69
8. Garbe C (1993) Chemotherapy and chemoimmunotherapy in disseminated malignant melanoma. Melanoma Res 3: 291-299
9. Lau JF, Horvath CM (2002) Mechanisms of Type I interferon cell signaling and STAT-mediated transcriptional responses. Mt Sinai J Med 69: 156-168
10. Caraglia M, Marra M, Pelaia G, Maselli R, Caputi M, Marsico SA, Abbruzzese A (2005) Alpha-interferon and its effects on signal transduction pathways. J Cell Physiol 202: 323-335
11. Platanias LC (2005) Mechanisms of type-I- and type-II-interferon-mediated signalling. Nat Rev Immunol 5: 375-386
12. Glue P, Fang JW, Rouzier-Panis R, Raffanel C, Sabo R, Gupta SK, Salfi M, Jacobs S (2000) Pegylated interferon-alpha2b: pharmacokinetics, pharmacodynamics, safety, and preliminary efficacy data. Hepatitis C Intervention Therapy Group. Clin Pharmacol Ther 68: 556-567
13. Motzer RJ, Rakhit A, Ginsberg M, Rittweger K, Vuky J, Yu R, Fettner S, Hooftman L (2001) Phase I trial of 40-kd branched pegylated interferon alfa-2a for patients with advanced renal cell carcinoma. J Clin Oncol 19: 1312-1319
14. Baker DE (2003) Pegylated interferon plus ribavirin for the treatment of chronic hepatitis C. Rev Gastroenterol Disord 3: 93-109
15. Fried MW, Shiffman ML, Reddy KR, Smith C, Marinos G, Goncales FL, Jr., Haussinger D, Diago M, Carosi G, Dhumeaux D, Craxi A, Lin A, Hoffman J, Yu J (2002) Peginterferon alfa-2a plus ribavirin for chronic hepatitis C virus infection. N Engl J Med 347: 975-982
16. Heathcote EJ, Shiffman ML, Cooksley WG, Dusheiko GM, Lee SS, Balart L, Reindollar R, Reddy RK, Wright TL, Lin A, Hoffman J, De Pamphilis J (2000) Peginterferon alfa-2a in patients with chronic hepatitis C and cirrhosis. N Engl J Med 343: 1673-1680
17. Manns MP, McHutchison JG, Gordon SC, Rustgi VK, Shiffman M, Reindollar R, Goodman ZD, Koury K, Ling M, Albrecht JK (2001) Peginterferon alfa-2b plus ribavirin compared with interferon alfa-2b plus ribavirin for initial treatment of chronic hepatitis C: a randomised trial. Lancet 358: 958-965
18. Marcellin P, Lau GK, Bonino F, Farci P, Hadziyannis S, Jin R, Lu ZM, Piratvisuth T, Germanidis G, Yurdaydin C, Diago M, Gurel S, Lai MY, Button P, Pluck N (2004) Peginterferon alfa-2a alone, lamivudine alone, and the two in combination in patients with HBeAg-negative chronic hepatitis B. N Engl J Med 351: 1206-1217
19. Zeuzem S, Feinman SV, Rasenack J, Heathcote EJ, Lai MY, Gane E, O'Grady J, Reichen J, Diago M, Lin A, Hoffman J, Brunda MJ (2000) Peginterferon alfa-2a in patients with chronic hepatitis C. N Engl J Med 343: 1666-1672
20. Baccarani M, Martinelli G, Rosti G, Trabacchi E, Testoni N, Bassi S, Amabile M, Soverini S, Castagnetti F, Cilloni D, Izzo B, de Vivo A, Messa E, Bonifazi F, Poerio A, Luatti S, Giugliano E, Alberti D, Fincato G, Russo D, Pane F, Saglio G (2004) Imatinib and pegylated human recombinant interferon-alpha2b in early chronic-phase chronic myeloid leukemia. Blood 104: 4245-4251
21. Bukowski R, Ernstoff MS, Gore ME, Nemunaitis JJ, Amato R, Gupta SK, Tendler CL (2002) Pegylated interferon alfa-2b treatment for patients with solid tumors: a phase I/II study. J Clin Oncol 20: 3841-3849
22. Motzer RJ, Rakhit A, Thompson J, Gurney H, Selby P, Figlin R, Negrier S, Ernst S, Siebels M, Ginsberg M, Rittweger K, Hooftman L (2002) Phase II trial of branched peginterferon-alpha 2a (40 kDa) for patients with advanced renal cell carcinoma. Ann Oncol 13: 1799-1805
23. Krepler C, Certa U, Wacheck V, Jansen B, Wolff K, Pehamberger H (2004) Pegylated and conventional interferon-alpha induce comparable transcriptional responses and inhibition of tumor growth in a human melanoma SCID mouse xenotransplantation model. J Invest Dermatol 123: 664-669
24. Certa U, Wilhelm-Seiler M, Foser S, Broger C, Neeb M (2003) Expression modes of interferon-alpha inducible genes in sensitive and resistant human melanoma cells stimulated with regular and pegylated interferon-alpha. Gene 315: 79-86
25. Grob JJ, Dreno B, de la SP, Delaunay M, Cupissol D, Guillot B, Souteyrand P, Sassolas B, Cesarini JP, Lionnet S, Lok C, Chastang C, Bonerandi JJ (1998) Randomised trial of interferon alpha-2a as adjuvant therapy in resected primary melanoma thicker than 1.5 mm without clinically detectable node metastases. French Cooperative Group on Melanoma. Lancet 351: 1905-1910
26. Kirkwood JM, Strawderman MH, Ernstoff MS, Smith TJ, Borden EC, Blum RH (1996) Interferon alfa-2b adjuvant therapy of high-risk resected cutaneous melanoma: the Eastern Cooperative Oncology Group Trial EST 1684. J Clin Oncol 14: 7-17

27. Kirkwood JM, Ibrahim JG, Sondak VK, Richards J, Flaherty LE, Ernstoff MS, Smith TJ, Rao U, Steele M, Blum RH (2000) High- and low-dose interferon alfa-2b in high-risk melanoma: first analysis of intergroup trial E1690/S9111/C9190. J Clin Oncol 18: 2444-2458

28. Kirkwood JM, Ibrahim JG, Sosman JA, Sondak VK, Agarwala SS, Ernstoff MS, Rao U (2001) High-dose interferon alfa-2b significantly prolongs relapse-free and overall survival compared with the GM2-KLH/QS-21 vaccine in patients with resected stage IIB-III melanoma: results of intergroup trial E1694/S9512/C509801. J Clin Oncol 19: 2370-2380

29. Pehamberger H, Soyer HP, Steiner A, Kofler R, Binder M, Mischer P, Pachinger W, Aubock J, Fritsch P, Kerl H, Wolff K (1998) Adjuvant interferon alfa-2a treatment in resected primary stage II cutaneous melanoma. Austrian Malignant Melanoma Cooperative Group. J Clin Oncol 16: 1425-1429

30. Cameron DA, Cornbleet MC, MacKie RM, Hunter JA, Gore M, Hancock B, Smyth JF (2001) Adjuvant interferon alpha 2b in high risk melanoma - the Scottish study. Br J Cancer 84: 1146-1149

31. Cascinelli N, Belli F, MacKie RM, Santinami M, Bufalino R, Morabito A (2001) Effect of long-term adjuvant therapy with interferon alpha-2a in patients with regional node metastases from cutaneous melanoma: a randomised trial. Lancet 358: 866-869

32. Eggermont AM, Suciu S, MacKie R, Ruka W, Testori A, Kruit W, Punt CJ, Delauney M, Sales F, Groenewegen G, Ruiter DJ, Jagiello I, Stoitchkov K, Keilholz U, Lienard D (2005) Post-surgery adjuvant therapy with intermediate doses of interferon alfa 2b versus observation in patients with stage IIb/III melanoma (EORTC 18952): randomised controlled trial. Lancet 366: 1189-1196

33. Hancock BW, Wheatley K, Harris S, Ives N, Harrison G, Horsman JM, Middleton MR, Thatcher N, Lorigan PC, Marsden JR, Burrows L, Gore M (2004) Adjuvant interferon in high-risk melanoma: the AIM HIGH Study–United Kingdom Coordinating Committee on Cancer Research randomized study of adjuvant low-dose extended-duration interferon Alfa-2a in high-risk resected malignant melanoma. J Clin Oncol 22: 53-61

34. Lens MB, Dawes M (2002) Interferon alfa therapy for malignant melanoma: a systematic review of randomized controlled trials. J Clin Oncol 20: 1818-1825

35. Wheatley K, Ives N, Hancock B, Gore M (2002) Need for a quantitative meta-analysis of trials of adjuvant interferon in melanoma. J Clin Oncol 20: 4120-4121

36. Wheatley K, Ives N, Hancock B, Gore M, Eggermont A, Suciu S (2003) Does adjuvant interferon-alpha for high-risk melanoma provide a worthwhile benefit? A meta-analysis of the randomised trials. Cancer Treat Rev 29: 241-252

37. Eggermont A (2002) Evaluation of intermediate dose interferon (EORTC 18952) and long-term therapy with PEG-Intron (EORTC 18991) in more than 2000 patients with very high risk melanoma. Melanoma Res 12: A5-A19

38. Eigentler TK, Caroli UM, Radny P, et al. (2003) Palliative therapy of disseminated malignant melanoma: a systematic review of 41 randomised clinical trials. Lancet Oncol 4:748-759

39. Keilholz U, Punt CJA, Gore M, Kruit W, Patel P, Lienard D, Thomas J, Proebstle TM, Schmittel A, Schadendorf D, Velu T, Negrier S, Kleeberg U, Lehman F, Suciu S, Eggermont AMM (2005). Dacarbazine, cisplatin and interferon-alpha-2b with or without interleukin-2 in metastatic melanoma: A randomized phase III trial (18951) of the EORTC Melanoma Group. J Clin Oncol 23: 6747-6755.

40. Helmbach H, Rossmann E, Kern MA, et al. (2001) Drug-resistance in human melanoma. Int J Cancer 93:617-622

41. Andreotti PE, Cree IA, Kurbacher CM, et al: Chemosensitivity testing of human tumors using a microplate adenosine triphosphate luminescence assay: clinical correlation for cisplatin resistance of ovarian carcinoma. Cancer Res 1995;55:5276-5282

42. Ugurel S, Schadendorf D, Pföhler C, Neuber K, Thoelke A, Ulrich J, Hauschild A, Spieth K, Kaatz M, Rittgen W, Delorme S, Tilgen W, Reinhold U (2006). In vitro drug sensivity predicts response and survival after individualized sensitivity-directed chemotherapy in metastatic melanoma – a multicenter phase II trial of the Dermatology Cooperative Oncology Group (DeCOG). Clin Cancer Res, 12(18):5454-63.

43. Food and Drug Administration Center for Drug Evaluation and Research: Oncologic Drugs Advisory Committee, Briefing Material: May 3, 2004 AM Session - Genasense. http://www.fda.gov/ohrms/dockets/ac/04/briefing/4037B1_02_FDA-Genasense.pdf

44. Fruehauf JP, Alberts DS: In vitro drug resistance versus chemosensitivity: two sides of different coins. J Clin Oncol 2005;23:3641-3643

45. Wiegand HS: Chemotherapy sensitivity and response assays: are the ASCO guidelines for clinical trial design too restrictive? J Clin Oncol 2005;23:3643-3644

46. Castro M: Resisting a fundamentalist policy. J Clin Oncol 2005;23:3645-3646

47. Cheson BD: Individualizing therapy for the hematologic malignancies: the stuff of genes and dreams. J Clin Oncol 23: 6283-6284, 2005

48. Lu J, Getz G, Miska EA, Alvarez-Saavedra E, Lamb J, Peck D, Sweet-Cordero A, Ebert BL, Mak RH, Ferrando AA, Downing JR, Jacks T, Horvitz HR, Golub TR: MicroRNA expression profiles classify human cancers. Nature 435:834-838, 2005
49. Mian S, Ugurel S, Parkinson E, Schlenzka I, Dryden I, Lancashire L, Ball G, Creaser C, Rees R, Schadendorf D: Serum proteomic fingerprinting discriminates between clinical stages and predicts disease progression in melanoma patients. J Clin Oncol 23: 5088-5093, 2005
50. Jansen B, Schlagbauer-Wadl H, Brown BD: Bcl-2 antisense therapy chemosensitizes human melanoma in SCID mice. Nat Med 4:232-234, 1998
51. Jansen B, Wacheck V, Heere-Ress E, Schlagbauer-Wadl H, Hoeller C, Lucas T, Hoermann M, Hollenstein U, Wolff K, Pehamberger H: Cehmosensitisation of malignant melanoma by BCL2 antisense therapy. Lancet 356: 1728-1733, 2000
52. Pao W, Miller VA: Epidermal growth factor receptor mutations, small-molecule kinase inhibitors, and non-small-cell lung cancer: current knowledge and future directions. J Clin Oncol 23: 2556-2568, 2005
53. Davies H, Bignell GR, Cox C, Stephens P, Edkins S, Clegg S: Mutations of the BRAF gene in human cancer. Nature 417: 949-954, 2002
54. Margolin K, Longmate J, Baratta T, Synold T, Christensen S, Weber J, Gajewski T, Quirt I, Doroshow JH: Cancer 104: 1045-1048, 2005
55. Mani A, Gelmann EP: The ubiquitin-proteasome pathway and its role in cancer. J Clin Oncol 21: 4776-4789, 2005
56. Markovic SN, Geyer SM, Dawkins F, Sharfman W, Albertini M, Maples W: A phase II study of bortezomib in the treatment of metastatic malignant melanoma. Cancer 103: 2584-2589, 2005
57. Ryan QC, Headlee D, Acharya M, Sparreboom A, Trepel JB, Ye J: Phase I and pharmacokinetic study of MS-275, a histone deacetylase inhibitor, in patients with advanced and refractory solid tumors or lymphoma. J Clin Oncol 23: 3912-3922, 2005
58. Gasparini G, Longo R, Fanelli M, Teicher BA: Combination of antiangiogenic therapy with other anticancer therapies: results, challenges, and open questions
59. Hwu WJ, Lis E, Menell JH, Panageas KS, Lamb LA, Merrell J: Temozolomide plus thalidomide in patients with brain metastases from melanoma: a phase II study. Cancer 103: 2590-2597, 2005
60. Miller KD, Chap LI, Holmes FA, Cobleigh MA, Marcom PK, Fehrenbacher L: Randomized phase III trial of capecitabine compared with bevacizumab plus capecitabine in patients with previously treated metastatic breast cancer. J Clin Oncol 23: 792-799, 2005
61. Hersey P, Sosman J, O'Day S, Richards J, Bedikian, Gonzalez R, Sharfman W, Weber R, Logan T, Kirkwood JM: A phase II, randomized, open-label study evaluating the antitumor activity of MEDI-522, a humanized monoclonal antibody directed against the human alpha v beta 3 8avb3) integrin ± dacarbazine (DTIC) in patients with metastatic melanoma (MM). J Clin Oncol 23, Suppl 16S: 711, 2005 (Abstract)

21. FUTURE PERSPECTIVES AND UNANSWERED QUESTIONS ON CANCER METASTASIS AND THE LYMPHOVASCULAR SYSTEM

STANLEY P. L. LEONG AND MARLYS H. WITTE*

University of California San Francisco, San Francisco, California, USA,
**Department of Surgery, University of Arizona, Tucson, Arizona, USA*

INTRODUCTION

For the clinical oncologist, the most humbling experience is when the cancer has spread and the disease is unresponsive to available therapy to curb progression. Paget developed the "seed and soil" hypothesis to explain the phenomenon of clinical cancer metastasis (1). Since the work of Paget, we have seen explosive advances in biological understanding of the mechanisms of metastasis. Numerous animal models have been applied to further understand the cellular and molecular mechanisms of cancer metastasis (2). But the translational link to the clinic from such basic science advances continues to remain elusive. It is important, therefore, to bring clinicians and basic scientists together to share their knowledge and perspectives on the phenomena surrounding cancer metastasis. For this reason, the first International Symposium on Cancer Metastasis and the Lymphovascular System was organized and successfully held in San Francisco in April 2005. The meeting highlights have been summarized in the June issue of 2006 Cancer Metastasis Reviews.

HISTORICAL BACKGROUND (3)

Since the 1890s and the work of physiologist Ernest Starling and embryologist Florence Sabin, substantial understanding has been gained on the anatomy, development, and physiology of the lymphovascular system. During the past two decades, further knowledge has accumulated in these areas and also in the cellular and, most recently, molecular aspects of the lymphovascular system. Using the melanoma and breast cancer models from the sentinel lymph node (SLN) era, it has been learned that about 80% of the time, metastasis from the primary site follows an orderly pattern of progression through the lymphatic network initially, whereas about 20% of the time systemic metastasis occurs without evidence of lymphatic invasion.

UNANSWERED QUESTIONS

Further progress is needed in unraveling the multifaceted aspects of micrometastasis including development of metastatic clones from the primary tumor site through proliferation and differentiation, acquisition of the surface molecules by the cancer cells to spread through either the lymphatic or blood vascular systems, and the host interaction with the invading cancer cells, so that more rational therapy can be developed to overcome these steps of progression from the primary site to the metastatic sites. Although the clinical patterns of cancer metastasis are well documented for many different types of cancer, the proximate molecular events linking each step from proliferation of the cancer within the tissue microenvironment to lymphatic or vascular invasion and widespread dissemination are not well understood. Recent studies suggest that stem cells (4–7) within the proliferating cancer cell population are the primary subset that metastasize from the tumor bulk, which continues to grow locally without subsequent spread. These stem cells need to be better characterized with respect to their phenotypic, genetic, and molecular profiles so that they can be selectively targeted for specific therapeutics.

On the other hand, the mechanisms of initiation and stimulation of lymphatic and blood vascular growth (both lymphangiogenesis and hemangiogenesis) within and around the tumor should be better understood (3); antiangiogenic therapy has already been used for specific molecular targeting. Can lymphangiogenesis be blocked as a therapeutic strategy? The functional role of SLNs and regional lymph nodes relating to cancer metastasis remains a crucial issue. Do the SLNs initially launch an immune response to the cancer cells and subsequently succumb to the invading cancer cells?

Tumor antigenic changes during metastasis should be further examined, whether these changes may result in tolerance of specific immune cells, allowing cancer cells to escape immune attack. New and improved technologies should be developed for dynamic noninvasive high resolution multimodal imaging to elucidate the microscopic and macroscopic events taking place in the lymphatic system during cancer development and spread. These techniques can form the basis for image-guided lymphatic-lymph node directed monitoring and selective treatment as molecular and cell-based therapies are developed. New approaches using nanoparticles to identify limited tumor burden should be explored (8). Molecular targeting against molecules involved in proliferation signaling pathways and apotosis may provide potential sites of intervention.

The recent identification of molecules on endothelial cells lining the lymphatic channels (3, 9) paves the way for future studies to analyze the important issue whether cancer cell entry into the lymphatic channels is an active vs. a passive process or both. If passive processes are involved, what are the influences of mechanical factors and anatomical structures on the facilitation of cancer cell transport through the lymphatic channel (Chap. 10). If the active process is operative, what are the endothelial cell receptor mechanisms operating between the cancer cell and the molecules of the lymphatic channels and the lining endothelial cells?

ONCOLYMPHOLOGY

This newly opening active field of so-called oncolymphology needs to be vigorously pursued. When the foregoing mechanisms and events are more fully understood, can new therapeutic strategies be developed to curb these processes? The development of nanotechnology is highly promising both from the imaging point of view for the detection of early metastatic foci and in the delivery of new nanoparticulate agents to these sites with more efficiency.

These important issues and questions and much else we do not know about cancer and the lymphatic system (10) will be addressed in our upcoming Second International Symposium on Cancer Metastasis and the Lymphovascular System: Basis for Rational Therapy to be held again in San Francisco from May 3–5, 2007. The thrust of the upcoming symposium is once more to bring basic and clinical scientists together on an international level to address these challenging issues of cancer metastasis, forge collaborations, and translate basic science advances to improve the outlook of patients with cancer.

REFERENCES

1. Paget S (1989) The distribution of secondary growths in cancer of the breast. Cancer Metastasis Rev 8: 98-101.
2. Hoon DS, Kitago M, Kim J, Mori T, Piris A, Szyfelbein K, Mihm MC Jr, Nathanson SD, Padera TP, Chambers AF, Vantyghem SA, MacDonald IC, Shivers SC, Alsarraj M, Reintgen DS, Passlick B, Sienel W, Pantel K (2006) Molecular mechanisms of metastasis. Cancer Metastasis Rev 25: 203-220.
3. Witte MH, Jones K, Wilting J, Dictor M, Selg M, McHale N, Gershenwald JE, Jackson DG (2006) Structure function relationships in the lymphatic system and implications for cancer biology. Cancer Metastasis Rev 25: 159-184.
4. Clarke MF, Becker MW (2006) Stem cells: the real culprits in cancer? Sci Am 295: 52-59.
5. Lapidot T, Sirard C, Vormoor J, Murdoch B, Hoang T, Caceres-Cortes J, Minden M, Paterson B, Caliguiri MA, Dick JE (1994) A cell initiating human acute myeloid leukaemia after transplantation into SCID mice. Nature 367: 645-68.
6. Hope KJ, Jin L, Dick JE (2003) Human acute myeloid leukemia stem cells. Arch Med Res 34: 507-514.
7. Al-Hajj M, Wicha MSA, Benito-Herdandez A, Morrison SJ, Clarke MF (2003) Prospective identification of tumorigenic breast cancer cells. Proc Natl Acad Sci USA 100: 3983-3988.

8. Roco MC (2006) Nanotechnology's future. Sci Am 295: 39.
9. Suri C (2006) The emergence of molecular and transgenic lymphology: what do we (really) know so far? Lymphology 39: 1-7.
10. Witte MH, Witte C (2999) What we don't know about cancer. In: Otter W, Root-Bernstein R, Koten JW (eds.) What is cancer? Anticancer Res 19: 4919-4934.

INDEX

Printed in the United States of America.